Identifying
and Treating Sex Offenders:
Current Approaches, Research,
and Techniques

Identifying and Treating Sex Offenders: Current Approaches, Research, and Techniques has been co-published simultaneously as *Journal of Child Sexual Abuse*, Volume 12, Numbers 3/4 2003.

The *Journal of Child Sexual Abuse* Monographic "Separates"

Below is a list of "separates," which in serials librarianship means a special issue simultaneously published as a special journal issue or double-issue *and* as a "separate" hardbound monograph. (This is a format which we also call a "DocuSerial.")

"Separates" are published because specialized libraries or professionals may wish to purchase a specific thematic issue by itself in a format which can be separately cataloged and shelved, as opposed to purchasing the journal on an on-going basis. Faculty members may also more easily consider a "separate" for classroom adoption.

"Separates" are carefully classified separately with the major book jobbers so that the journal tie-in can be noted on new book order slips to avoid duplicate purchasing.

You may wish to visit Haworth's website at . . .

http://www.HaworthPress.com

. . . to search our online catalog for complete tables of contents of these separates and related publications.

You may also call 1-800-HAWORTH (outside US/Canada: 607-722-5857), or Fax 1-800-895-0582 (outside US/Canada: 607-771-0012), or e-mail at:

docdelivery@haworthpress.com

Identifying and Treating Sex Offenders: Current Approaches, Research, and Techniques, edited by Robert Geffner, PhD, Kristina Crumpton Franey, PsyD, Teri Geffner Arnold, MSSW, and Robert Falconer, MA (Vol. 12, No. 3/4, 2003). *Address the assessment and treatment issues when working with adult sex offenders, exploring current issues, research, and theory behind sex offending, as well as the implications for new policies.*

Misinformation Concerning Child Sexual Abuse and Adult Survivors, edited by Charles L. Whitfield, MD, FASAM, Joyanna Silberg, PhD, and Paul J. Fink, MD (Vol. 9, No. 3/4, 2001). *"A thorough, intellectually stimulating, and compelling primer. . . . This collection of scholarly articles represents a comprehensive view of the issues. This is a must for everyone's bookshelf." (Ann Wolbert Burgess, RN, DNSc, CS, Professor of Psychiatric Nursing, School of Nursing, Boston College)*

Robert Geffner, PhD
Kristina Crumpton Franey, PsyD
Teri Geffner Arnold, MSSW
Robert Falconer, MA
Editors

Identifying and Treating Sex Offenders: Current Approaches, Research, and Techniques

Identifying and Treating Sex Offenders: Current Approaches, Research, and Techniques has been co-published simultaneously as *Journal of Child Sexual Abuse*, Volume 12, Numbers 3/4 2003.

More Pre-publication
REVIEWS, COMMENTARIES, EVALUATIONS . . .

"AN EXCEPTIONAL BOOK that should be on the shelf of every practitioner and researcher working with adult sex offenders. THOUGHT- FUL AND TIMELY . . . . Provides the reader with a solid foundation of current knowledge regarding assessment, practice, and policy . . . . At the same time, this edited book is much more than a basic primer–it offers important insights and cutting-edge information in a number of areas. Valuable for practitioners and researchers."

Keith Kaufman, PhD
Psychology Professor and Chair
Portland State University
Oregon

HMTP

The Haworth Maltreatment & Trauma Press®
An Imprint of The Haworth Press, Inc.

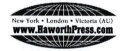

New York • London • Victoria (AU)
www.HaworthPress.com

Identifying and Treating Sex Offenders: Current Approaches, Research, and Techniques

Robert Geffner, PhD
Kristina Crumpton Franey, PsyD
Teri Geffner Arnold, MSSW
Robert Falconer, MA
Editors

Identifying and Treating Sex Offenders: Current Approaches, Research, and Techniques has been co-published simultaneously as *Journal of Child Sexual Abuse*, Volume 12, Numbers 3/4 2003.

HMTP
The Haworth Maltreatment & Trauma Press
An Imprint of
The Haworth Press, Inc.
New York • London • Oxford

Published by

The Haworth Maltreatment & Trauma Press, 10 Alice Street, Binghamton, NY 13904-1580 USA

The Haworth Maltreatment & Trauma Press is an imprint of The Haworth Press, Inc., 10 Alice Street, Binghamton, NY 13904-1580 USA.

Identifying and Treating Sex Offenders: Current Approaches, Research, and Techniques has been co-published simultaneously as *Journal of Child Sexual Abuse*, Volume 12, Numbers 3/4 2003.

The development, preparation, and publication of this work has been undertaken with great care. However, the publisher, employees, editors, and agents of The Haworth Press and all imprints of The Haworth Press, Inc., including The Haworth Medical Press® and The Pharmaceutical Products Press®, are not responsible for any errors contained herein or for consequences that may ensue from use of materials or information contained in this work. Opinions expressed by the author(s) are not necessarily those of The Haworth Press, Inc.

Cover design by Marylouise E. Doyle

Library of Congress Cataloging-in-Publication Data

Identifying and treating sex offenders : current approaches, research, and techniques / Robert Geffner . . . [et al.], editors.
     p. cm.
     "Co-published simultaneously as Journal of child sexual abuse, volume 12, numbers 3/4, 2003."
     Includes bibliographical references and index.
     ISBN 0-7890-2506-X (hard cover : alk. paper) – ISBN 0-7890-2507-8 (soft cover : alk. paper)
     1. Sex offenders–Rehabilitation. 2. Psychosexual disorders–Diagnosis. 3. Child sexual abuse–Prevention. I. Geffner, Robert. II. Journal of child sexual abuse.
RC560.S47I335 2004
616.85'83–dc22   2003027732

Indexing, Abstracting & Website/Internet Coverage

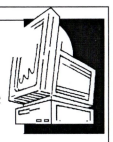

This section provides you with a list of major indexing & abstracting services. That is to say, each service began covering this periodical during the year noted in the right column. Most Websites which are listed below have indicated that they will either post, disseminate, compile, archive, cite or alert their own Website users with research-based content from this work. (This list is as current as the copyright date of this publication.)

Abstracting, Website/Indexing Coverage . . . . Year When Coverage Began

- *Academic Search Elite (EBSCO)* **1996**
- *Academic Search Premier (EBSCO)* **1996**
- *Applied Social Sciences Index & Abstracts (ASSIA)*
  (Online: ASSI via Data-Star) (CDRom: ASSIA Plus)
  <http://www.csa.com> **1992**
- *Behavioral Medicine Abstracts* **1992**
- *Cambridge Scientific Abstracts (Health & Safety Science*
  Abstracts/Risk Abstracts) is a leading publisher of
  scientific information in print journals, online databases,
  CD-ROM and via the Internet <http://www.csa.com> **1992**
- *CareData: the database supporting social care*
  management and practice
  <http://www.elsc.org.uk/caredata/caredata.htm> **1994**
- *Child Development Abstracts & Bibliography (in print & online)*
  <http://www.ukans.edu> **1994**
- *CINAHL (Cumulative Index to Nursing & Allied Health*
  Literature), in print, EBSCO, and SilverPlatter, Data-Star,
  and PaperChase. (Support materials include Subject Heading List,
  Database Search Guide, and instructional video).
  <http://www.cinahl.com> **1993**
- *CNPIEC Reference Guide: Chinese National Directory*
  of Foreign Periodicals **1995**

(continued)

(continued)

(continued)

  *Exact start date to come.

Special Bibliographic Notes related to special journal issues (separates) and indexing/abstracting:

- indexing/abstracting services in this list will also cover material in any "separate" that is co-published simultaneously with Haworth's special thematic journal issue or DocuSerial. Indexing/abstracting usually covers material at the article/chapter level.
- monographic co-editions are intended for either non-subscribers or libraries which intend to purchase a second copy for their circulating collections.
- monographic co-editions are reported to all jobbers/wholesalers/approval plans. The source journal is listed as the "series" to assist the prevention of duplicate purchasing in the same manner utilized for books-in-series.
- to facilitate user/access services all indexing/abstracting services are encouraged to utilize the co-indexing entry note indicated at the bottom of the first page of each article/chapter/contribution.
- this is intended to assist a library user of any reference tool (whether print, electronic, online, or CD-ROM) to locate the monographic version if the library has purchased this version but not a subscription to the source journal.
- individual articles/chapters in any Haworth publication are also available through the Haworth Document Delivery Service (HDDS).

Identifying and Treating Sex Offenders: Current Approaches, Research, and Techniques

CONTENTS

ABOUT THE EDITORS

Robert Geffner, PhD, is the Founder and President of the Family Violence and Sexual Assault Institute located in San Diego, CA. Dr. Geffner is a Clinical Research Professor of Psychology at the California School of Professional Psychology, Alliant International University in San Diego, and is also a Licensed Psychologist and a Licensed Marriage & Family Therapist in California and in Texas. He was the clinical director of a large private practice mental health clinic in East Texas for over 15 years; one of his roles was the supervision of the sex offender assessment and treatment programs. Dr. Geffner is the Editor-in-Chief of The Haworth Maltreatment & Trauma Press, which includes being the Editor of the *Journal of Child Sexual Abuse* and *Journal of Aggression, Maltreatment, & Trauma*, and co-editor of the *Journal of Emotional Abuse*, all internationally disseminated. He also is Senior Editor of the Maltreatment, Trauma, and Interpersonal Aggression book program for The Haworth Press. He has a Diplomate in Clinical Neuropsychology from the American Board of Professional Neuropsychology. He served as an adjunct faculty member for the National Judicial College from 1990 - 2000, and was a former Professor of Psychology at the University of Texas at Tyler for 16 years. Dr. Geffner has published extensively and given presentations and workshops world-wide in the areas of family violence, sexual assault, child abuse, family and child psychology, custody issues, forensic psychology, neuropsychology, and diagnostic) assessment. He has served on several national and state committees dealing with various aspects of family psychology, family violence, child abuse, and family law. In addition, he has served as a consultant for various agencies and centers of the federal government, including the Department of Health & Human Services, National Center for Child Abuse & Neglect, Department of Defense, and different branches of the military.

Kristina Crumpton Franey, PsyD, received her doctorate in Psychology from the California School of Professional Psychology at Alliant International University in San Diego, CA, with specialized training in child and adolescent psychology. Her research has focused on the experiences of adolescent sexual offenders who have re-entered society following treatment. Dr. Franey is currently working with juvenile sex offenders at the Sexual Treatment and Recovery Program in San Diego, and is working with Forensic Psych Consultants in San Diego, CA. She has worked with the Family Violence and Sexual Assault Institute (FVSAI) since 1998, and co-edited *The Cost of Child Maltreatment: Who Pays? We All Do*, published in 2001 by FVSAI.

Teri Geffner Arnold, MSSW, received her Bachelor of Arts in Psychology from the University of Texas at Austin, and her Master of Science in Social Work, also from UT Austin. Since 2001, Ms. Geffner Arnold has been an assistant editor with the Family Violence & Sexual Assault Institute (FVSAI) for the *Journal of Child Sexual Abuse*, the *Journal of Emotional Abuse*, and the *Family Violence & Sexual Assault Bulletin.* She has provided editing assistance on three prior books and treatment manuals for the FVSAI in the past four years. Her primary interest lies in clinical practice with both adults and children. She has recently completed a social work internship providing services to children in a school setting.

Robert Falconer, MA, is currently the executive director of the Institute for Trauma Oriented Psychotherapy. He has been involved in the child maltreatment arena for over a decade, has been the President of a foundation, and has supported numerous intervention and educational projects concerning child sexual abuse. He has previously co-edited two books in this field: *Trauma, Amnesia, & the Denial of Abuse*, and *The Cost of Child Maltreatment: Who Pays? We All Do*, published as joint projects by FVSAI and the Institute for Trauma Oriented Psychotherapy.

About the Contributors

Mirza S. A. Baig, MD, CCHP, completed his medical degree at Osmania University in Hyderabad, India. He has served as the medical director, chief of staff, and president of the medical staff at facilities operated by the Illinois Department of Human Services. Dr. Baig is an Associate Professor of Psychiatry at Southern Illinois University School of Medicine. He currently teaches both residents and fellows in forensic psychiatry. Dr. Baig has previously served as the corporate medical director of psychiatric services for Health Professionals, Ltd. based in Peoria, IL. He has numerous publications in the field of psychiatry. He is currently practicing forensic psychiatry at Menard Correctional Center in Menard, IL, which is the largest maximum-security prison in the state.

Fred S. Berlin, MD, PhD, is the Director of the National Institute for the Study, Prevention and Treatment of Sexual Trauma, and Founder of The Johns Hopkins Sexual Disorders Clinic. Today the clinic continues the tradition of providing care to patients with a variety of sexual disorders and to some victims of sexual trauma, as well. Dr. Berlin has written extensively on paraphilias for numerous distinguished journals, such as *The American Journal of Psychiatry*, *The New England Journal of Medicine*, and *The American Journal of Forensic Psychiatry*. Dr. Berlin is listed in the Best Doctors in America; he was an invited participant at a White House Conference on Child Sexual Abuse, and as a "national leader in law and health" for the National Symposium on the Child Victim of Sexual Abuse (National Council of Juvenile and Family Court Judges).

Mark S. Carich, PhD, is employed with the Illinois Department of Corrections at Big Muddy River CC and is an adjunct faculty member of the Adler School of Professional Psychology in Chicago. Dr. Carich specializes in sex offender assessment and treatment and currently coordinates the sexually dangerous persons program. He provides training and consultation on the subject. He has recently co-authored with Martin Calder (2003) *Contemporary Treatment of Adult Sex Offenders* published by Russell House, and co-edited the *Handbook for Sexual Abuse Assessment and Treatment* (2001, Safer Press).

Clark R. Clipson, PhD, is a licensed psychologist in private practice specializing in psychological and neuropsychological assessment. The majority of his practice involves either criminal or civil evaluations. He has been evaluating sexual offenders since 1983, and has been a member of the evaluator panel for the California Department of Mental Health Sex Offender Commitment Program since 1998. He is also Adjunct Professor of Psychology at the California School of Professional Psychology at Alliant International University in San Diego.

Joseph J. Harper, LCSW, MBA, CCHP, is employed by the Illinois Department of Corrections and practices in the state's largest maximum security correctional facility. He is a Fellow of the Wisconsin Sex Offender Treatment Network. Mr. Harper is licensed as a clinical social worker in the states of Illinois and Missouri. Mr. Harper received his Master of Social Work degree from the George Warren Brown School of Social Work at Washington University in St. Louis, Missouri. Mr. Harper has co-authored several articles related to sex offender treatment. A recent article entitled "A Brief Review of Contemporary Sex Offender Treatment" appeared in *The Forensic Therapist.* Mr. Harper was also a speaker at the Association for the Treatment of Sexual Abusers 21st Annual Research and Treatment Conference.

Richard I. Hooper, LCSW, PhD, is a licensed clinical social worker and Assistant Professor of Social Work at Weber State University. He earned his MSW from the University of Georgia and PhD from Portland State University. His clinical experience includes working inpatient and outpatient psychiatry, dual diagnosis PTSD and drug and alcohol treatment. In private practice since 1994, he has worked with client problems ranging from agoraphobia, depression, chronic pain, forensic police work, and sex offender treatment. He was nominated for outstanding professor of the year in Utah by the National Association of Social Workers, Utah Chapter in 2002.

Toni Cavanagh Johnson, PhD, is a licensed clinical psychologist in private practice in South Pasadena, California. She has been working in the field of child abuse for 24 years as a researcher, trainer and clinician. She has written five books, two booklets, two therapeutic games, published numerous articles in refereed journals and book chapters on child sexual abuse and children with sexual behavior problems. As chairperson of a task force of the California Professional Society on the Abuse of Children (CAPSAC), Dr. Johnson assisted in the development of Guidelines for Monitored (Supervised) Visits. Dr. Johnson has lectured on child abuse and domestic violence throughout the world.

Ron Kokish, PhD, is a Licensed Family Therapist and Board Certified Clinical Social Worker with 17 years of experience in government operated Child Protective Services. He was in private practice from 1987 through 2000, treating victims and perpetrators of sexual, physical and emotional abuse, preparing forensic evaluations, serving as an expert witness, and training social workers, psychologists, probation and parole officers, teachers, and counselors through various accredited human services programs. He has been using polygraph in treatment since 1987. His present practice specializes in consultation, training, and evaluations.

Jill S. Levenson, PhD, is a faculty member at Florida International University School of Social Work. A licensed clinical social worker, Dr. Levenson has over 16 years of clinical practice experience with abused children, perpetrators, adult survivors, and non-offending parents. She has lectured locally and internationally on the topic of sexual abuse, and has published several articles and book chapters. She has co-authored three books, *Treating Nonoffending Parents in Sexual Abuse Cases* and the *Connections Workbook*, both published by Sage, and *The Road to Freedom*, a workbook for sex offenders in treatment, distributed by Wood and Barnes. Dr. Levenson's research interests include sexual violence policy, therapeutic engagement, and the practice of sex offender risk assessment.

Carole K. Metzger, LCSW, received her Master of Social Work degree from the University of Illinois in Champaign-Urbana, and now practices at Chester Mental Health Center, a maximum-security forensic hospital. Prior to accepting a unit director position at Chester Mental Health Center, Ms. Metzger worked for the Illinois Department of Corrections. At Big Muddy Correctional Center, she held two positions in a nine-year period; her first position was a sex offender treatment therapist and second as the mental health professional for both Big Muddy and the DuQuion Impact Incarceration Program. She has written fifteen professional publications on sex offender assessment and treatment. She has also provided training on psychiatric care, sex offender treatment and assessment, and forensic psychiatric assessment and treatment since 1992. She has provided training at the annual Association for the Treatment of Sexual Abusers conference.

Ray E. Quackenbush, PsyD, practices with Affiliated Psychologists, Ltd., Chicago, Illinois. His work involves assessment of Sexually Violent Persons, probation clients and others, as well as treatment and frequent court testimony. He holds a Masters in Family Therapy from the University of Houston-Clear Lake, together with a Masters and Doctorate in Clinical Psychology from the California Institute of Integral Studies. The author of several articles, Dr. Quackenbush lectures and consults internationally concerning forensic psychology. His research interests include actuarial risk assessment and the dynamics of sexual abuse.

Fabian M. Saleh, MD, received his medical degree at the University of Florence Medical School, Italy. In 1996, Dr. Saleh came to the United States to pursue residency training in Psychiatry at Case Western Reserve University and University Hospitals of Cleveland. On completing his residency at Case Western Reserve University, he pursued a residency in psychiatry at Johns Hopkins Hospital and Johns Hopkins University School of Medicine. At Johns Hopkins, Dr. Saleh enhanced his expertise in a wide range of psychopathology, in particular, the phenomenology of sexually deviant behaviors. Dr. Saleh was named a member of the Sexual Offenders Committee of the American Academy of Psychiatry and the Law. Working with Dr. Berlin, Dr. Saleh has evaluated and treated children, adolescents, and adults engaging in paraphilic behaviors and performed research on their sexually deviant behaviors. He is now in the process of implementing a multi-site study of the use of two different medications (leuprolide acetate and sertraline) for paraphilias. Recently, Dr. Saleh was the recipient of the Richard Rosner Award for the Best Paper by a Fellow in Forensic Psychiatry or Forensic Psychology, awarded by the American Academy of Forensic Sciences.

Pamela M. Yates, PhD, RPsych, has her doctorate degree in psychology and is the National Manager for Sex Offender Programs at the Correctional Service of Canada. She was formerly senior researcher for the Assessment and Treatment of Sex Offenders Research Team at the Muriel McQueen Fergusson Centre for Family Violence Research at the University of New Brunswick. She has researched sex offender risk, recidivism, treatment, substance abuse, and violence prevention, and has collaborated on numerous reports and presentations in the areas of prevention of sexual assault, sex offender risk assessment, phallometric assessment, treatment for sexual offenders, and sexual sadism. She has worked both within correctional systems with offenders, including with high-risk sexual offenders, as well as in community settings with victims of violence. She is presently developing and provides training in treatment programs for sexual offenders.

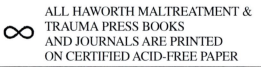

INTRODUCTION AND THEORETICAL ISSUES

Adult Sexual Offenders:
Current Issues and Future Directions

Robert Geffner
Kristina Crumpton Franey
Robert Falconer

SUMMARY. Sex offender research is still in its infancy, but our knowledge about adult sex offenders has increased in the last several decades. However, public interest in the issues of assessment, treatment, and recidivism with respect to risk and safety has increased substantially during this time. This article provides an introduction to the significant issues involved in the assessment, treatment, and current state-of-the-science for adult sex offenders. Prevalence rates are discussed, but these are more difficult to narrow down due to definitional problems. In addition, controversial issues involving diagnoses, classification, public notification, and risk as-

Address correspondence to: Robert Geffner, PhD, 6160 Cornerstone Court East, San Diego, CA 92121 (E-mail: bgeffner@alliant.edu).

[Haworth co-indexing entry note]: "Adult Sexual Offenders: Current Issues and Future Directions." Geffner, Robert, Kristina Crumpton Franey, and Robert Falconer. Co-published simultaneously in *Journal of Child Sexual Abuse* (The Haworth Maltreatment & Trauma Press, an imprint of The Haworth Press, Inc.) Vol. 12, No. 3/4, 2003, pp. 1-16; and: *Identifying and Treating Sex Offenders: Current Approaches, Research, and Techniques* (ed: Robert Geffner et al.) The Haworth Maltreatment & Trauma Press, an imprint of The Haworth Press, Inc., 2003, pp. 1-16. Single or multiple copies of this article are available for a fee from The Haworth Document Delivery Service [1-800-HAWORTH, 9:00 a.m. - 5:00 p.m. (EST). E-mail address: docdelivery@haworthpress.com].

sessment are introduced, and the goals of this volume are described. The purpose of this volume is to provide current information regarding what is known about sex offenders so that appropriate assessment, treatment, and prevention techniques can be developed and utilized. *[Article copies available for a fee from The Haworth Document Delivery Service: 1-800-HAWORTH. E-mail address: <docdelivery@haworthpress.com> Website: <http://www.HaworthPress.com> © 2003 by The Haworth Press, Inc. All rights reserved.]*

KEYWORDS. Sex offender assessment, sex offender treatment, risk assessment, sex offender policies

Sexual violence remains prevalent in today's society. Finkelhor (1994), in a review of studies in the United States and Canada, concluded that approximately 20-25% of women and 5-15% of men experienced some type of unwanted sexual contact in their lifetime. These figures are similar but somewhat lower than the estimates reported 10 years earlier by Russell (1984). Russell and others have estimated rates of sexual violence to be between 16-44% of women and 5-25% of men, depending upon definitions, sampling, and study methodology. In a review of research and methods for detecting adult rape prevalence, Koss (1993) found that 10-25% of adult women, depending upon methodology and definitions, report an adult rape experience. According to recent statistics and research, there are approximately 100,000 cases of child sexual abuse substantiated by various child protective services (CPS) agencies annually in the United States (U.S. Department of Health & Human Services, 2003). However, this only includes those cases that are reported to and investigated by CPS. There are also substantial numbers of women who are sexually assaulted by acquaintances and strangers (Bureau of Justice Statistics, 2002).

The above statistics may not include all of the recent reports of children and adolescents sexually abused by members of the clergy, as has been reported in recent months in several newspapers and television news shows. A recent report estimated that as many as 1,000 children were abused by priests during the past few decades in one state alone (Robinson & Rezendes, 2003). Further, since it has been widely known that most sexual assaults are never reported to official agencies, the statistics are estimated by the various criminal justice agencies to be grossly under-reported.

While the term "sex offender" typically conjures up an image of a stranger in a trench coat, in reality the offender is often known by the victim (Greenfield, 1997; Tjaden & Thoennes, 1998). Yet, even when the victim knows the offender, many times the abuse goes unreported and not prosecuted. An area of specific concern in this respect is marital rape. In their national sample, Tjaden and Thoennes (2000) found that 0.2% of men and 4.5% of women indicated that they had been forcibly raped by a current or former intimate partner. When this is extrapolated to the population of married or co-habiting couples at a national level, a large number of women and men are involved. Thus, we do not actually know how many women, men, boys, and girls are sexually assaulted each year, or during their lifetime.

Regardless of the exact numbers, it is clear that sexual offending occurs at high rates, is usually not reported to agencies or even friends/family members, and few of the offenders are actually prosecuted. In fact, Abel and colleagues reported that only 3% of any sexual offenses are ever criminally adjudicated (Abel, Becker, Cunningham-Rathner, Mittleman, Murphy, & Rouleou, 1987); Warshaw (1988) suggests in an investigative report for the media that an even lower percentage of cases are adjudicated since only 5% of rape cases are ever reported to law enforcement. In addition, it is clear that we know much more about the victims of sexual assault and their prevalence than we do about sex offenders.

DEFINITIONS OF SEX OFFENDERS AND RECENT CONTROVERSIES

The definition of a sex offender has been problematic. Legally, different jurisdictions define sexual assault in various ways, and these definitions usually involve such issues as consent, ages of the parties and age differences when minors are involved, marital or co-habiting relationships, and degree of force or pressure with acquaintances. The notion that all sex offenders are either "fixated" or "regressed" has become obsolete as we learn more about the variations in typologies, especially when dealing with a serial rapist on one hand and a single incident incest offender on the other. Some professionals believe that diagnoses may not even be appropriate in dealing with sex offenders (e.g., Doren, 2002). When discussing sexual deviations from a mental health/mental illness perspective, various distinctions are made.

Most sexual deviations come under the heading of paraphilias (American Psychiatric Association, 2000). When the offense involves an adult and a child, the subheading is pedophilia. However, the categories are further broken down by gender preference (attracted to males, attracted to females, or attracted to both; the latter is most common in pedophiles), specificity within the family unit only (i.e., incest) or nonspecific, and exclusivity (i.e., exclusively attracted to children or nonexclusivity, where the offender is also attracted to or in sexual relationships with adults). These variations are important in classifying sex offenders so that appropriate interventions can be ascertained and implemented. Unfortunately, inexperienced or untrained individuals conducting sex offender assessments often appear unaware of the important distinctions in the types of offenders.

In addition, there is a recent movement that desires to have pedophilia and other paraphilias removed from the recognized psychiatric/psychological diagnoses (e.g., Green, 2002). This new movement suggests that paraphilias represent sexual behavior, not mental health problems. That is, the proponents argue that, like homosexuality, paraphilic behaviors represent sexual preferences or orientation, not a mental illness. According to this group, paraphilic behaviors, especially pedophilia, should be controlled by legal sanctions and not seen as an illness or a mental health issue (Green, 2002).

This is somewhat similar to the arguments being made in several arenas that there should not even be a diagnosis of pedophilia, but it should instead be called adult-child sex (e.g., Rind, Tromovitch, & Bauserman, 1998). This argument stems from two mistaken views: one, that minor children even as young as age 12 can consent to sexual interactions; and two, that sexual interactions between adults and children may not be harmful. This is not a new advocacy position, but has been put in more sophisticated terms under the umbrella of "research" and "academic freedom" issues (for a good review of the fallacy of these views and their distortion of the research findings, see Dallam, 2001; Whittenburg, Tice, Baker, & Lemmy, 2001). A recent book focuses on the above controversies relating to child sexual abuse as well as other areas of misinformation concerning sexual behavior and abuse (Whitfield, Silberg, & Fink, 2001).

LEGAL ISSUES AND PUBLIC POLICIES

Changes in laws and public policy attempt to address society's growing concern about sexual violence. When an offender is caught and convicted of sexually offending, his or her average amount of time spent in prison varies depending upon the type of sexual assault, the specific victim(s) (i.e., adult or child), whether the offender has repeated incidents, the particular jurisdiction, and the pre-sentence investigation (for reviews of sex offender supervision, criminal justice issues, and systemic responses, see Flora, 2001; Holmes & Holmes, 2002; Kercher, 1998). While incarcerated, an offender may receive sex offense specific treatment. Yet society realizes that just as treatment is not completely effective in preventing future offenses, neither is incarceration (Malesky & Keim, 2001). What has been shown in the research is that treatment effectiveness (as measured by reoffense rates) is dependent on a number of variables. For instance, the method of treatment offered, the type of offender (e.g., adult rapist vs. child molester vs. incest offender), and the treatment settings are important factors (Crow, 2001; Flora, 2001; Freeman-Longo, 2000; Holmes & Holmes, 2002). Nonetheless, small treatment effects have been found when comparing recidivism rates between those who have received treatment versus those who have not (Blanchette, 1996; Hanson & Harris, 2000). However, it is not clear what percentage of offenders, incarcerated or on probation, receives the treatment that has been shown to be more effective in reducing reoffense rates (for reviews of the research and issues regarding recidivism in sex offenders, see Doren, 2002; Quinsey & Lalumiere, 2001; as well as the articles by Quackenbush and Clipson in this volume). It is also not clear how many victims most sex offenders abuse before being caught or stopped.

Lawmakers have attempted to address society's increasing concern by creating public policy called "sexually violent predator statutes." These civil commitment laws allow for those declared sexually violent predators to be held after they have completed their prison terms (for a review of civil commitment issues, see Levenson, in this volume). To date, 16 states have adopted these laws. Once declared a sexually violent predator, the offender is confined to a treatment facility until it is determined that s/he has benefited from treatment and is no longer dangerous. Whereas the laws have been challenged in the courts, to date no state's civil commitment legislation has been successfully overturned (Talbot, Gilligan, Carter, & Matson, 2002). However, once the appropriate authorities or program agree that the offender is rehabilitated, they are then freed. This often results in a public outcry (e.g., Moran, 2003). We still do not have adequate data that indicate whether the civil commitment laws decrease the recidivism rates once the offender is released, even though a variety of studies and reports raise these issues (for reviews, see Doren, 2002; Flora, 2001; Levenson, in this volume).

Upon release, most of those convicted of such offenses are required to register with local authorities and be listed as a sex offender. These registries have made public the names of more than 450,000 convicted sex offenders according to Megan's Law statutes (Hughes, 2001; Willing, 2003). The idea behind these laws is that the public may gain access to the names and general vicinity of the offender's residence by going to the local sheriff's department or, in some states, by gaining access to a Web site. It is commonly believed that knowing where an offender lives will assist the public in keeping their children safe (this of course does not apply to rapists who sexually assault other adults). Some have argued that such notifications are a form of community justice (for a past review of these issues, see Presser & Gunnison, 1999). However, recent lawsuits have challenged the legality of these registries based upon rights of privacy as well as cruel and unusual punishment. Since we do not have definitive research to support one position or the other, the debate of individual rights versus society's need to protect its children and citizens is likely to continue for many years.

In addition to registries, some states in the United States have attempted to decrease public anxiety by enacting laws that dictate where the offender can work and live. These so-called "child safety zones" prohibit an offender from living or spending time within 500 to 2,000 feet (depending on the state) of schools and day care centers. In the state of Oregon, for example, a convicted offender cannot go to areas where teens would normally spend time. The city of Albuquerque, New Mexico, is requesting that convicted sex offenders register with their landlords and employers in addition to their local law enforcement (Willing, 2003). The city and state statutes requiring registration are based upon the public's fear and outrage over sexual exploitation of children. However, it is again unclear whether the registries are effective in preventing future abuse of children.

In addition, a recent article by Curtis (2003) points out that these registries are not always enforced. In the newspaper article, Curtis reported that the State of California lost track of at least 33,000 sex offenders, or 44% of those who registered with the state at least once. The sex offenders, including child molesters, seemed to have "vanished" after registering with their local criminal justice departments (Curtis, 2003). The article also points out that the 44% does not represent the total number of sex offenders whose whereabouts are unknown. That is, this number does not include those offenders who failed to register after leaving prison or those who were not required to register at all. The registry may give the public a false sense of security: People may assume that if no offenders are listed for their neighborhood, their children will be safe.

The situation has recently become more complicated with the U.S. Supreme Court ruling that California and other states cannot retroactively prosecute sex offenders for cases that had passed the original statute of limitations (see *Stogner v. California*, 2003). Many states enacted new laws extending the period during which those accused of sexual offending against children could then be prosecuted, especially after the scandals within the Catholic Church became publicly known. As a result of the Court's decision, California was forced to release hundreds of confessed or convicted sex offenders, 24 of whom were released in Los Angeles, CA, on one day alone (Guccione & Winton, 2003).

The public outcry against adult sex offenders suggests that changes in public policy should be made. However, policies should be based upon research data or a sound theoretical framework, not just public anxiety. It is important to ensure that those who commit sexual offenses are stopped and prevented from committing additional assaults, and that policies that will protect society are established based on the best research. By providing an underlying understanding of the assessment, treatment, and polices related to adult sex offenders, this volume seeks to inform those who make decisions regarding this population.

THIS VOLUME

The purpose of this volume is to provide current information regarding what is known about sex offenders so that appropriate assessment, treatment, and prevention techniques can be developed and utilized. Too much misinformation exists in this field, which can lead to policies that are based on ideology and myth rather than accurate information. In addition, too many people are treating or assessing sex offenders in various settings and contexts without having an adequate understanding of the research and appropriate protocols. This volume therefore first discusses the controversial public policies briefly mentioned above. Next, it looks at the importance of thorough assessment when attempting to determine who is a sex offender and whether s/he is treatable in various settings. Finally, we address treatment options, including therapy as well as medical intervention. The specific articles are described below.

The beginning articles of this volume explore theoretical issues regarding sexual offenders. The first article, "Policy Interventions Designed to Combat Sexual Violence: Community Notification and Civil Commitment" by Levenson, provides an updated review of the literature regarding community notification and civil commitment as interventions designed to combat sexual violence. The history and context of each policy are discussed, as is a review of available research evaluating the impact of each policy. Driving the new civil commitment laws are people's beliefs that sex offenders are not treatable, and therefore they are not willing to take the risk that an offender may re-offend. Levenson therefore presents the various legal statutes as well as a brief introduction to recidivism and risk assessment. These latter issues are then discussed in more depth in later articles.

Saleh and Berlin's article entitled "Sexual Deviancy: Diagnostic and Neurobiological Considerations" reviews the clinical and neurobiological characteristics of paraphilias. In addition to addressing basic information on paraphilias, Saleh and Berlin provide an examination of the most recent relevant research findings. The issue of diagnosis plays an important role in the ongoing debate about sex offenders. The public, as well as some mental health, social work, and criminal justice professionals, still seem to believe that an adult who molests a female child within a family setting could not do a similar act with a male child or a stranger. As stated above, the purpose of the differential diagnoses listed in the *Diagnostic and Statistical Manual of Mental Disorders-IV R* (American Psychiatric Association, 2000) was to distinguish among exclusive and nonexclusive, preferential and nonpreferential offenders. Thus, the assessment of paraphilias in sex offenders becomes a key aspect of sex offender assessment, which is covered in the next section.

Quackenbush addresses the challenges in risk assessment. Research on risk assessment with this population continues to grow, and yet researchers have yet to find a method of risk assessment that specifically predicts who will re-offend, or when. In his article entitled "The Role of Theory in the Assessment of Sex Offenders," Quackenbush asserts that there is no generally accepted theory of sex offender behavior that currently exists. He examines prominent theories of assessment and discusses the uses and limitations of each theory and various measures, based upon various research studies.

Moving from theory to practice, the articles then address practical issues regarding assessment and forensic considerations in working with adult sex offenders. This includes more specialized topics such as family boundaries. In their article, "Boundaries and Family Practices: Implications for Assessing Child Abuse," Johnson and Hooper interview mental health professionals to obtain their views of acceptable family boundaries, with the goal of establishing what clinicians believe is normal behavior versus abuse. Family practices related to bathing, expression of affection, and privacy are studied, including what age it is acceptable for parents and children of the same gender and mixed gender to engage in certain family practices. The article concludes by discussing the implications of the substantial differences of opinion found among these professionals. This is an important issue since assessment interpretations are usually based on comparisons to normative data. If the norms are not clear or not agreed upon, this impacts the assessment protocols and interpretation.

Clipson, in "Practical Considerations in the Interview and Evaluation of Sexual Offenders," discusses the ramifications of sex offender assessment. He points out that most clinicians are not properly trained to complete evaluations and assessment of adult sex offenders. He contends that working with this population is unlike any other type of work. His article in this volume addresses the clinical and ethical issues particular to the interview, assessment, and evaluation of adult sex offenders. As Clipson and others point out, too often in forensic settings, clinicians licensed as psychologists, psychiatrists, or social workers evaluate a person accused of child sexual abuse using the typical intake questionnaires or assessment batteries that they use for their general clinical populations. After finding no significant pathology on standardized measures of personality, for example, these clinicians without sufficient training in sex offender dynamics or research conclude that the person is not a sex offender and/or is not at risk for sexual offending. It is clear that such absolute statements, even when an appropriate evaluation had been conducted, are not justifiable or appropriate.

It is important that sex offender evaluations include specific measures designed for this population, such as the Multiphasic Sex Inventory (Nichols & Molinder, 1984), the Abel-Becker Cognitions Scale (in Abel, Gore, Holland, Camp, Becker, & Rathner, 1989), the Clarke Sex History Questionnaire (Langevin, Paitich, Russon, Handy, & Langevin, 1990), or the Psychopathy Checklist–Revised (Hare, 1991), as well as other instruments and questionnaires, to specifically assess for attitudes, beliefs, and behaviors consistent with sexual offending (see Clipson in this volume, and for other recent reviews of such techniques and measures, see Doren, 2002; Quinsey & Lalumiere, 2001). Therefore, Clipson also reviews the various measures and inventories that can be used to specifically assess sex offenders.

However, it is important to note that even with the appropriate techniques and protocols administered and interpreted by someone specifically trained in sex offending dynamics and assessment, the state-of-the-science does not support a definitive ability to determine whether someone is or is not a sex offender based primarily on such an assessment (American Psychological Association, 1996, 1997). Methods of ascertaining certainty of sex offending behaviors include a confession, DNA matches, someone actually observing the behavior, or in the case of child sexual abuse, the evaluation of the child (for excellent reviews of the appropriate guidelines, techniques, and procedures involved in the latter, see Faller, 2003; Myers, Berliner, Briere, Hendrix, Jenny, & Reid, 2002; Righthand, Kerr, & Drach, 2003). Clipson (in this volume) also points out the ethical issues related to the assessment of those accused of sexual offending, and reviews the various actuarial and other risk assessment instruments that can be used (e.g., the VRAG, the SORAG, the RRASOR, etc.). An important issue in this process is psychopathy (e.g., see Hare, 1991; Porter, Fairweather, Drugge, Herve, Birt, & Boer, 2000). Both Quackenbush and Clipson include this issue and related research in their articles in this volume.

Continuing with forensic issues, the next article reviews the application of polygraph technology to the treatment of sex offenders. Kokish, in his article "The Current Role of Post-Conviction Sex Offender Polygraph Testing in Sex Offender Treatment," discusses clinical and ethical implications in the use of polygraphy. Overcoming denial plays a key role in the treatment of sex offenders (Barbaree & Cortoni, 1993). The use of polygraphy can assist in countering denial. Kokish also discusses the controversy surrounding the use of polygraphy in sex offender treatment. Rather than providing a definitive answer, Kokish completes his article by allowing readers to decide the wisdom and ethics of using polygraph testing in their own practices. It should be noted, however, that there is an important distinction between using polygraphy as part of treatment to determine whether relapses or additional offending has occurred, and as a major part of the assessment to determine whether someone is a sex offender. The former has support in the literature whereas the latter has not been shown to be sufficiently reliable to be used in court (also, see the past review by Cross & Saxe, 1992, and the rebuttal by Williams, 1995).

Once assessment and evaluation have been completed, treatment is usually warranted and recommended. Yet sex offender treatment programs are often under-funded and unpopular, even though one year of community-based treatment and close supervision is less expensive than a year of incarceration without treatment (e.g., Freeman-Longo, 2000). Likewise, a meta-analysis of 43 studies showed sexual recidivism rates are lower among offenders who receive treatment (12.3%) versus those who go without treatment (16.8%), and that the same is true for nonsexual crimes after release from prison (Hanson et al., 2002). While 4.5% may not be a large difference, when percentages are translated into victims of crimes that may have been prevented, any difference becomes meaningful and suggests that additional research is warranted. A comprehensive meta-analysis that looked at recidivism of adult sexual offenders found a 13.4% sexual recidivism rate 4-5 years after treatment (Hanson & Bussiere, 1998). In their landmark study, Hanson and Bussiere reviewed 61 studies that met stringent inclusion criteria (longitudinal studies with comparison groups). In addition to reporting overall and sexual specific recidivism rates, the authors point out that not completing treatment (either while incarcerated or on an outpatient basis) is a moderate predictor of sexual recidivism. Therefore, the belief that sex offenders cannot be treated is a fallacy: Those who go without treatment are more apt to re-offend upon their release. This major study is discussed in more depth by many of the authors in this volume.

It should be noted, though, that there is also controversy about the definition of recidivism. Many studies, as the one above, rely on re-arrests as the main indicator of recidivism. This may underestimate the true incidence of repeat offending since many offenders may not have been caught. The very purpose of risk assessment and evaluation is to achieve estimates of the probability of re-offense as well as the circumstances under which an offender is most likely to re-offend (Hudson, Wales, Bakker, & Ward, 2002).

Therapists who work with this population face many obstacles, including changes in public policy, public perception of the "evil sex offender," as well as trying to find empirically based assessment and treatment tools. Accordingly, the next section of this volume addresses various aspects of treatment of adult sex offenders, including cognitive-behavioral treatment, medical treatment, and enhancing empathy for victims of sexual offense. Some believe that the mere presence of a paraphilia makes sex offenders untreatable (Tucker, 2003). As mentioned above, more recent meta-analyses suggest that treatment can be effective for some sex offenders. It is not yet clear which treatment approaches work best with which offenders, and under which conditions. Unquestionably, more research is needed. However, guidelines for treatment of this population have now been created by two organizations: the Association for Treatment of Sexual Abusers (ATSA; see their Web site for more information: www.atsa.org) and the International Conference on the Treatment of Sex Offenders (Coleman et al., 2001).

Various treatment approaches have been described in the literature (e.g., Crow, 2001; Kercher, 1998). One common technique involves cognitive-behavioral intervention specifically geared toward sex offenders. In her article entitled "Treatment of Adult Sexual Offenders: A Therapeutic Cognitive-Behavioural Model of Intervention," Yates reviews components of cognitive-behavioral treatment with sexual offenders, including recent developments in intervention and the importance of therapist characteristics required for treatment.

Likewise, Saleh and Berlin, in "Sex Hormones, Neurotransmitters, and Psychopharmacological Treatments in Men with Paraphilic Disorders," provide a discussion of prominent medical treatments for sexual deviance. Their article begins with two case reports that reflect the benefit and effectiveness of pharmacotherapy in paraphilic clients. Subsequently, they review the key concepts of the serotonin and catecholamine systems, as well as the sex hormones. The article concludes with a review of the pertinent neurobiological and psychopharmacological studies relevant to the paraphilias.

Finally, Carich, Metzger, Baig, and Harper examine a treatment modality that seeks to increase empathy among offenders for the victims of sexual abuse. In their article, "Enhancing Victim Empathy for Sex Offenders," the authors assert that victim empathy can be learned and is a useful and necessary component of sex offender treatment. They define victim empathy as well as the key elements in the development of empathy. Writing from a clinically applicable approach, the authors next provide readers with the basic principles of empathy enhancement in addition to covering different techniques utilized to enhance victim empathy skills in sex offenders.

CONCLUSION

The assessment and treatment of adult sex offenders is an emerging field. It is hoped that this volume will assist clinicians who assess or work with sex offenders, as well as those who set public policy and researchers interested in continuing work in the field. Ideally, future work can begin to focus on ways to prevent sexual abuse from occurring in the first place. Until that time, research must continue to focus on developing a more thorough understanding of the offender's choice to offend, as well as predictors of future violence and abuse. Sexual violence continues to exist. Enhancing risk assessment and treatment effectiveness as well as developing public polices that emphasize accountability and rehabilitation will be crucial in lowering overall sexual abuse rates as well as actual recidivism.

REFERENCES

Abel, G. G., Becker, J. V., Cunningham-Rathner, J., Mittleman, M. S., Murphy, M. S., & Rouleou, J. L. (1987). Self-reported crimes of nonincarcerated paraphiliacs. *Journal of Interpersonal Violence, 2*, 3-25.

Abel, G. G., Gore, D. K., Holland, C. L., Camp, N., Becker, J. V., & Rathner, J. (1989). The measurement of the cognitive distortions of child molesters. *Annals of Sex Research, 2*, 135-153.

American Psychiatric Association. (2000). *Diagnostic criteria from DSM-IV-R*. Washington, DC: Author.

American Psychological Association. (1996). *Violence and the family: A report of the presidential task force on violence and the family*. Washington, DC: Author.

American Psychological Association. (1997). *Potential problems for psychologists working with the area of interpersonal violence*. Washington, DC: Author.

Barbaree, H. E., & Cortoni, F. A. (1993). Treatment of the juvenile sexual offender within the criminal justice and mental health systems. In H. E. Barbaree, W. L. Marshall, & S. Hudson (Eds.), *The juvenile sex offender* (Vol. 1, pp. 243-263). New York: The Guilford Press.

Blanchette, K. (1996). *Sex offender assessment, treatment and recidivism: A literature review*. Technical Research report, Correctional Service of Canada. Retrieved September 3, 2003, from http://www.csc-scc.gc.ca/text/pblct/forum/e093/e093vv_e.shtml.

Bureau of Justice Statistics. (2002). *Rape and sexual assault: Reporting to police and medical attention, 1992-2000*. Retrieved September 3, 2003, from http://www.ojp.usdoj.gov/bjs/pub/pdf/rsarp00.pdf.

Carich, M. S., Metzger, C. K., Baig, M. S. A., & Harper, J. J. (2003). Enhancing victim empathy for sex offenders. *Journal of Child Sexual Abuse, 12*(3/4), 257-278.

Clipson, C. R. (2003). Practical considerations in the interview and evaluation of sexual offenders. *Journal of Child Sexual Abuse, 12*(3/4), 127-173.

Coleman, E., Dwyer, S. M., Abel, G., Berner, W., Breiling, J., Eher, R. et al. (2001). Standards of care for the treatment of adult sex offenders. *Journal of Psychology and Human Sexuality, 13*(3/4), 115-121.

Cross, T. P., & Saxe, L. (1992). A critique of the validity of polygraph testing in child sexual abuse cases. *Journal of Child Sexual Abuse, 1*(4), 19-33.

Crow, I. (2001). *The treatment and rehabilitation of offenders*. Thousand Oaks, CA: Sage.

Curtis, K. (2003, February 6). *California loses track of more than 30,000 sex offenders*. Retrieved February 6, 2003, from AP Online.

Dallam, S. J. (2001). Science or propaganda? An examination of Rind, Tromovitch and Bauserman (1998). *Journal of Child Sexual Abuse, 9*(3/4), 109-134.

Doren, D. M. (2002). *Evaluating sex offenders: A manual for civil commitments and beyond.* Thousand Oaks, CA: Sage.

Faller, K. C. (2003). *Understanding and assessing child sexual maltreatment* (2nd ed.). Thousand Oaks, CA: Sage.

Finkelhor, D. (1994). Current information on the scope and nature of child sexual abuse. *Future of Children, 4,* 31-53.

Flora, R. (2001). *How to work with sex offenders: A handbook for criminal justice, human service, and mental health professionals.* Binghamton, NY: The Haworth Clinical Practice Press.

Freeman-Longo, R. (2000). *Myths and facts about sex offenders.* Center for Sex Offender Management Website retrieved September 3, 2003, from http://www.csom.org/pubs/mythsfacts.html.

Green, R. (2002). Is pedophilia a mental disorder? *Archives of Sexual Behavior, 31*(6), 467-471(5).

Greenfield, L. (1997). *Sex offenses and offenders: An analysis of data on rape and sexual assault.* Washington, DC: Bureau of Justice Statistics.

Guccione, J., & Winton, R. (2003, July 24). 24 child molesters released. *Los Angeles Times,* p. B1.

Hanson, R. K., & Bussiere, M. T. (1998). Predicting relapse: A meta-analysis of sexual offender recidivism studies. *Journal of Consulting and Clinical Psychology, 66,* 348-362.

Hanson, R. K., Gordon, A., Harris, A. J. R., Marques, J., Murphy, W., Quinsey, V. L., & Seto, M. C. (2002). First report of the collaborative outcome data project on the effectiveness of psychological treatment for sex offenders. *Sexual Abuse: A Journal of Research and Treatment, 14*(2), 169-194.

Hanson, R. K., & Harris, A. J. R. (2000). Where should we intervene? Dynamic predictors of sexual offense recidivism. *Criminal Justice and Behavior, 27*(1), 6-35.

Hare, R. D. (1991). *Manual for the Psychopathy Checklist-Revised.* Toronto, Ontario, Canada: Multi-Health Systems.

Holmes, S. T., & Holmes, R. M. (2002). *Sex crimes: Patterns and behavior* (2nd ed.). Thousand Oaks, CA: Sage.

Hudson, S., Wales, D., Bakker, L., & Ward, T. (2002). Dynamic risk factors: The Kia Marama evaluation. *Sexual Abuse: A Journal of Research and Treatment, 14*(2), 103-119.

Hughes, T. (2001). The creation of and considerations surrounding Megan's Law: The D.A. can't get no relief. In R. M. Holmes, & S. T. Holmes (Eds.), *Current perspectives on sex crimes* (pp. 135-142). Thousand Oaks, CA: Sage.

Johnson, T. C., & Hooper, R. I. (2003). Boundaries and family practices: Implications for assessing child abuse. *Journal of Child Sexual Abuse, 12*(3/4), 103-125.

Kercher, G. A. (1998). *Supervision and treatment of sex offenders* (Rev. ed.). Holmes Beach, FL: Learning Publications.

Kokish, R. (2003). The current role of post conviction sex offender polygraph testing in sex offender treatment. *Journal of Child Sexual Abuse, 12*(3/4), 175-195.

Koss, M. P. (1993). Detecting the scope of rape: A review of prevalence research methods. *Journal of Interpersonal Violence, 8,* 198-222.

Langevin, R., Paitich, D., Russon, A., Handy, L., & Langevin, A. (1990). *Clarke Sex History Questionnaire for Males manual.* Oakville, Ontario, Canada: Juniper Press.

Levenson, J. S. (2003). Policy interventions designed to combat sexual violence: Community notification and civil commitment. *Journal of Child Sexual Abuse, 12*(3/4), 17-52.

Malesky, A., & Keim, J. (2001). Mental health professionals' perspectives on sex offender registry web sites. *Sexual Abuse: A Journal of Research and Treatment, 13*(1), 53-63.

Moran, G. (2003, August 17). Public incensed as sex offender goes free. *San Diego Union Tribune,* p. A1, A19.

Myers, J. E. B., Berliner, L., Briere, J., Hendrix, C. T., Jenny, C., & Reid, T. A. (2002). *The APSAC handbook on child maltreatment* (2nd ed.). Thousand Oaks, CA: Sage.

Nichols, H. R., & Molinder, I. (1984). *Multiphasic Sex Inventory manual.* Tacoma, WA: Author.

Porter, S., Fairweather, D., Drugge, J., Herve, H., Birt, A., & Boer, D. P. (2000). Profiles of psychopathy in incarcerated sexual offenders. *Criminal Justice and Behavior, 27*(2), 216-233.

Presser, L., & Gunnison, E. (1999). Strange bedfellows: Is sex offender notification a form of community justice? *Crime & Delinquency, 45*(3), 299-315.

Quackenbush, R. E. (2003). The role of theory in the assessment of sex offenders. *Journal of Child Sexual Abuse, 12*(3/4), 77-102.

Quinsey, V. L., & Lalumiere, M. (2001). *Assessment of sexual offenders against children* (2nd ed.). APSAC Study Guide. Thousand Oaks, CA: Sage.

Righthand, S., Kerr, B., & Drach, K. (2003).*Child maltreatment risk assessments: An evaluation guide.* Binghamton, NY: The Haworth Maltreatment & Trauma Press.

Rind, B., Tromovitch, P., & Bauserman, R. (1998). A meta-analytic examination of assumed properties of child sexual abuse using college samples. *Psychological Bulletin, 124*, 22-53.

Robinson, W. V., & Rezendes, M. (2003, July 24). Abuse scandal far deeper than disclosed, report says: Victims of clergy may exceed 1,000, Reilly estimates. *The Boston Globe,* p. A1.

Russell, D. E. H. (1984). *Sexual exploitation: Rape, child sexual abuse, and workplace harassment.* Newbury Park, CA: Sage.

Saleh, F. M., & Berlin, F. S. (2003). Sexual deviancy: Diagnostic and neurobiological considerations. *Journal of Child Sexual Abuse, 12*(3/4), 53-76.

Saleh, F. M., & Berlin, F. S. (2003). Sexual hormones, neurotransmitters, and psychopharmacological treatment in men with paraphilic disorders. *Journal of Child Sexual Abuse, 12*(3/4), 235-256.

Stogner v. California (01-1757), 93 Cal. App. 4th 1229, 114 Cal. Rptr. 2d 37 (rev'd, U.S. June 26, 2003). U.S. Supreme Court decision retrieved September 3, 2003, from http://www.supremecourtus.gov/opinions/02pdf/01-1757.pdf.

Talbot, T., Gilligan, L., Carter, M., & Matson, S. (2002, July). An overview of sex offender management. Retrieved September 3, 2003, from www.csom.org/pubs/csom_bro.pdf.

Tjaden, P., & Thoennes, N. (1998). *Prevalence, incidence, and consequences of violence against women: Findings from the National Violence Against Women Survey.* Washington, DC: U.S. Department of Justice, National Institute of Justice.

Tjaden, P., & Thoennes, N. (2000). Prevalence and consequences of male-to-female and female-to-male intimate partner violence as measured by the National Violence Against Women Survey. *Violence Against Women, 6*(2),142-161.

Tucker, J. (2003, January 21). Giving treatment to child molesters: Reformers say offenders need help to stop from molesting again–and the numbers back them up. *San Mateo County Times*, http://www.sanmateocountytimes.com.

U.S. Department of Health & Human Services, Administration for Children and Families, Administration on Children, Youth and Families, Children's Bureau. (2003). Child maltreatment 2001. Washington, DC: U.S. Government Printing Office.

Warshaw, R. (1988). *I never called it rape: The Ms. report on recognizing, fighting, and surviving date and acquaintance rape.* New York: Sarah Lazin.

Whitfield, C. L., Silberg, J., & Fink, P. J. (2001). *Misinformation concerning child sexual abuse and adult survivors.* Binghamton, NY: The Haworth Maltreatment & Trauma Press.

Whittenburg, J. A., Tice, P. P., Baker, G. L., & Lemmy, D. E. (2001). A critical appraisal of the 1998 meta-analytic review of child sexual abuse outcomes reported by Rind, Tromovitch, and Bauserman. *Journal of Child Sexual Abuse, 9*(3/4), 135-155.

Williams, V. L. (1995). Response to Cross and Saxe's "A critique of the validity of polygraph testing in child sexual abuse cases." *Journal of Child Sexual Abuse, 4*(3), 55-71.

Willing, R. (2003, May 11). Laws tighten on sex offenders. *USA Today*, p. A1.

Yates, P. M. (2003). Treatment of adult sexual offenders: A therapeutic cognitive-behavioural model of intervention. *Journal of Child Sexual Abuse, 12*(3/4), 197-234.

Policy Interventions Designed to Combat Sexual Violence: Community Notification and Civil Commitment

Jill S. Levenson

SUMMARY. Much attention has been given to the problem of sexual predators and the struggles of the legal-justice system to contain them. In response to public outcry over high-profile sex crimes, federal and state legislators have responded in the past decade with innovative but controversial public policy initiatives, called "sexually violent predator statutes." In 1996 President Clinton signed "Megan's Law," mandating all 50 states to develop requirements for convicted sex offenders to register with local law enforcement agencies and to notify communities when a sex offender lives in close proximity. Less publicized have been the civil commitment statutes introduced by 16 states which allow convicted sex offenders to be evaluated for involuntary and indefinite confinement in a psychiatric hospital following their release from prison. This article will review the literature regarding community notification and civil commitment as interventions designed to combat sexual violence. The his-

---

Address correspondence to: Jill S. Levenson, PhD, Florida International University School of Social Work, 11200 SW 8th Street, ECS 460, Miami, FL 33199 (E-mail: levenson@fiu.edu).

[Haworth co-indexing entry note]: "Policy Interventions Designed to Combat Sexual Violence: Community Notification and Civil Commitment." Levenson, Jill S. Co-published simultaneously in *Journal of Child Sexual Abuse* (The Haworth Maltreatment & Trauma Press, an imprint of The Haworth Press, Inc.) Vol. 12, No. 3/4, 2003, pp. 17-52; and: *Identifying and Treating Sex Offenders: Current Approaches, Research, and Techniques* (ed: Robert Geffner et al.) The Haworth Maltreatment & Trauma Press, an imprint of The Haworth Press, Inc., 2003, pp. 17-52. Single or multiple copies of this article are available for a fee from The Haworth Document Delivery Service [1-800-HAWORTH, 9:00 a.m. - 5:00 p.m. (EST). E-mail address: docdelivery@haworthpress.com].

http://www.haworthpress.com/web/JCSA
Digital Object Identifier: 10.1300/J070v12n03_02

tory and context of each policy will be discussed, as will a review of available research evaluating the impact of each policy. Implications for future research and social policy will be examined. *[Article copies available for a fee from The Haworth Document Delivery Service: 1-800-HAWORTH. E-mail address: <docdelivery@haworthpress.com> Website: <http://www.HaworthPress. com> © 2003 by The Haworth Press, Inc. All rights reserved.]*

KEYWORDS. Civil commitment, community notification, Megan's Law, sex offender, sexually violent predator statutes

THE PROBLEM OF SEXUAL VIOLENCE

Over the past 20 years, sexual assault has been increasingly recognized as a significant social problem with complex and far-reaching consequences for victims, families, and society. The National Center on Child Abuse Prevention Research reported that in 1997, 223,650 children were reported to child welfare agencies in alleged child sexual abuse cases (Wang & Daro, 1998). Self-report victimization surveys have found that 23% of adults reported that they were sexually abused before the age of 18 (Finkelhor, Moore, Hamby, & Straus, 1997). It is estimated, based on national surveys, that 302,091 women have experienced rape or attempted rape during their lifetime–a rate of 8.7 per 1,000 women (Satcher, 2001). Other studies estimate that 22% of women and 2% of men have been victims of a forced sexual act and that 104,000 children are victims of sexual abuse each year (Satcher, 2001). Almost invariably, researchers caution that official reports of sexual assault are underestimates and may not fully represent the scope of the problem.

Sex offenders make up a substantial portion of the population of prison inmates. Among 906,000 inmates confined in state prisons across the U.S. in 1994, 88,000, or nearly 10%, were violent sex offenders (Bureau of Justice Statistics, 1997). Despite the high proportion of sex offenders in the prison population, Abel et al. (Abel, Becker, Cunningham-Rathner, Mittleman, Murphy, & Rouleou, 1987), based on research soliciting anonymous admissions of sexual crimes, speculated that only 3% of sex offenses are ever criminally adjudicated.

In response to public outcry over high-profile sex crimes, federal and state legislators have responded in the past decade with innovative but controversial public policy initiatives, called "sexually violent predator statutes." In 1996 President Clinton signed "Megan's Law" following the tragic New Jersey murder of Megan Kanka by a recently released child molester. This federal statute mandated all 50 states to develop requirements for convicted sex offenders to register with local law enforcement agencies and to notify communities when a sex offender lives in close proximity. Less publicized have been the civil commitment statutes introduced by 16 states which allow convicted sex offenders to be evaluated for involuntary confinement in a psychiatric hospital following their release from prison. The intent of these laws is to remove dangerous sex offenders from society even after they have served a prison sentence and can no longer be held by the criminal justice system. The purposes of post-incarceration commitment are both rehabilitation and incapacitation.

Much attention has been given to the problem of sexual predators and the struggles of the legal-justice system to contain them. Driven by revulsion, anger, and fear that far exceed responses to other types of crimes in our society, sexually violent predator statutes may succeed in providing an illusion of public safety. The true efficacy of these laws, however, remains undetermined.

This article will review the literature regarding community notification and civil commitment as interventions designed to combat sexual violence. The history and context of each policy will be discussed, as will a review of available research. Implications for future research and social policy will also be examined.

COMMUNITY NOTIFICATION

In October of 1989, while riding his bike in his Minnesota neighborhood with two other boys, 11-year-old Jacob Wetterling was abducted by a stranger, and was never to be found again. Following the event, Jacob's parents became vocal advocates for a national networking system by which known sex offenders could be tracked. In 1994, the Jacob Wetterling Crimes Against Children and Sexually Violent Offender Registration Act was passed, creating sex offender registries in all 50 states and requiring sex offenders to register with local law enforcement agencies so that their current whereabouts are known (Petrosino & Petrosino, 1999).

In July 1994, a 7-year-old New Jersey child named Megan Kanka was lured into the home of a convicted sex offender with promises that she could play with his puppy. She was then sexually assaulted and strangled. Following her tragic death, Megan's parents and 100,000 other New Jersey residents petitioned the New Jersey legislature to create a law requiring communities to be told of the presence of a convicted sex offender. Only three months after Megan's murder, Governor Whitman signed the nation's first community notification law, known as "Megan's Law" (Lotke, 1997). In 1996, President Clinton signed the Federal version of Megan's law, requiring all states to implement community notification as part of the sex offender registration requirements designated in the 1994 Wetterling Act (Petrosino & Petrosino, 1999). Financial incentives are offered to states that comply with federal guidelines.

Because community notification was first proposed in response to the sexually motivated murder of a child, it was originally conceived as a strategy designed to combat predatory child sexual abuse. As legislation evolved, it became inclusive of all sexual perpetrators, including incestuous offenders, rapists of adults, non-contact offenders such as exhibitionists, and child pornographers. Notification is intended to enhance community protection from sexual violence through public awareness and education as well as through vigilant surveillance and collaboration between law enforcement agents and citizens. The commonly cited goal of these statutes is to prevent sexual victimization by notifying potential victims that a convicted sex offender lives nearby.

In a review of notification laws in all 50 states and in other countries, Matson and Lieb (1996) found that each state implements notification differently. The methods used to inform citizens of the locations where sex offenders reside include press releases, flyers, phone calls, door-to-door contact, neighborhood meetings, and Internet access. Many states assign offenders to one of three risk levels and notify differentially according to risk. Other states employ broad community notification, notifying communities and organizations (e.g., schools and day care centers) about the presence of all sex offenders without regard for risk assessment (Matson & Lieb, 1996).

Community notification statutes have been challenged on issues related to rights to privacy as well as the constitutionality of the lifetime notification requirements in some states. In *Connecticut Department of Public Safety v. Doe* (2003), the U.S. Supreme Court ruled that states can put the names of sex offenders on a registry without first holding a hearing to determine their dangerousness to the community, concluding that offenders receive all the process that is constitutionally required when they are given the opportunity to contest their guilt in the criminal proceedings. In an Alaska case, *Smith v. Doe* (2003), the Court ruled that the public identification on Internet Websites of registered sex offenders who have successfully completed their probation does not amount to unconstitutional retroactive punishment.

Although the literature pertaining to community notification is vast, the overwhelming majority of publications address legal issues such as the constitutionality of notification laws and procedures. Some theoretical, descriptive, and anecdotal literature exists, but few writers offer evidence-based conclusions regarding community notification, particularly around its commonly cited goal of reducing or preventing sexual assault. Empirical evidence is also lacking in the investigation of which types of notification strategies, if any, are most successful at preventing sexual abuse.

Sex Offense Recidivism

Community notification statutes are clear political winners. They were created in an attempt to prevent repeat sexual offenses, a noble goal that most constituents would undoubtedly support. The popular media routinely portrays sexual offenders as having extraordinary rates of recidivism, which ostensibly justifies community notification statutes and the public's "right to know." However, this very foundation on which notification legislation is built may be flawed. The notion "once a sex offender, always a sex offender" incites fear, but may represent a misleading and inaccurate myth. In fact, the recidivism base rate for child molesters was found in a recent meta-analysis to be much lower than is commonly believed–12.7% over a 5-year follow up period (Hanson & Bussiere, 1998). This finding may be surprisingly low because incestuous offenders, who tend to have lower recidivism rates than predatory pedophiles, were included in the study (Doren, 1998). In studies that more narrowly defined the type of offender and used longer follow-up periods of 25 and 31 years, base rates for extra-familial child molesters were found to be approximately 52% (Hanson, Scott, & Steffy, 1995; Prentky, Lee, Knight, & Cerce, 1997). Prentky et al. (1997) found the 25-year recidivism rate for rapists to be 39%, but noted that rapists showed higher reconviction rates than child molesters within their first five years at risk.

Although these findings represent high recidivism rates, they are much lower than the commonly accepted myth that "all sex offenders re-offend." Of course, recidivism rates underestimate true re-offense rates, because many sex crimes are not reported or prosecuted

(Hanson & Bussiere, 1998). Overall, however, sex offenders have consistently lower recidivism rates than perpetrators of non-sexual crimes (Hanson et al., 1995).

The widely held belief that sex offender treatment does not work has further fueled public outrage and demands for protective legislation following high-profile sexual offenses. This common belief is based largely on a study (Furby, Weinrott, & Blackshaw, 1989) that determined, in a review of 42 sex offender recidivism studies, that "there is as yet no evidence that clinical treatment reduces rates of sex re-offenses in general" (p. 27). Widely cited, these conclusions are often misrepresented and used to dismiss less restrictive treatment interventions as completely ineffective.

Furby et al. (1989) did not in fact conclude that sex offender treatment is futile, but that due to the methodological inadequacies of the studies they examined, they were unable to find a statistically significant treatment effect on recidivism. The authors cited several methodological deficiencies that rendered the researchers unable to draw conclusions using conventional meta-analytical techniques for combining results from different studies. Some of the identified flaws included short follow-up periods, small sample sizes, unclear operationalization of important variables such as recidivism, failure to evaluate data separately for different types of offenders, and widely variable treatment protocols (Furby et al., 1989). Given the skepticism generated from this highly publicized study, it is perhaps less surprising that legislative initiatives to reduce sexual violence have become more extreme.

A more recent meta-analysis (Hanson et al., 2002), conducted in a collaborative project by leading researchers in the field of sexual offending, has found reductions in both sexual recidivism and general recidivism when contemporary cognitive-behavioral relapse prevention treatment approaches are evaluated with methodologically sound research designs. The 43 studies reviewed included programs in which 80% of the 9,454 subjects had received treatment since 1980. Overall, treated groups sexually recidivated at a rate of 12% compared with a 17% recidivism rate for untreated control groups. Cognitive-behavioral and systemic treatment programs reduced sexual offense recidivism from 17.4% to 10%, reducing recidivism by almost 40%. Recidivism rates were based on an average 46-month follow-up period (Hanson et al., 2002).

Community Notification: The Emperor's New Clothes?

Freeman-Longo (1996) suggested that public notification is an emotionally driven response to sexual violence, and that it provides a false sense of security to citizens, as exemplified in a Florida case. Howard Steven Ault was on the "list," publicly identified as a sexual predator in one of Florida's earliest notification efforts. His photo, name, and past sexual crimes were distributed to thousands via a newspaper specially designed for the purpose of notifying communities of the presence of sex offenders. Despite this publicity, in November of 1996, just three months later, Ault was arrested for sexually assaulting and strangling a Fort Lauderdale child and also murdering her sister, who had witnessed the molestation. The two girls, daughters of a homeless woman who lived in a park, had been befriended by Ault and lured to his home with promises of Halloween candy. A week after their disappearance, police found their bodies hidden in Ault's attic.

Although stranger abductions receive a great deal of media attention, Jones (1999) pointed out among the flaws of notification, the fact that most offenses are committed by a family member or acquaintance rather than the strangers implied in notification laws. Importantly, *U.S. News & World Report* (Shenk, 1998) advised parents that fear of strangers is misplaced because the vast majority of sexual perpetrators are known to their victims. Others have expressed concern that community notification may increase the resistance of victims of family members or acquaintances to report sexual abuse, ultimately interfering with the child protection system and decreasing the likelihood that the victim will receive therapeutic intervention (Edwards & Hensley, 2001; Freeman-Longo, 1996; Lotke, 1997).

Critics (Freeman-Longo, 1996; Jones, 1999; Levi, 2000; Lotke, 1997; Prentky, 1996) argue that because notification is typically restricted to the geographical community in which the offender resides, offenders can easily seek victims in communities other than their own. Most offenders, however, appear to commit new crimes in the same area in which notification occurred (Lieb, 1996). As seen in the Ault case, notification may not reach potential victims who may be most vulnerable to the grooming tactics of a predatory pedophile. Even when notification does occur, a "nice man" who is so attentive to children that he does not seem dangerous might fool naïve parents.

Freeman-Longo (1996) and Lotke (1997) agreed that there are other complex issues involved in notification, such as its potential negative impact on offenders' family members and the inadvertent identification of victims. Community notification may violate the constitutional rights to privacy of offenders, their families, and their victims. For instance, some communities distribute flyers to schoolchildren when a sex offender moves in to a neighborhood. The child of an identified sex offender might, as a result, be subject to humiliation, scorn, and alienation from playmates.

Notification also creates the potential for vigilantism, despite the fact that all state laws warn citizens that such behavior will not be tolerated and allow for the prosecution of those who use notification as an excuse to harass or harm sex offenders (Freeman-Longo, 1996; Lotke, 1997). Although serious harassment incidents such as arson are rare (Lieb, 1996), many sex offenders report verbal harassment, eviction, and minor destruction to property (Zevitz & Farkas, 2000b).

Freeman-Longo (1996) proposed that notification sends a mixed message to offenders in treatment by placing responsibility for abuse prevention on the public rather than on the individual offender himself. Furthermore, notification may undermine pro-social and rehabilitative efforts by offenders, inadvertently reducing the effectiveness of interventions more likely to protect the community. Notification itself may actually negatively affect its ability to achieve its stated goal of reducing and preventing sexual assault (Edwards & Hensley, 2001). Specifically, notification may exacerbate the stressors (e.g., isolation, disempowerment, shame, depression, anxiety, lack of social supports) that often trigger sexual offenders to relapse. Jones (1999) advocated for humanistic treatment and rehabilitation of sex offenders by mental health professionals in an attempt to counteract the punitive and rejecting approach of the community response. Community notification is a costly endeavor. The costs of community notification vary with the notification method and the size of the community (Poole & Lieb, 1995). Costs include equipment (e.g., computer systems), personnel (for background checks, risk assessment, neighborhood meetings, information development and distribution, registration verification, and violation sanctions), printing, and postage. Because resources are prioritized for notification efforts, treatment and primary prevention strategies may suffer due to under-funding.

Berliner (1996) suggested that notification is a supplement to, not a substitute for, sexual abuse prevention efforts, and should be seen as only one component of a social response to the problem of sexual violence. Although not yet empirically shown to reduce sexual recidivism, Berliner asserted that notifying communities about sex offenders seems to be a reasonable endeavor in helping parents protect their children.

Sex Offender Notification Outcome Research

Notification strategies include alerting organizations (e.g., schools, housing authorities, churches), residents, and the media through door-to-door contact, distribution of flyers, telephone calls, neighborhood meetings, press releases, direct mailing, and Websites. Each state or local community can decide how community notification should be implemented. Finn (1997) discussed the advantages and drawbacks of allowing local jurisdictions to establish criteria for notification. While jurisdictional discretion encourages ownership of the program, allows for case-by-case decisions, and makes individual law enforcement agencies accountable for their decisions, it may also result in inequitable or inconsistent notification procedures. Many states use some form of risk level criteria based on empirically derived risk factors, but others employ broad notification laws in which all offenders are subject to aggressive notification regardless of risk (Matson & Lieb, 1996).

Few empirical studies have been conducted, leaving speculation as to the effectiveness of community notification or particular notification strategies in reducing sex offense recidivism. Berliner (1996) pointed out, however, that science and outcome data do not necessarily drive legislation, and that because citizens believe that awareness of the presence of a sex offender will afford them the opportunity to protect themselves, outcome research might be a moot point.

The only study evaluating the impact of notification on sex offense recidivism was conducted in Washington State by the Washington Institute for Public Policy (Schram & Milloy, 1995). The study compared 125 released adult sex offenders who were subject to Washington's highest level of notification with a randomly selected control group of 90 offenders released before the law went into effect. Follow-up periods ranged from one to four years.

Schram and Milloy (1995) found no statistically significant difference in recidivism rates between offenders who were subject to notification (19% recidivism) and those who were not (22% recidivism). However, sex offenders who were subject to community notification were arrested more quickly for new sex crimes than those not subject to notification. It was found that 63% of the new sex offenses occurred in the jurisdiction where notification took place. Based on the findings, the authors concluded that community notification had little effect on sex offense recidivism (Schram & Milloy, 1995).

An unusual research design retroactively speculated upon the public safety potential of Megan's Law in Massachusetts (Petrosino &

Petrosino, 1999). The researchers randomly selected 136 of 400 sexual psychopaths confined in a maximum-security institution and collected data from their case files. Ultimately, the 36 offenders who would have met registration and notification criteria (a prior sex offense conviction) at the time of their last sex offense were selected for the study. The research design did not include a control group. Of the 36 offenders who met notification eligibility, 12 had committed predatory (non-incestuous) offenses, and these 12 cases were examined to determine if notification might have prevented the new sex offense.

The authors assumed that the 12 selected offenders would all be subject to the most aggressive notification due to their high-risk level, and that all would comply with registration requirements. The proximity of the offender's residence and employment (the neighborhoods that would be notified) to the location of the crime was analyzed. The crimes were then evaluated for the potential of notification reaching the victim and coded as improbable, poor to moderate, or good. Results determined that in 6 of the 12 cases, the crime occurred within the area where notification would have taken place, suggesting that in those 6 cases there was a chance that notification might have prevented the assault.

Impact on Communities. Most studies have focused on community notification's impact on those affected by it. Surveys were conducted in Wisconsin to determine the impact of notification laws on neighborhood residents (Zevitz & Farkas, 2000b). Results indicated that 38% of citizens reported increased anxiety due to notification and the lack of alternatives for dealing with sex offenders living in communities. Caputo (2001) also found, through telephone surveys of 250 residents in Tuscaloosa, that those most fearful of sex offenders were women and parents, but that few crime-specific coping strategies were used by respondents. Caputo (2001) suggested the development of community interventions geared toward specific empowerment against sexual victimization.

Matson and Lieb (1996) surveyed 45 police officers in Washington who used community notification meetings to inform neighborhoods of the release of a sex offender. Meetings included a discussion of the law, a description of offenders' crimes, education regarding the characteristics and behaviors of a pedophile, sex offender facts versus myths, and prevention and protection information for parents. Meeting attendees' reactions (as reported by the law enforcement officers) were "generally positive" and highly supportive of the community notification process. Negative reactions to the offender and the idea of him living in the neighborhood were also reported. Advantages of the meetings were identified by law enforcement agents as enhanced community surveillance, public awareness, promotion of child safety, and deterrence.

In a study examining the effectiveness of neighborhood meetings (Zevitz, Crim, & Farkas, 2000a), attendees at all community notification meetings held throughout Wisconsin were surveyed during a nine-month period. Community meetings provided information about the released sex offender, his release conditions, and correctional supervision strategies. Victim advocates were also present to provide information regarding preventive measures to protect community members from sexual victimization and to educate the public about the nature of sex offending behavior. The intent of the meetings was to reduce criminal opportunity through awareness and deterrence, although the researchers were unable to test whether that goal was met. However, attendees indicated that they were generally willing to work with police and probation to "keep track" of sex offenders. Survey results showed that neighborhood meetings left most participants feeling more concerned rather than less concerned. Anxiety appeared to be related to the manner in which attendees were notified of meetings, how clearly the purpose of the meeting was conveyed, and how organized the meeting was.

In New York City, 300 discharged jurors were asked to rate their potential willingness to participate in crime prevention activities when notified that a criminal plans to move into their neighborhood (Blain, 2000). Results determined that participants were more willing to engage in reactive behaviors when notified of the presence of a sex offender rather than a non-sex offender.

Impact on Law Enforcement. When law enforcement officers and probation agents in Wisconsin were surveyed about the impact of community notification on their job duties, 66% of law enforcement agencies reported concerns about increased labor and expenditures (Zevitz & Farkas, 2000b). Probation officers also reported increased workload and costs associated with maximizing surveillance. A similar study in Washington cited the disadvantages of community notification as additional workload, overreaction by the public, difficulties with data collection, and harassment of sex offenders (Matson & Lieb, 1996). The National Criminal Justice Association (1997) examined implementation of community notification in Alaska, Louisiana, New Jersey, and Washington through interviews with officials charged with enforcing and implementing the laws. Implementation problems were found to focus on the lack of resources and funding.

Zevitz and Farkas (2000a) surveyed 77 Wisconsin probation officers and found that community notification had added more work to already overworked agents, including time-consuming duties such as electronic monitoring, periodic polygraph examination, monitoring of treatment compliance, and paperwork associated with revocation sanctions. Other difficulties identified included finding housing for offenders, dealing with media attention, lags in obtaining timely information, and pressure from superiors due to the high-profile nature of high risk sex offender cases. Zevitz and Farkas concluded that community safety comes at a high cost in terms of personnel, time and budgetary resources.

Impact on Sex Offenders. Other researchers have studied the social and psychological impact of community notification on sex offender reintegration. Data were collected through interviews with 30 convicted sex offenders throughout Wisconsin who were designated as high risk and therefore subject to notification through media releases, distribution of flyers, and neighborhood meetings (Zevitz, Crim, & Farkas, 2000b). Offenders reported that inability to maintain stable housing and employment were among the most disruptive effects of notification. The majority of participants also reported ostracism, harassment, and emotional harm to family members. Psychological impact included despair and hopelessness–"no one believes I can change, so why even try?" Although some offenders expressed interest in attending a neighborhood meeting to show a demonstration of responsibility and to try to reduce negative perceptions, the three respondents who did attend a meeting reported the experience to be unproductive, with attendees "shouting insults" and causing them to fear for their safety. Zevitz and Farkas (2000b) found that over 90% of the 30 sex offenders interviewed reported being adversely affected by notification, including facing ostracism, harassment or threats, loss of employment, reintegration problems, expulsion from a residence, and the breakup of personal relationships.

Summary of Community Notification Research

Thus far, little empirical evidence exists to support community notification as an effective strategy for reducing sex offense recidivism. In the only controlled study to date, Schram and Milloy (1995) found no appreciable difference in actual recidivism rates between offenders who were subject to notification and those who were not. Schram and Milloy did find, however, that offenders subject to notification were arrested more quickly for new sex crimes. Petrosino and Petrosino (1999) suggested that in half of the cases in their study, notification might have prevented the sexual assault that occurred. This study had some important limitations, however. The extremely small sample size ($n = 12$) certainly limits the generalizability of this study to other populations. Perhaps more importantly, the study only speculated retrospectively as to the ability of notification to warn the communities in which these offenders resided and worked. Even if, as the authors suggest, in 6 of 12 cases, citizens were aware of the presence of the sex offender, it seems unreasonable to conclude that this awareness would have prevented the sex crimes from occurring.

Other studies have suggested that community notification, while supported by citizens, increases the anxiety of parents and fails to empower potential victims to protect themselves. Community notification has created excessive fiscal and workload costs for law enforcement agencies. It has had an overwhelmingly negative impact on sex offenders, potentially compromising their community adjustment and treatment success.

In summary, it can be concluded that there is very little evidence to support that community notification enhances community safety from sex crimes. Although there is some agreement that community notification has enhanced the tracking and monitoring of sex offenders (Matson & Lieb, 1996; Zevitz & Farkas, 2000b), the empirical evidence is too limited to be considered conclusive. Both Lotke (1997) and Freeman-Longo (1996) cite the lack of empirical evidence supporting the impact of notification on reducing recidivism, as well as the high costs of implementation, as considerations that should be seriously reviewed.

IMPLICATIONS FOR FUTURE RESEARCH

More data are needed to determine whether community notification accomplishes its stated goal of reducing and preventing sexual assault, and more specifically, to determine which, if any, notification strategies are most successful in accomplishing this goal. Replication in other states of the research design utilized by Schram and Milloy (1995) in Washington would be valuable in providing a larger-scale evaluation of community notification efforts across the nation.

Critics of community notification point out that sex offenders can avoid increased scrutiny by venturing outside of their notification area to seek victims. Therefore, further study is needed to explore whether repeat sex crimes occur within the communities in which notification takes place, or whether sex offenders do indeed travel outside of their own communities to commit new crimes. This task might be accomplished by studying the police reports of sex crimes committed by known sex offenders subject to notification to determine the proximity of the crime to the notification area.

Time series analysis might be helpful in determining whether Megan's Law has been successful in reducing sex crime rates. The mean sex crime rate in the largest municipalities in a particular state can be compared before and after the law was implemented. Confounding and interactive variables, such as the concurrent implementation of other types of sexually violent predator legislation (e.g., civil commitment or "three strikes" laws) would need to be controlled in order to determine the independent effect of Megan's Law.

A comparative analysis might be employed to address the question of whether specific notification procedures are more or less successful in bringing about reductions in sex crimes. A survey of law enforcement agencies might be conducted to seek data regarding which notification strategies are used (e.g., flyers, press releases, community meetings) in each jurisdiction. The different types of notification strategies used might then be correlated with each city's sex crime rate before and after the law's implementation. Of course, numerous confounding variables exist and would need to be controlled.

Studying the effect of community notification on sex offense recidivism presents many methodological complexities. Ultimately, however, empirical evidence must inform the development, implementation, and evaluation of social policy. The public's "right to know" must be balanced with the potential social and fiscal costs of Megan's Law to individuals, families, and communities.

CIVIL COMMITMENT OF SEXUALLY VIOLENT PREDATORS

Historical Context

Civil commitment has historically been recognized as the process by which mentally ill individuals who are considered dangerous to themselves or others are detained in an inpatient facility and forced to receive mental health care (King, 1999). Civil commitment has traditionally been clearly distinguished from criminal punishment in that its primary purposes have been treatment and protective isolation from society for those individuals who were dangerous as a result of an existing psychiatric condition (King, 1999). Involuntarily confined persons are entitled to periodic review of their condition and released when deemed to have recovered sufficiently (i.e., they are no longer considered an acute threat to themselves or others). Civil interventions emphasize a prospective danger, and seek to protect against future harm (Janus, 2000). In contrast, criminal interventions are intended to punish a past act for which the individual is responsible while also preventing future harm through incapacitation (Janus, 2000). Legislation allowing the civil commitment of sexual offenders first evolved in the 1930s. Sexual psychopath laws were designed to offer alternatives to prison for sexual offenders thought to be morally insane and at high risk for recidivism but amenable to treatment (Janus, 2000). Between 1930 and 1970, coinciding with the growing influence of psychiatry and the therapeutic ideal, these laws were enacted with the belief that sexual psychopaths could be treated, and once cured, could be safely released (Lieb & Matson, 1998). Many states eventually abolished these laws due to claims that the ability to assess and predict propensity for violence lacked scientific validity, and that treatment for sex offenders was ineffective (Janus, 2000). After the commission of a series of brutal sex crimes by "treated" sexual psychopaths during the 1960s and early 1970s, a criminal justice model of managing dangerous offenders was emphasized (Janus & Walbeck, 2000; Lieb & Matson, 1998).

In 1990, Washington State enacted the nation's first "second generation" sexual predator commitment statute in response to the acts of a sex offender with a 24-year history of murder and sexual assaults. In 1987, as the offender prepared to complete a 10-year prison sentence for kidnapping and assaulting two teenage girls, officials learned that he had plans to torture children following his release. Efforts to detain him through traditional psychiatric commitment failed and he was released from prison. Two years after his release, he abducted and violently sexually assaulted a 7-year-old boy. As a result, Washington's Community Protection Act of 1990 was enacted to provide for increased penalties and stricter post-release supervision of sexual offenders. It also contained the "Sexually Violent Predator Statute," a law mandating the civil commitment, following criminal incarceration, of convicted offenders found to be sexually violent predators (Lieb & Matson, 2000).

In contrast to the "first generation" sexual psychopath laws, which allowed for treatment of sex offenders as an alternative to traditional sentencing, new sexual predator statutes allow for civil confinement and treatment following the completion of a criminal sentence. This philosophical and political change resulted from both the feminist agenda to alter societal attitudes about sexual violence and the public perception that sentences for sex offenders were often too short (Janus, 2000). Thus, new sex offender commitment laws were designed to increase the ability to manage risk by incapacitating violent sexual offenders. This risk-management model was ostensibly adopted to reduce the threat that sex offenders pose to public safety (Winick, 1998), as opposed to being driven by the therapeutic optimism that led to original sexual psychopath laws.

Judicial History of Contemporary Sexually Violent Predator Statutes

The U.S. Supreme Court addressed the constitutionality of new sex offender civil commitment statutes in 1997 in the case of *Kansas v. Hendricks* (1997). In this case, Leroy Hendricks, a Kansas man convicted seven times between 1955 and 1984 for sexually abusing children, was found, prior to his release from prison in 1994, to meet the criteria for Kansas' newly enacted Sexually Violent Predator Act. Despite his own statement that the only way that he would stop abusing children would be to die, Hendricks motioned the trial court to dismiss the state's petition to confine him, arguing that the Act violated the Constitution's due process, double jeopardy, and ex post facto clauses (Rollman, 1998). The court found probable cause to define Hendricks as a sexually violent predator and ordered a psychological evaluation, after which a jury found beyond reasonable doubt that he should be committed.

Hendricks appealed his commitment to the Kansas Supreme Court, which overturned the trial court's finding and ruled that the Act violated the Due Process Clause of the Constitution. The State of Kansas petitioned the U.S. Supreme Court for clarification. The U.S. Supreme Court voted 5-4 in 1997 to reverse the judgment of the Kansas Supreme Court, holding that the state's Sexually Violent Predator Act meets substantive due process requirements and violates neither the double jeopardy nor ex post facto clause. Clarence Thomas, for the majority, wrote:

> The Kansas Act . . . requires a finding of future dangerousness, and then links that finding to the existence of a 'mental abnormality' or 'personality disorder' that makes it difficult, if not impossible, for the person to control his dangerous behavior . . . The pre-commitment requirement of a 'mental abnormality' or 'personality disorder' . . . narrows the class of persons eligible for confinement to those who are unable to control their dangerousness. (p. 7)

The Hendricks decision pointed out that the existence of a particular paraphilic or personality disorder does not, by itself, make an individual a predator or a danger to society. Thus, sexually violent predator statutes must set four criteria for commitment: (a) a history of sexual violence, (b) a current mental disorder or abnormality, (c) a likelihood of future sexual crimes, and (d) a link between the first two elements and the third (Janus, 2000). The Supreme Court ruling (*Kansas v. Hendricks*, 1997) led the way for more states to initiate civil commitment statutes.

In October 2001, the U.S. Supreme Court again visited the issue of sex offender civil commitment in the case of *Kansas v. Crane* (2001). The Kansas Supreme Court found that in 2000, the state violated federal due process when Crane was committed in the absence of showing that he could not control his dangerous conduct. Specifically, the Kansas court reasoned that commitment should be restricted only to those individuals unable to control their "irresistible impulses" and petitioned the U.S. Supreme Court for clarification. In an amicus brief, the Association for the Treatment of Sexual Abusers (ATSA) submitted that the "cannot control" standard is untenable, as it is not supported by scientific research and is a standard impossible for practitioners to assess (ATSA, 2000). ATSA argued that sex offenders intend to commit sexual crimes, and that in virtually all cases, claims of volitional impairment should be rejected (ATSA, 2000). Janus (2000) agreed that "inability to control" is a "highly confused concept with little or no meaningful content" (p. 14).

In January 2002 the Supreme Court issued a majority opinion vacating the Kansas Supreme Court ruling in the *Crane* case, stating that Kansas interpreted the *Hendricks* decision in an overly restrictive manner. The finding that a dangerous individual must be completely unable to control his behavior is, said the Supreme Court, too rigid, but they established that there must be a finding of some inability to control behavior. The dissenting opinion, however, argued that the majority opinion was redundant because the *Hendricks* ruling had already prohibited the commitment of sex offenders that have no volitional impairment and that the requirement of a mental abnormality, by definition, implies "difficulty if not impossibility" in controlling behavior (*Kansas v. Crane*, 2002).

Civil commitment statutes have also been the subjects of judicial scrutiny in other states. Most notably, the case of *Turay v. Seling/Weston* (2000) in Washington challenged the conditions of confinement as well as deficiencies in the treatment program, resulting in an injunction that appointed a special master to oversee the statute's implementation. In November 2001 an appellate court in Tampa, Florida, ruled that many sex offenders were being held pending civil commitment trials without sworn testimony upholding probable cause (Keough, 2001). The ruling resulted in the release of over a dozen sex offenders, while state attorneys across the state scrambled to petition for probable cause hearings in which experts could testify to the potential dangerousness of sex offenders awaiting trial.

Who Is a Sexually Violent Predator?

In many states the label "sexual predator" applies specifically to sex offenders who target strangers or acquaintances with whom a relationship has been established primarily for the purpose of victimization, who have multiple victims, or who commit especially violent offenses (Lieb & Matson, 1998). Other states, such as Florida, broadly define sexually violent predators (SVP) as a "small but extremely dangerous number of offenders who are highly likely to sexually re-offend" (Jimmy Ryce Act, 1998). It is important to note that the term "sexually violent predator" is a legal term rather than a clinical one. Sex offenders will usually lack the severe mental illness requirement necessary in traditional psychiatric commitment where one is considered a danger to self or others (Lieb & Matson, 1998). Instead, they must be found to exhibit only a "mental abnormality" or "personality disorder" which predisposes them to commit sexually violent crimes (*Kansas v. Hendricks*, 1997). Translated into clinical terms, these individuals are most commonly diagnosed with Paraphilia or Antisocial Personality Disorder as defined by the *Diagnostic and Statistical Manual of Mental Disorders, Fourth Edition (DSM-IV)* (American Psychiatric Association, 1994).

Society appears to feel most threatened by sex offenders who prey on children. The sexual deviance literature makes a clear distinction between predatory pedophiles and other types of child molesters (Barbaree & Seto, 1997). Pedophiles present clinically as men with a clear sexual preference for children rather than adults, while child molesters are described as individuals who have committed a sexual offense against a child victim (Barbaree & Seto, 1997). Although virtually all pedophiles are child molesters, not all child molesters are pedophiles. Pedophiles may abuse family members, but the majority of their offenses are predatory–directed towards vulnerable children whom they court or groom for the purpose of victimization. Offenders who seek out children to victimize by placing themselves in positions of trust, authority, and easy access to youngsters, for example, can have hundreds of victims over the course of their lifetimes. Abel et al. (1987), in their survey of 561 incarcerated sex offenders who were encouraged to disclose past offenses through guaranteed anonymity and criminal immunity, found that the average number of victims for pedophiles who molested girls was 20; for pedophiles who preferred boys, the average number of victims was over 100.

Adults can also be victims of sexually violent predators. Research has found that rapists, like their pedophilic counterparts, have often committed many more crimes than those for which they have been arrested. When 37 convicted, incarcerated rapists were guaranteed anonymity, they admitted to an average of nearly 12 rape victims, a sharp contrast to their mean number of arrests, which was less than two (Weinrott & Saylor, 1991). Freeman-Longo (1985) found that 23 rapists admitted to an astonishing mean of 221 sex crimes each, including rapes, child molestations, and other sexual offenses.

Rapists have also been found to have more antisocial qualities than other types of sex offenders. Abel, Mittleman, and Becker (1985) found that 29% of a sample of 89 rapists met the DSM-II criteria for Antisocial Personality Disorder (APD), and Marques, Day, Nelson, and Miner (1989) found that 75% of their rapists had APD. Antisocial qualities render a person undeterred by the threat of punishment, less likely to inhibit sexual aggression, and more likely to obtain sexual gratification opportunistically (Quinsey, Lalumiere, Rice, & Harris, 1995). Among individuals with deviant sexual preferences, antisocial personality disorder has been found to increase the likelihood of sexual reconviction (Hanson & Bussiere, 1998; Quinsey et al., 1995).

Sexually violent predator statutes seek to prevent the recurrence of sexual victimization by repeat sexual offenders. Although definitional ambiguity exists, most state laws appear to exclude from their definitions those offenders who have had only incestuous victims or those who have not had physical contact with a victim (e.g., exhibitionists) (Doren, 2002). Generally, sexually violent predators are legally and clinically defined as those offenders who pose the greatest threat to public safety.

Goals of Civil Commitment

The goals of sex offender civil commitment statutes have been the subject of considerable debate among both mental health professionals and legal scholars. Although the civil commitment of sexually violent predators implies rehabilitation, Winick (1998) asserts that it is punishment, isolation and incapacitation that appear to be its dominant purposes.

The U.S. Supreme Court, in its opinion upholding the constitutionality of civil commitment of sexually violent offenders (*Kansas v. Hendricks*, 1997), stated that incapacitation and treatment are both legitimate aims of SVP statutes. Although the primary goal of civil commitment of SVPs has been described as preventive detention (LaFond, 2000), Winick (1998) interprets the Supreme Court as saying that the civil aspect of the laws requires the state to provide treatment as an ancillary goal. Critics have argued that the intended goal of civil commitment is further incarceration, with treatment existing only as a red herring to hide its punitive intent (Rollman, 1998; Winick, 1998). Because the Supreme Court (*Kansas v. Hendricks*, 1997) allowed for states to commit individuals for whom no effective treatment exists, some say that civil confinement amounts to little more than disguised punishment (Janus, 2000).

Mad or Bad? Sexually violent predator laws have inspired debate as to whether sexual deviancy, as identified for example by a diagnosis of a paraphilia (American Psychiatric Association, 1994), meets the criteria of "mental illness" previously established by courts to justify traditional civil commitment. Critics contend that they do not, questioning the Supreme Court's requirement that sexually violent predators be diagnosed with a "mental abnormality" or personality disorder (LaFond, 2000). The term "mental abnormality" has no scientific or clinical meaning, but rather represents only a "deviation from the normal" (Janus, 2000, p. 15).

Civil rights advocates have attacked SVP laws as disingenuous and unconstitutional (Rollman, 1998) and contend that their intent is to simply warehouse society's most hated criminals. If sex offenders are truly mentally ill, as some argue, they should have qualified for an insanity defense or traditional psychiatric commitment in lieu of criminal sentencing (Schopp & Slain, 2000). If sex offenders are responsible moral agents and were therefore appropriately tried and punished through the criminal justice system, then sex offender civil commitment undermines the foundation of our criminal justice system–culpability–and distorts the primary function of the civil commitment system–therapeutic treatment (Presley, 1999).

Mental health researchers and legal scholars alike raise this paradigmatic question of "sick" versus "evil." Alexander (1997) discussed the reconstruction of sex offenders as mentally ill from a labeling perspective, concluding that the medicalization of sexual predation allows states to exert more control by extending their confinement beyond criminal sentencing. Schopp and Slain (2000) argue that psychopathy, a combination of interpersonal, affective, and behavioral characteristics (Hare, 1991, 1999) that interferes with empathy, conscience, and moral reasoning, does not undermine the capacities of practical reasoning required to function as an accountable agent to the criminal justice system. Schopp and Slain conclude that civil commitment and criminal justice are therefore mutually exclusive and offer this interpretation as a fundamental flaw of sexual predator statutes.

Interestingly, Florida's SVP law, in its legislative intent, states that "sexually violent predators generally have antisocial personality features which are not amenable to existing mental illness treatment modalities" (Jimmy Ryce Act, 1998). This wording has inspired debate among Florida's legal advocates as to the genuine motivation of a state to provide "treatment and care" for a population that is not amenable to existing treatment protocols (Presley, 1999). The U.S. Supreme Court, however, in *Kansas v. Hendricks* (1997), opined that the Constitution does not prevent civil detainment for those for whom no treatment is available but who pose a threat to others. They added that there are many forms of mental illness that are not fully understood and for which no effective "cure" has been discovered, and that low likelihood of recovery does not preclude civil commitment.

The *Hendricks* decision (1997) did note that provision of treatment is an obligation of states in a civil commitment, although amenability to treatment is not an essential criterion. The ruling mandated treatment "where possible" and allowed states to commit individuals for whom no effective treatment exists (Janus, 2000). This paradox has led critics to refer to treatment as a "fig leaf" designed to obscure the punitive nature of SVP commitment (Perlin, 1998), especially in light of the speculation that the most dangerous SVPs may be among those least likely to benefit from available treatments (Schwartz, 1999). Further, the requirement that only a "mental abnormality" exist may preclude the diagnosis of a treatable mental illness, leaving "nothing to treat" (Janus, 2000, p. 16).

Who Is Being Committed, and How? A survey conducted in June 2000 revealed that nationwide, 894 individuals had been committed throughout the U.S., with another 822 detained pending trial (Lieb & Matson, 2000). Each state varies in its criteria for eligibility for commitment. For instance, California requires that individuals evaluated for commitment have two or more victims, while Florida screens any offender with history of a past conviction for a sexual crime–even if the sexual crime is not the instant offense for which the inmate is currently incarcerated (Jimmy Ryce Act, 1998). Some states, such as Illinois, Washington, and Wisconsin, allow juveniles to be considered for commitment, while Florida allows juvenile sex offenders to be evaluated for civil commitment only if they are over 18 at the time of release (Lieb & Matson, 1998). New Jersey requires a "pattern of repetitive, compulsive behavior" and Minnesota requires a "psychopathic personality" (Lieb & Matson, 1998). Most states allow females to be considered for commitment.

Other differences in criteria also emerge when comparing state statutes. Most states require "beyond reasonable doubt" as the burden of proof in commitment trials, but others, such as Florida, use the lower standard of "clear and convincing evidence" and require only that a sex offender is "likely" to re-offend (Lieb & Matson, 1998). California law allows only a 2-year confinement, while all other states allow indeterminate periods of commitment with yearly review hearings (Lieb & Matson, 1998).

SVP civil commitment is generally a multi-step process. First, a screening team, usually administered by a state's mental health department, receives referrals of sex offenders due to be released from prison. The team determines which inmates meet statutory criteria, and these inmates are then referred for face-to-face evaluation and risk assessment. If, after evaluation, an individual is determined to be at high risk for sexually violent re-offense, a prosecutor determines whether there is sufficient evidence to file the case. If so, a hearing is held in which a court determines whether probable cause exists to believe the person is a sexually violent predator. If probable cause exists, a trial is held in which both the state and the individual present evidence that is heard by a judge or a jury. If found to be a sexually violent predator, the individual is confined within the bounds of the state statute until such time he or she is deemed to no longer be a danger to the community (Lieb & Matson, 1998). Across the states, approximately 5-12% of all eligible individuals are referred to prosecutors (Lieb & Matson, 1998).

Nationally, child molesters comprise approximately 51-76% of individuals committed under SVP statutes, with the remainder being rapists (Doren & Epperson, 2001). A descriptive study of commitments in Minnesota revealed that 37% of offenders had committed sex crimes against adults only, with the remainder molesting children. Some of the offenders defined as child molesters had also committed rapes of adults, but the rapists were defined as those offenders having only victims over the age of 18 (Janus & Walbeck, 2000).

The Costs of Civil Commitment

The monetary costs of civil commitment are extraordinarily high, as they include funding for screening, evaluation, trials and appeals, treatment, confinement, release programs, community training programs, and post-release supervision (LaFond, 2000). Yearly costs for civil commitment programs are estimated to range from $70,000 per client in Washington to $103,000 in California (Lieb & Matson, 1998). Legal costs range from $60,000 per case in Washington to nearly $100,000 per case in Minnesota (LaFond, 2000). LaFond (2000) contends that most states have grossly underestimated the number of sexually violent predators to be evaluated and treated as well as the length of institutionalization and associated costs.

Despite the growing numbers of committed offenders, release from commitment programs is rare. As of June 2000, only about 20 offenders had been released nationwide (Lieb & Matson, 2000) since the first commitment law passed in Washington in 1990. The difficulty in determining when an offender should be released is a factor in cost effectiveness. LaFond (2000) notes that prosecutors resist recommendations for release and that the public is understandably frightened by the prospect of an offender's release. Because the attrition rate in civil commitment programs is so low, states should expect an incrementally growing treatment population with costs that will increasingly exceed budgeted allowances.

A less costly alternative to civil commitment that has been proposed by Washington and California, and implemented in Colorado, is to legislate lengthier criminal sentences for offenders deemed likely to re-offend and to provide treatment during incarceration. Another alternative, lifetime probation, costs approximately $1,400 per year per offender in Arizona (LaFond, 1998), and provides intensive supervision of sex offenders while allowing them to live in the community, obtain treatment, and work. LaFond (1998) cited research by the Arizona Judicial Department suggesting low recidivism rates of sex offenders on lifetime probation.

Janus (2000) questioned whether the costs of civil commitment divert resources from community and correctional programs, noting that prisons provide the greatest opportunity for providing treatment for large numbers of sex offenders. The enormous costs of civil commitment should be justified by research demonstrating its effectiveness in reducing recidivism by comparison to less costly alternatives such as lengthier prison sentences and extended probation. If SVP laws do not result in lower recidivism rates, then resources might be better spent on alternative strategies for increasing public safety.

Civil commitment has other costs for the individuals in question and society in general. Civil rights advocates argue that a possible increase in public safety is not worth the potential costs to civil liberty (Morse, 1998). Suggesting that hysteria often drives social policy, Morse (1998) claimed that the Supreme Court went too far to protect the public from sex offenders, ultimately threatening the liberty, dignity and constitutional rights of all of us. At the same time, it is hard to imagine a parent who would not support a political agenda promising to protect children from abduction and sexual assault. Civil rights advocates say the most immediate concern is the danger of denying an offender his freedom based only on the chance that he may re-offend. Conversely, the danger to potential victims of releasing a prisoner who is deemed likely to re-offend through a valid risk assessment process must also be considered.

Civil commitment legislation may have emotional appeal to citizens, victim advocates, and policy makers. It remains to be seen, however, whether these initiatives are ultimately cost effective in reducing (a) the incidence of sexual assault in general, (b) the occurrence of the most "serious" sexual offenses, or (c) the frequency of sexual victimization.

Impact of Civil Commitment on Sexual Offense Recidivism

An exhaustive literature and Internet search revealed that no studies have been published that evaluate whether civil commitment impacts the rate of sexual offense recidivism or, more specifically, the rate of the most seriously injurious sexual crimes. During the first six years following the passage of Washington's sexually violent predator statute, a related study conducted by the Washington State Institute for Public Policy (Schram & Milloy, 1998) tracked 61 sexual offenders who were referred for possible commitment but were released because they did not meet legal criteria. Recidivism among this group, defined as new arrests or convictions, was tracked through the Washington State Patrol reports, the Department of Corrections, and the National Crime Information Center. Patterns were then analyzed using survival curves. Schram and Milloy (1998) found that 28% of these released offenders were arrested for a new sex offense within the 6-year follow-up period.

Schram and Milloy (1998) concluded that the members of the screening team "appeared discerning in their selection and referral of sex offenders as possible predators requiring civil commitment" (p. 13). Most of the 61 offenders had two or more prior sexual offense convictions that involved victims who were physically harmed or threatened with harm. It is noteworthy that these offenders were evaluated prior to the development of actuarial sex offender risk assessment instruments. The cases were declined for civil commitment proceedings by prosecuting attorneys who reviewed these cases and considered them, for a variety of reasons, to fail to meet legal standards. Schram and Milloy's (1998) study was descriptive in nature, describing only the characteristics and recidivism rates of offenders considered for commitment but for whom proceedings were declined. Their study did not compare the sample with a control group, nor did they attempt to draw conclusions regarding the impact of civil commitment on recidivism. In fact, their conclusions supported newly enacted "persistent offender statutes" in Washington, which will require life sentences without parole for sex offenders with multiple convictions.

The Wisconsin Department of Corrections is in the process of conducting a study examining the recidivism rates over a 4-year follow up period of sex offenders who were screened for commitment but released. Studies being undertaken in California evaluate the civil commitment screening and selection process but have no recidivism study as of yet. Minnesota researchers are reportedly tracking probation revocations and recidivism since implementing the current procedures for community notification and civil commitment, and plan to analyze the data once a sufficient sample size is reached.

Analysis of civil commitment legislation is currently quite limited and offers little information regarding the impact of sexually violent predator statutes. Janus (2000) argued that selective incapacitation is based on the assumption that the most dangerous predators can be identified. Janus acknowledged the "intuitive simplicity" (p. 18) of the claim that detaining this group is an effective way to reduce sexual violence, but emphasized the need for empirical studies that examine the effect of these statutes on sexual offense recidivism. This would inform policy makers about the long-term outcomes of civil commitment of sex offenders. The true efficacy of these laws presumably depends on the ability to assess risk and select for commitment those sexual offenders most likely to commit future sexually violent crimes.

Risk Assessment and Civil Commitment

Historically, the ability of the mental health practitioner to predict future violence has been a subject of considerable debate. Although the Hendricks decision cited a need to identify those likely to commit future sexually violent crimes, there was surprisingly little discussion in it of the risk assessment process or its validity (Hanson, 1998). This omission is undoubtedly related to the tradition of courts to leave that task to experts, despite evidence that the clinical judgment of mental health professionals is inadequate in predicting dangerousness (Monahan, 1981). The American Psychiatric Association (1994) concluded that the ability of psychiatrists to predict dangerousness had not been established and declared that psychiatrists should avoid drawing conclusions about the risk of future violence. A landmark 1983 Supreme Court decision (*Barefoot v. Estelle*), however, upheld the constitutionality of clinical predictions of violence despite research demonstrating their low accuracy rates.

John Monahan's (1981) review of research on clinical judgment found that across studies, only one out of three persons predicted to be dangerous by mental health professionals actually engaged in criminal or violent behavior. These studies imply that clinicians make inaccurate predictions up to two-thirds of the time, tending to over-predict violent behavior (Monahan, 1981). Otto (1994) countered that less widely cited are the findings that many subjects predicted not to be dangerous did not go on to commit violent crimes. He further argued that, because all violent behavior does not come to the attention of authorities, in some unknown number of cases violent behavior that would have confirmed predictions was not detected.

Studies comparing clinical judgment with statistical, or actuarial predictions based on known outcomes have consistently found that the actuarial method is equal to or superior to informal clinical judgment (Grove & Meehl, 1996). Grove and Meehl (1996) reviewed a meta-analysis of 136 studies comparing actuarial methods with clinical judgment by a variety of professionals concerning a range of medical, behavioral, and mental health phenomena. They reported that 64 studies favored the actuary, 64 showed approximately equivalent accuracy, and 8 favored the clinician. They noted that experience or education of the clinician seemed to make no difference in predictive accuracy, but the type of mechanical prediction used did seem to matter. The best results were obtained by actuarial instruments constructed through weighted linear prediction such as multiple linear regression (Grove & Meehl, 1996).

Statistical prediction can raise the accuracy of predictions by setting statistical thresholds for decision-making and by standardizing factors that professionals readily recognize as key diagnostic features (Swets, Dawes, & Monahan, 2000a, 2000b). This process, known as the actuarial method, estimates the likelihood of a certain outcome by referring to the known (actual) outcomes of individuals with similar characteristics. The actuarial method cannot be used to predict with certainty that any given individual will act in a particular way. It can, however, provide important probability data with which to inform one's expectations regarding a particular individual. The identification of variables associated with violent re-offending has improved our ability to predict it.

Over the past decade, prompted in large part by sexually violent predator statutes, empirical inquiry has focused on the prediction of sexual offense recidivism. The need for clinicians to integrate the science of prediction into the art of interviewing and assessment has led several researchers (Epperson, Kaul, Huot, Hesselton, Alexander, & Goldman, 1999b; Hanson, 1997; Hanson & Bussiere, 1998; Hanson & Thornton, 1999; Quinsey, Harris, Rice, & Cormier, 1998) to conduct studies identifying pertinent risk factors and then develop actuarial risk assessment instruments. These researchers have found that it is not only possible to identify risk factors that are correlated with sexual recidivism (Hanson & Busierre, 1996, 1998), but it is also possible to identify a subset of sexual offenders at highest risk for sex offense recidivism (Hanson, 1997; Hanson & Thornton, 2000). Hanson (1998) opined that it is therefore feasible, prudent, and cost-effective to develop public policies that apply the most intensive interventions to the highest risk offenders while managing lower-risk offenders with less restrictive alternatives.

Hanson (1998) discussed three plausible approaches to conducting risk assessments of sex offenders. In a guided clinical approach, practitioners consider a wide range of empirically validated risk factors and then form an educated opinion concerning the offender's risk. Pure actuarial prediction allows the clinician to evaluate the offender on a set of known predictors and to combine the variables using a predetermined weighting system. The adjusted actuarial approach (a combination of the first two) begins with actuarial prediction but is then adjusted after considering other important factors that were not included in the actuarial equation, for example, access to children in the case of pedophilic sex offenders. Hanson (1998) concluded that as research advances, actuarial measures will continue to surpass clinical assessments in their predictive ability, but that clinical assessment can still provide useful information. Others caution that clinical judgment is so poor that adjusting actuarial assessment dilutes the predictive validity of the actuarial scale (Quinsey et al., 1998).

Prediction of Sexual Offense Recidivism

Observed sex offense recidivism rates are always considered to be underestimates because of the large number of sexual crimes that go undetected, unreported, or do not result in arrests or convictions (Doren, 1998; Quinsey et al., 1998). Contrary to public opinion and current legislation, average sex offender recidivism rates of 13.4% (Hanson & Bussiere, 1998) are consistently lower than recidivism base rates of 61-83% for nonsexual criminals (Hanson et al., 1995). However, this difference may be partly related to the difficulty of detecting and effectively prosecuting sexual crimes.

The ability to predict sexual dangerousness is crucial to the identification of those offenders who meet the criteria for civil commitment, and therefore to the effectiveness of civil commitment as a policy designed to protect society's most vulnerable members from repeat offenders. For a more detailed description of risk factors of sexual offender recidivism and assessment, see Quackenbush (this volume) and Clipson (this volume). The predictive validity of the risk assessment instruments used by evaluators in civil commitment proceedings is crucial in determining the credibility of civil commitment evaluation procedures. Predictive validity refers to the degree to which actual outcomes match predicted outcomes (Quinsey et al., 1998; Swets et al., 2000a). Measures and instruments used in such assessments are described more fully in Clipson's article (in this volume).

The actuarial risk assessment instruments do have some important limitations. They cannot assess the severity, frequency, or imminence of sex offense recidivism (Doren, 2002). Although the instruments can predict with moderate accuracy whether a sex offender will re-offend, they cannot predict the degree of harm the offender will cause. They cannot predict the type of offense that might be committed, although, in general, past patterns are usually indicative of future behavior. In other words, even if a sex offender is assessed to be likely to re-offend, it is not possible to predict whether that offense will involve a child or an adult, whether it will be a "hands-on" or "hands-off" offense, or if it will involve physical injury to the victim. The frequency of future offending, or number of offenses committed by a particular individual, also cannot be predicted. However, all sex offender civil commitment laws implicitly define risk simply as the likelihood of at least one more sex offense (Doren, 2002). In SVP statutes, the relevant time frame for the risk assessment is whether or not the offender will re-offend in his or her lifetime (Doren, 2002). Risk assessment instruments, however, have been validated using finite time frames ranging from 5 to 15 years. Therefore, they are unable to predict recidivism beyond the time frames for which they are validated or to determine when an offense might occur.

Evaluating Readiness for Release from Civil Commitment

The ability to predict sexual dangerousness is well ahead of the ability to predict safety (Hanson, 1998). Although the actuarial risk assessment instruments used to predict sexual recidivism have clearly demonstrated improvements over clinical judgment, they are based primarily on static factors, which are by definition, unchangeable. Thus, while they have demonstrated utility in predicting future sexual dangerousness for the purposes of civil commitment evaluation, they are not applicable in assessing treatment progress or in evaluating readiness for release from commitment facilities. The lack of ability to evaluate successful treatment completion is another source of controversy in the civil commitment debate. Janus (2000) emphasized that research measuring treatment-induced changes is sorely lacking but is essential to the integrity of civil commitment policy.

Research into dynamic risk factors has identified variables that can be changed through treatment and can therefore modify risk level. Not surprisingly, access to victims has been found to increase the likelihood of sexual re-offense (Hanson & Harris, 1998). The individuals most likely to recidivate also have poor social supports, attitudes tolerant of sexual assault, antisocial lifestyles, and poor self-management strategies (Hanson & Harris, 1998). Although a history of substance abuse is not related to sexual offense recidivism (Hanson & Bussiere, 1998), Hanson and Harris (1998) found that ongoing substance abuse problems were common among recidivists. Because substance use can impair judgment and impulse control, it may be a particularly important factor to consider when monitoring ongoing risk.

Recidivists tend to show an increase in anger and subjective distress just prior to re-offending, are more likely to have past treatment failures, and are generally less cooperative with probationary and child protective services supervision (Hanson & Harris, 1998). Dynamic factors can be used to assess the timing and imminence of re-offense (Hanson & Harris, 2001).

To date, only one actuarial scale, the Sex Offender Needs Assessment Rating (SONAR), has been established to evaluate change in risk among treated offenders (Hanson & Harris, 2001). Designed to measure both stable and acute dynamic risk factors, the SONAR showed adequate internal consistency and moderate ability to differentiate recidivists from non-recidivists (Hanson & Harris, 2001). However, the SONAR was validated on samples of offenders in community-based treatment and therefore cannot be used to assess the reduction of dynamic risk in incarcerated or civilly committed offenders. Hanson and Harris (2001) suggest that considering dynamic factors may help to improve the predictions of actuarial instruments, but only for offenders under community supervision.

Thus, risk assessment based on static variables creates a conundrum. Because static factors are unchangeable, change is logically impossible, and risk assessment scores cannot be reduced over time or after treatment. Therefore, while current risk assessment protocols are useful for identifying factors that justify commitment, they cannot be used to justify release.

Implications for Future Research

Inquiry into the effectiveness of civil commitment is especially problematic due to the extremely small number of individuals released from commitment programs and the long follow-up periods necessary to efficiently evaluate recidivism rates after involuntary treatment. Confounding this issue is the difficulty in determining whether any observed reduction in recidivism is due to treatment effect, maturation, concurrent implementation of other legislative initiatives, the decreasing trend in violent crime rates, or other factors.

An avenue by which to explore the efficacy of civil commitment as a social policy might be to track the recidivism rates of those rejected for civil commitment and released as "low risk." By comparing those individuals assessed as low risk to a control group of individuals released without any risk assessment at all (e.g., prior to implementation of commitment statutes), it might be possible to determine if, by committing the most dangerous offenders, a significant number of sex crimes are successfully eliminated. However, low base rates, under-reporting of sex crimes, and the need for long follow-up periods are methodological problems that make this type of study difficult at best. Predictive validity studies that follow released SVPs to determine whether their re-offense rates were accurately predicted by actuarial assessment is vital.

The cost-effectiveness of civil commitment remains a serious concern. Commitment is known to be a very costly solution with little research available to justify those expenditures. Caseload growth due to extraordinarily low attrition rates, along with the expense of programming, litigation, and physical plant requirements, have been cited as critical concerns for the fiscal viability of sex offender commitment programs. Studies are needed to compare less restrictive alternatives such as lifetime probation, prison-based treatment, and community-based treatment with civil commitment in an effort to determine the wisdom of diverting dwindling resources into the ever-growing fiscal demands of commitment programs.

CONCLUSION

Many questions remain unanswered about policy initiatives intended to combat sexual perpetration. The legal foundations of both community notification and civil commitment are issues for continued exploration. Two recent cases (*Connecticut Department of Public Safety v. Doe*, 2003; *Smith v. Doe*, 2003) decided by the Supreme Court upheld the constitutionality of community notification. Although the U.S. Supreme Court has twice upheld sex offender commitment laws, legal challenges continue to be raised concerning the implementation of the statutes.

Perhaps the most pressing need is the importance of establishing empirical evidence that community notification and civil commitment achieve their goal of reducing sexual violence. Identified as a pertinent issue is the role of risk assessment technology in the implementation of notification and commitment laws. Although empirical evidence supports the predictive validity of current actuarial risk assessment instruments, they are not perfect and thus inherently create the risks of both over-prediction and under-prediction. Dangers exist at both ends of the continuum–enlisting more restrictive interventions for those who might not re-offend is as problematic as employing less restrictive interventions for those who may continue to commit sexually violent offenses. Confounding this issue is the tendency of mental health professionals to "adjust" actuarial scales to include variables excluded from the prediction equation. Quinsey et al. (1998) maintains that clinical judgment is so poor that any deviation from the actuarial scheme decreases its predictive validity.

Sex offender legislation should be grounded in empirical evidence and informed by theoretical literature. However, in the wake of emotionally charged reactions to sexual violence, legislation is not always driven by data or science but rather by outrage and fear. Scientists and practitioners have a responsibility to assist lawmakers to respond to the problem of sexual violence by advocating for well-planned strategies that empower women and children as well as rehabilitate perpetrators.

REFERENCES

Abel, G. G., Becker, J. V., Cunningham-Rathner, J., Mittleman, M. S., Murphy, M. S., & Rouleou, J. L. (1987). Self-reported crimes of nonincarcerated paraphiliacs. *Journal of Interpersonal Violence, 2*, 3-25.

Abel, G. G., Mittleman, M. S., & Becker, J. V. (1985). Sexual offenders: Results of assessment and recommendations for treatment. In M. R. Ben-Aron, S. J. Huckle, & C. D. Webster (Eds.), *Clinical criminology: The assessment and treatment of criminal behavior* (pp. 191-205). Toronto: M & M Graphic Ltd.

Alexander, R. (1997). Reconstructing sex offenders as mentally ill: A labeling explanation. *Journal of Sociology and Social Welfare, 24*(2), 65-76.

American Psychiatric Association. (1994). *Diagnostic and statistical manual of mental disorders* (4th ed.). Washington, DC: Author.

Association for the Treatment of Sexual Abusers (ATSA). (2000). Brief for the Association for the Treatment of Sexual Abusers as Amicus Curiae in support of petitioner. *Kansas v. Crane.*

Barbaree, H. E., & Seto, M. C. (1997). *Pedophilia: Assessment and treatment.* New York: Guilford Press.

Barefoot v. Estelle, 463 U.S. 107 (1983).

Berliner, L. (1996). Community notification: Neither a panacea nor a calamity. *Sexual Abuse: A Journal of Research & Treatment, 8*(2), 101-104.

Blain, N. (2000). Self-reported potential community response to sexual offender release notification: An analysis of New Jersey's Megan's law procedures. *Dissertation Abstracts International, 61*(93-B).

Bureau of Justice Statistics. (1997). *Sex offenses and offenders: An analysis of Data on rape and sexual assault.* (NCJ-163392). Washington, DC: U.S. Department of Justice.

Caputo, A. A. (2001). Community notification laws for sex offenders: Possible mediators and moderators of citizen coping. *Dissertation Abstracts International, 61*(9-B).

Clipson, C. R. (2003). Practical considerations in the interview and evaluation of sexual offenders. *Journal of Child Sexual Abuse, 12*(3/4), 127-173.

Connecticut Department of Public Safety v. Doe, 123 S. Ct. 1160 (2003).

Doren, D. M. (1998). Recidivism base rates, predictions of sex offender recidivism, and the "sexual predator" commitment laws. *Behavioral Sciences and the Law, 16*, 97-114.

Doren, D. M. (2002). *Evaluating sex offenders: A manual for civil commitments and beyond.* Thousand Oaks, CA: Sage Publications.

Doren, D. M., & Epperson, D. L. (2001). Great analysis, but problematic assumptions: A critique of Janus and Meehl (1997). *Sexual Abuse: A Journal of Research & Treatment, 13*(1), 45-52.

Edwards, W., & Hensley, C. (2001). Contextualizing sex offender management legislation and policy: Evaluating the problem of latent consequences in community notification laws. *International Journal of Offender Therapy and Comparative Criminology, 45*(1), 83-101.

Epperson, D. L., Kaul, J. D., Huot, S. J., Hesselton, D., Alexander, W., & Goldman, R. (1999b). *Minnesota sex offender screening tool-revised (MnSost-R): Development performance, and recommended risk level cut scores.* Retrieved May 5, 2002, from http://psych-server.iastate.edu/faculty/epperson/MnSOST-R.htm.

Finkelhor, D., Moore, D., Hamby, S. L., & Straus, M. A. (1997). Sexually abused children in a national survey of parents: Methodological issues. *Child Abuse & Neglect, 21*, 1-9.

Finn, P. (1997). *Sex offender community notification.* Washington, DC: U.S. Department of Justice.

Freeman-Longo, R. E. (1985). *Incidence of self-reported sex crimes among incarcerated rapists and child molesters.* Unpublished manuscript.

Freeman-Longo, R. E. (1996). Prevention or problem? *Sexual Abuse: A Journal of Research & Treatment, 8*(2), 91-100.

Furby, L., Weinrott, M., & Blackshaw, L. (1989). Sex offender recidivism: A review. *Psychological Bulletin, 105*(1), 3-30.

Grove, M. G., & Meehl, P. E. (1996). Comparative efficiency of informal and formal prediction procedures: The clinical-statistical controversy. *Psychology, Public Policy and Law, 2*(2), 293-323.

Hanson, R. K. (1997). *The development of a brief actuarial scale for sexual offense recidivism.* Ottawa: Department of the Solicitor General of Canada.

Hanson, R. K. (1998). What do we know about sex offender risk assessment? *Psychology, Public Policy and Law, 4*(1/2), 50-72.

Hanson, R. K., & Bussiere, M. T. (1996). *Predictors of sexual offender recidivism: A meta-analysis.* (1996-04). Ottawa: Department of the Solicitor General of Canada.

Hanson, R. K., & Bussiere, M. T. (1998). Predicting relapse: A meta-analysis of sexual offender recidivism studies. *Journal of Consulting and Clinical Psychology, 66*, 348-362.

Hanson, R. K., Gordon, A., Harris, A. J. R., Marques, J. K., Murphy, W., Quinsey, V. L., & Seto, M. C. (2002). First report of the collaborative outcome data project on the effectiveness of treatment for sex offenders. *Sexual Abuse: A Journal of Research & Treatment, 14*(2), 169-194.

Hanson, R. K., & Harris, A. J. R. (1998). *Dynamic predictors of sexual recidivism.* Ottawa, Canada: Department of the Solicitor General of Canada.

Hanson, R. K., & Harris, A. J. R. (2001). A structured approach to evaluating change among sexual offenders. *Sexual Abuse: A Journal of Research & Treatment, 13*(2), 105-122.

Hanson, R. K., Scott, H., & Steffy, R. A. (1995). A comparison of child molesters and nonsexual criminals: Risk predictors and long-term recidivism. *Journal of Research in Crime and Delinquency, 32*, 325-337.

Hanson, R. K., & Thornton, D. (1999). *Static 99: Improving actuarial risk assessments for sex offenders.* (User report 1999-02). Ottawa: Department of the Solicitor General of Canada.

Hanson, R. K., & Thornton, D. (2000). Improving risk assessments for sex offenders: A comparison of three actuarial scales. *Law and Human Behavior, 24*, 119-136.

Hare, R. D. (1991). *The Hare Psychopathy Checklist-Revised.* Toronto, Canada: Multi-Health Systems.

Hare, R. D. (1999). *Without conscience: The disturbing world of psychopaths among us.* New York: Simon & Shuster.

Janus, E. S. (2000). Sexual predator commitment laws: Lessons for law and the behavioral sciences. *Behavioral Sciences and the Law, 18*, 5-21.

Janus, E. S., & Walbeck, N. (2000). Sex offender commitments in Minnesota: A descriptive study of second generation commitments. *Behavioral Sciences and the Law, 18*, 343-374.

Jimmy Ryce Involuntary Civil Commitment for Sexually Violent Predators' Treatment and Care Act, Florida Statute 394.912 (1998).

Jones, K. D. (1999). The media and Megan's law: Is community notification the answer? *Journal of Humanistic Counseling, Education and Development, 38*(2), 80-88.

Kansas v. Crane, 534 U.S. S. Ct. 407 (2001).

Kansas v. Hendricks, 117 S. Ct. 2072 (1997).

Keough, C. J. (2001, November 27). As law is tested, many sex offenders may go free. *Miami Herald*, p. 1A.

King, C. A. (1999). Fighting the devil we don't know: Kansas v. Hendricks, a case study exploring the civilization of criminal punishment and its ineffectiveness in preventing child sexual abuse. *William and Mary Law Review, 40*(4), 1427-1458.

LaFond, J. Q. (1998). The costs of enacting a sexual predator law. *Psychology, Public Policy and Law, 4*(1/2), 468-504.

LaFond, J. Q. (2000, November). *The costs of sexual predator laws and their impact on participants and policy.* Paper presented at the 19th Annual Research and Treatment Conference of the Association for the Treatment of Sexual Abusers, San Diego, CA.

Levi, R. (2000). Community notification laws: A step toward more effective solutions. *Journal of Interpersonal Violence, 11*(6), 298-300.

Lieb, R. (1996). Community notification laws: A step toward more effective solutions. *Journal of Interpersonal Violence, 11*(2), 298-300.

Lieb, R., & Matson, S. (1998). *Sexual predator commitment laws in the United States.* (38). Olympia, WA: Washington State Institute for Public Policy.

Lieb, R., & Matson, S. (2000). *Sexual predator commitment laws in the United States.* Olympia, WA: Washington State Institute for Public Policy.

Lotke, E. (1997). Politics and irrelevance: Community notification statutes. *Federal Sentencing Reporter, 10*(2), 64-68.

Marques, J. K., Day, D. M., Nelson, C., & Miner, M. H. (1989). *The sex offender treatment and evaluation project: California's relapse prevention program.* New York: Guilford Press.

Matson, S., & Lieb, R. (1996). *Community notification in Washington state: A 1996 survey of law enforcement.* Olympia, WA: Washington State Institute for Public Policy.

Monahan, J. (1981). *Predicting violent behavior: An assessment of clinical techniques.* Beverly Hills, CA: Sage Publications.

Morse, S. J. (1998). Fear of danger, flight from culpability. *Psychology, Public Policy and Law, 4*(1/2), 250-267.

National Criminal Justice Association. (1997). *Sex offender community notification: Policy report.* Washington, DC: Author.

Otto, R. K. (1994). On the ability of mental health professionals to "predict dangerousness": A commentary on interpretations of the "dangerousness" literature. *Law & Psychology Review, 18*(43), 43-68.

Perlin, M. (1998). There's no success like failure/and failure is no success at all: Exposing the pretextuality of Kansas v. Hendricks. *Northwestern University Law Review, 92*(1247), 1247.

Petrosino, A. J., & Petrosino, C. (1999). The public safety potential of Megan's law in Massachusetts: An assessment from a sample of criminal sexual psychopaths. *Crime and Delinquency, 45*(1), 140-158.

Poole, C., & Lieb, R. (1995). *Community notification in Washington state: Decision-making and costs.* Olympia, WA: Washington State Institute for Public Policy.

Prentky, R. A. (1996). Community notification and constructive risk reduction. *Journal of Interpersonal Violence, 11*(6), 295-298.

Prentky, R. A., Lee, A. F., Knight, R. A., & Cerce, D. (1997). Recidivism rates among child molesters and rapists: A methodological analysis. *Law and Human Behavior, 21*(6), 635-659.

Presley, M. M. (1999). Jimmy Ryce involuntary civil commitment for sexually violent predators' treatment and care act: Replacing criminal justice with civil commitment. *Florida State University Law Review, 26*(2), 488-516.

Quackenbush, R. E. (2003). The role of theory in the assessment of sex offenders. *Journal of Child Sexual Abuse, 12*(3/4), 77-102.

Quinsey, V. L., Harris, G. T., Rice, M. E., & Cormier, C. A. (1998). *Violent offenders: Appraising and managing risk.* Washington, DC: American Psychological Association.

Quinsey, V. L., Lalumiere, M. L., Rice, M. E., & Harris, G. T. (1995). Predicting sexual offenses. In J. C. Campbell (Ed.), *Assessing dangerousness: Violence by sexual offenders, batterers, and child abusers* (pp. 114-137). Thousand Oaks, CA: Sage Publications.

Rollman, E. M. (1998). Mental illness: A sexually violent predator is punished twice for one crime. *Journal of Criminal Law and Criminology, 88,* 985-1014.

Satcher, D. (2001). *The surgeon general's call to action to promote sexual health and responsible sexual behavior.* Washington, DC: U.S. Department of Health and Human Services.

Schopp, R. F., & Slain, A. J. (2000). Psychopathy, criminal responsibility, and civil commitment as a sexual predator. *Behavioral Sciences and the Law, 18,* 247-274.

Schram, D., & Milloy, C. D. (1995). *Community notification: A study of offender characteristics and recidivism.* Olympia, WA: Washington Institute for Public Policy.

Schram, D., & Milloy, C. D. (1998). *A study of the characteristics and recidivism of sex offenders considered for civil commitment but for whom proceedings were declined.* Olympia, WA: Washington State Institute for Public Policy.

Schwartz, B. (1999). The case against involuntary commitment. In C. Cohen, & A. Schlank (Eds.), *The sexual predator: Law, policy, evaluation and treatment,* Chapter 4. Princeton, NJ: Civic Research Institute.

Shenk, J. W. (1998, March 9). Do "Megan's laws" make a difference? *U.S. News & World Report,* p. 27.

Smith v. Doe, 123 S. Ct. 1140 (2003).

Swets, J. A., Dawes, R. M., & Monahan, J. (2000a, October). Better decisions through science. *Scientific American,* 82-87.

Swets, J. A., Dawes, R. M., & Monahan, J. (2000b). Psychological science can improve diagnostic decisions. *Psychological Science in the Public Interest, 1*(1), 1-26.

Turay v. Seling/Weston, 108 F. Supp. 2d 1148 (WD Wash. 2000).

Wang, C. T., & Daro, D. (1998). *Current trends in child abuse reporting and fatalities: The results of the 1997 annual fifty state survey.* Chicago: National Center on Child Abuse Prevention Research.

Weinrott, M., & Saylor, M. (1991). Self-report of crimes committed by sex offenders. *Journal of Interpersonal Violence, 6*(3), 286-300.

Winick, B. J. (1998). Sex offender law in the 1990's: A therapeutic jurisprudence analysis. *Psychology, Public Policy and Law, 4*(1/2), 505-570.

Zevitz, R. G., Crim, D., & Farkas, M. A. (2000a). Sex offender community notification: Examining the importance of neighborhood meetings. *Behavioral Sciences and the Law, 18,* 393-408.

Zevitz, R. G., Crim, D., & Farkas, M. A. (2000b). Sex offender community notification: Managing high risk criminals or exacting further vengeance? *Behavioral Sciences and the Law, 18,* 375-391.

Zevitz, R. G., & Farkas, M. A. (2000a). The impact of sex offender community notification on probation/parole in Wisconsin. *International Journal of Offender Therapy and Comparative Criminology, 44*(1), 8-21.

Zevitz, R. G., & Farkas, M. A. (2000b). *Sex offender community notification: Assessing the impact in Wisconsin.* Washington, DC: U.S. Department of Justice.

Sexual Deviancy: Diagnostic and Neurobiological Considerations

Fabian M. Saleh
Fred S. Berlin

SUMMARY. Individuals who engage in sexual offenses may be afflicted with a paraphilic disorder or sexual deviation syndrome. Paraphilias are psychiatric disorders characterized by deviant and culturally non-sanctioned sexual fantasies, thoughts, and/or behaviors. A proportion of these individuals may also suffer from symptoms of mental illness that can go unrecognized. Although the etiology and pathophysiology of paraphilic disorders continue to be under investigation, data from empirical, biomedical, and psychopharmacological studies suggest abnormalities at a biological level. This article will discuss and review clinical and neurobiological characteristics of the paraphilias. To this end, we will begin with a general exploration and overview of basic principles that are germane to the subject matter and will conclude with an examination of the most recent relevant research findings. *[Article copies available for a fee from The Haworth Document Delivery Service: 1-800-HAWORTH. E-mail address: <docdelivery@haworthpress.com> Website: <http://www.HaworthPress.com> © 2003 by The Haworth Press, Inc. All rights reserved.]*

[Haworth co-indexing entry note]: "Sexual Deviancy: Diagnostic and Neurobiological Considerations." Saleh, Fabian M., and Fred S. Berlin. Co-published simultaneously in *Journal of Child Sexual Abuse* (The Haworth Maltreatment & Trauma Press, an imprint of The Haworth Press, Inc.) Vol. 12, No. 3/4, 2003, pp. 53-76; and: *Identifying and Treating Sex Offenders: Current Approaches, Research, and Techniques* (ed: Robert Geffner et al.) The Haworth Maltreatment & Trauma Press, an imprint of The Haworth Press, Inc., 2003, pp. 53-76. Single or multiple copies of this article are available for a fee from The Haworth Document Delivery Service [1-800-HAWORTH, 9:00 a.m. - 5:00 p.m. (EST). E-mail address: docdelivery@haworthpress.com].

Digital Object Identifier: 10.1300/J070v12n03_03

KEYWORDS. Paraphilia, diagnosis, co-morbidity, HPG-axis, genetics, neurobiology

We will begin this article with two commonly raised questions. The first question asked: Are all sexually offending men afflicted with a sexual disorder or are they just misbehaving people who act out sexually? The second and somewhat more complex question: What is the nature of sexual deviancy? In answering these questions three illustrative case reports will be reviewed, followed by a discussion pertaining to the various aspects of the paraphilias.

CASE 1

"I've been a person that, whatever I wanted, I took. I felt that if it was there and I needed it, I would take it. I took that route instead of the more conventional one of working . . . I knew the difference between right and wrong, and I made the choice to go into the street and to break the laws . . . I knew the difference between what I was doing and what I should be doing, but there was always that feeling that nobody's going to give it to me, and if I want it I'm going to have to take it . . . no matter who I hurt . . . This rape was so spontaneous; I see this woman and I say to myself, I want her, and I took her . . . The motivation was selfish. I wouldn't consider another human being's right to own property, to live without the fear of somebody intruding upon their reality . . . I saw her and I just raped her in her apartment . . . I knew that I could use the psychology of her fear to make her do what I wanted her to do and I did that . . . I think that if that woman had . . . fought me, or showed more resistance, I would have either run away or forced her, been really obnoxiously forceful" (Berlin et al., 1997, p. 15).

CASE 2

". . . This urge began to . . . get very strong, very intense. At first it was just . . . voyeurism again, but then it progressed . . . I would go out the evening to peek into windows . . . [It] began to go into an all-night thing. As I was out on these all-night excursions, it became looking for doors that were unlocked, to where maybe I could go into the house to see someone.

If I found . . . a woman that . . . for example, fell asleep while watching TV on the couch, let me draw a picture for you . . . She is lying there, she is in her nightgown. [I would be tempted] to go in and maybe lift the nightgown to peek underneath it. Then it progressed to actually going upstairs to bedrooms to look for females that were alone, and then progressed from that to actually touching them.

At this time . . . if they would wake up, I would immediately just run out of the house, back to my car, and take off. But it then progressed . . . if they woke up, to trying to persuade them to take their clothes off. [. . .] I felt really sick inside that I had done something like that to another person. Not just emotionally sick, but most times I would be physically sick. I would have diarrhea, be sick to my stomach. It's, you know, I hated what I did. I hated it. I just couldn't stop it at that time . . ." (Berlin et al., 1997, pp. 26-27).

CASE 3

"Mr. A., a 40-year-old white male, was referred by his attorney for assessment as a consequence of the patient's sexual involvement with a 13-year-old boy. Having been charged five years earlier with a similar offense, at the time of his assessment the patient was on court-mandated probation. Though apprehended only once before, he had been sexually active almost exclusively with young males, most ranging between the ages 14 and 17 (but some as young as age 8), since he himself was 7 years old. Sexual activity, which included undressing, fondling, mutual masturbation, and oral-genital contact occurred frequently with a variety of partners, sometimes as often as several times per month. In almost all cases the children were persuaded rather than coerced, but in two instances, while intoxicated, Mr. A. threatened the victims with a paring knife. The patient indicated that he had begun to drink frequently 'to get up the courage to approach potential partners.' After each incident the patient felt ashamed and guilty, vowing that he would try not to act similarly in the future. However, in time, as his sexual urges began once again to intensify, he would give in to temptation. The mere happenstance of watching young boys in television commercials would sometimes elicit a strong urge to focus his attention towards the child's genitalia area . . . 'If I have seen an exceptionally nice looking boy I get aroused. I want to go over there, but then again I don't. I see him, and I want to get out of there because I know I am going to start fantasizing. I have noticed that the first thing is I drop my eyes to his genitals. It gets more intense, the fantasies, that is . . .' " (Berlin, 1983, pp. 84-85).

DEFINITIONS AND DIAGNOSIS

The term paraphilia derives from ancient Greek and means love (philia) beyond the usual (para) or attraction (philia) to deviance (para). The category of the paraphilias was first discussed in the third edition of the *Diagnostic and Statistical Manual of Mental Disorders* (DSM-III; American Psychiatric Association [APA], 1980). The revised fourth edition of the DSM (DSM-IV-TR; APA, 2000) lists the paraphilic disorders under the rubric of "Sexual and Gender Identity Disorders." In DSM-IV-TR paraphilias are defined categorically as sexual deviation syndromes characterized by "recurrent, intense sexual urges, fantasies, or behaviors that involve unusual objects, activities, or situations and cause clinically significant distress or impairment in social, occupational, or other important areas of functioning." Per definition, the deviant sexual phenomena have to be present over a period of at least six months in order to meet criteria for one of the following nine listed paraphilic categories: (a) exhibitionism (exposure of one's genitals to an unsuspecting stranger), (b) pedophilia (sexual attraction towards children and/or activity with prepubescent children), (c) fetishism (erotic arousal through inanimate/inert objects), (d) frotteurism (rubbing and/or touching against a non-consenting person), (e) sexual masochism (suffering physical and/or mental pain from a partner), (f) sexual sadism (infliction of physical and/or mental pain upon a partner), (g) transvestic fetishism (cross-dressing), and (h) voyeurism (observation of an unsuspecting person who is disrobing, naked or engaging in sexual activity).

Additional and less common paraphilias are included in the *Not Otherwise Specified* (N.O.S.) category. This category encompasses but is not limited to conditions such as necrophilia (having sex with corpses), telephone scatologia (obscene phone calls), zoophilia (incorporation of animals in sexual acts), klismaphilia (the use of enemas), partialism (an exclusive focus on specific parts of the body), and autoerotic asphyxia (enhancement of orgasm through the restriction of oxygen) (see Table 1).

John Money (1984) recognized 32 phenomenologically different and distinct paraphilias. Based on the predominant phenomenological feature, he defined six categories or subtypes: (a) the sacrificial, (b) the predatory, (c) the mercantile, (d) the fetish, (e) the eligibility, and (f) the allurement type, respectively (see Table 2).

TABLE 1. Categories of Paraphilias and Their Distinguishing Features as Listed in DSM-IV-TR

Exhibitionism (exposing of one's genitals to a stranger)

Fetishism (using inert objects)

Frotteurism (rubbing or touching)

Pedophilia (involving children age 13 or younger)

Sexual masochism (suffering of pain)

Sexual sadism (inflicting of pain)

Transvestic fetishism (cross-dressing)

Voyeurism (observing of unsuspected person)

Paraphilia N.O.S.

Martin Kafka first introduced the term "paraphilia-related disorders" (PRD). PRD embraces a group of sexual syndromes characterized mainly by hypersexual but culturally sanctioned behaviors. Analogous to the DSM-IV-TR criteria for paraphilic disorders, PRD have a duration of at least six months and generally cause significant interpersonal and psychosocial impairment and/or distress. They comprise the following types: (a) compulsive masturbation, (b) protracted promiscuity, (c) pornography dependence, (d) telephone/cyber sex, (e) severe sexual desire incompatibility, and (f) the paraphilia-related disorder not otherwise specified category (see Table 3) (Kafka, 1994; Kafka & Prentky, 1992).

Despite recent improvements and advancements in the taxonomy of the sexual deviances, many clinicians continue to be critical of the available nomenclatures, particularly of the DSM. O'Donohue, Regev, and Hagstrom (2000), for example, questioned in a recently published paper the taxonomic adequacy of DSM-IV diagnostic criteria of pedophilia. Numerous psychiatrists, including the authors of this article, recognize the shortcomings of the current classification systems, which often fail to take into account the complexity of the relevant mental phenomena. Irrespective of these deficiencies, it is important to note that classifying and categorizing sexual phenomena as such does not represent a mere codification of social customs and traditions as some authors thought to suggest at earlier times (Suppe, 1984).

TABLE 2. Paraphilias as Enumerated by Money (1984)

Displacement/Allurement Types:

      Aspyxiophilia (self-strangulation)

      Autagonistophilia (on stage)

      Autassassinophilia (own murder staged)

      Frotteurism (rub against stranger)

      Narratophilia (erotic talk)

      Peidoeiktophilia (penile exhibitionism)

      Pictophilia (pictures)

      Scoptophilia (watching coitus)

      Telephone scatophilia (lewdness)

      Voyeurism or peepingtomism

Eligibility Types:

      Acrotomohilia (amputee partner)

      Apotemnophilia (self-amputee)

      Ephebophilia (youth)/age discrepancy paraphilias

      Gerontophilia (elder)/age discrepancy paraphilias

      Necrophilia (corpse)

      Pedophilia (child)/age discrepancy paraphilias

      Stigmatophilia (piercing; tattoo)

      Zoophilia (animal)

Fetish Types:

      Coprophilia (feces)

      Fetishism

      Hyphephilia (fabrics)

      Klismaphilia (enema)

      Mysophilia (filth)

      Urophilia or undinidm (urine)

      Merchantile

      Troilism (couple + one)

Predatory Types:

    Erotophonophilia (lust murder)

    Kleptophilia (stealing)

    Rapism or Biastophilia (violent assault)

    Somnophilia (sleeper)

Sacrificial Types:

    Masochism (suffering pain)

    Sadism (inflicting of pain and suffering)

    Symphorophilia (disaster)

TABLE 3. Categories of Paraphilia-Related Disorders (PRD)

Compulsive masturbation

Protracted promiscuity

Pornography dependence

Telephone sex dependence

Cyber sex dependence

Severe sexual desire incompatibility

Paraphilia-Related Disorder N.O.S.

Epidemiological Data

Although the true incidence and prevalence of the paraphilias are not known, these disorders appear to be more common in men than in women (Balon, 1998; Bradford, 1998; Bradford, Boulet, & Pawlak, 1992; Kafka, 1996; Money, 1984). Though assumed to be rare in women, some studies seem to suggest the contrary. Indeed, a recent survey conducted by Anderson (1996) showed that approximately 21% of young female college students acknowledged a history of sexually offending behaviors. Although quite interesting, these data did not elaborate and report on the individuals' mental status at the time of the behaviors. As the reader can appraise, this point is worth mentioning, given our discussion on behavioral/paraphilic disorders.

Once established, paraphilic disorders typically tend to run a chronic and stable course (Berlin, 1983; Bradford, 1993; Money, 1984; Seligman &

Hardenburg, 2000). The natural history of the syndrome and the age at which deviant sexual behaviors are first acted on seems to vary from person to person, and to some extent appears to be influenced by the type of paraphilia in question. Paraphiliacs commonly report a first awareness of their deviant sexual proclivities around the time of puberty.

In accordance with the findings of some authors, pedophiles, particularly homosexual pedophiles, entertain deviant sexual fantasies and thoughts at an earlier age when compared to non-pedophilic paraphiliacs (Berlin, 1983; Frosch & Bromberg, 1939). Though the inception of deviant sexual thoughts appears to be around the time of puberty, patients typically do not engage in sexually offending behaviors until several years later, and patterns of sexual deviancy as they relate to behaviors are not established until late adolescence or early adulthood (Abel, Becker, Cunningham-Rathner, Mittelman, & Roul, 1988; Abel & Rouleau, 1990; Bradford, 1993).

A certain percentage of these individuals may also suffer from symptoms of mental illness that can go unrecognized (Allnutt, Bradford, Greenberg, & Curry, 1996; Brown et al., 1996; Kafka & Hennen, 2001). Raymond, Coleman, Ohlerking, Christenson, and Miner (1999), for instance, conducted structured interviews in a group of 44 male pedophiles and found high lifetime prevalence rates of psychiatric disorders which included mood disorders (67%), anxiety disorders (64%), substance abuse disorders (60%), paraphilic disorders (53%) as well as sexual dysfunction disorders (24%). If left untreated, these co-morbid conditions seem to have unfavorable bearings on the course and prognosis of the specific sexual disorder (Seligman & Hardenburg, 2000). Though co-occurrence with non-related psychiatric disorders appears to be rather common, the data on co-morbidity with a second or third paraphilic disorder, notwithstanding the above cited studies, continue to be somewhat conflicting and inconsistent (Abel, Becker, & Mittelman, 1987; Abel et al., 1988; Bradford et al., 1992; Money, 1984).

The Importance of an Astute Assessment

Albeit relatively uncommon in the general population, the number of people referred for the evaluation and management of sexually offending behaviors is steadily increasing (Meyer, 1995; Rosler, 2000). Regrettably, few patients with paraphilic proclivities seek professional help voluntarily and preemptively. The preponderance of patients is referred by the courts and is mandated to attend sex offender specific programs as a condition of probation or parole (Kelly & Cavanaugh, 1982; Packard & Rosner, 1985). With either group of patients, a comprehensive psychiatric and psychosexual evaluation is mandatory. This should always encompass a meticulous query about sexual phenomenology in general and deviant and unconventional sexual thoughts and behaviors in particular. An inquiry about masturbatory fantasies and behaviors may also be enlightening since sexual arousal for the purpose of masturbation may be difficult for these patients in the absence of erotic mental imagery (Evans, 1968).

Given the content and the nature of the query, few patients will volunteer embarrassing sexual information. Therefore, an empathic but proactive approach is recommended when inquiring about sexual experiences and sexual phenomena. In addition to the individual evaluation, pertinent and relevant corroborative data should always be obtained from auxiliary sources, such as primary care physicians, legal authorities, and/or relatives. Because of the aforesaid, some clinicians recommend the routine use of assessment tools, such as phalloplethysmography (volumetric or circumferential) and/or the Abel Assessment for Sexual Interest Screen. Limitations notwithstanding (Fischer & Smith, 1999; Marshall & Fernandez, 2000; Smith & Fischer, 1999), these devices help to appraise and measure sexual arousal and sexual interest, respectively. Given that an in-depth discussion of these methods is beyond the scope of this article, the reader is advised to review the listed references for a more detailed analysis (Abel, Huffman, Warberg, & Holland, 1998; Blanchard, Klassen, Dickey, Kuban, & Blak, 2001; Seto, Lalumiere, & Blanchard, 2000).

In the authors' judgment it is imperative to be cognizant of those neuropsychiatric disorders and/or mental states which have been shown to be associated with hypersexual behaviors or sexual deviancy. Clinicians should judiciously review differential diagnostic aspects of normative and deviant sexual behaviors before offering a diagnosis of a paraphilia in an individual who engaged in sexually offending behaviors (see Table 4).

Smith and Taylor (1999), for example, after reviewing the records of 84 schizophrenic men convicted for a sex offense, found that nearly all patients (80 out of 84) were psychotic at the time of the index offense. Ward (1975) reported the case of a patient with a history of bipolar disorder whose sexually offending behaviors reportedly occurred in the context of a manic episode. This proposed approach to diagnosis ought not to be considered germane to the psychiatric profession only, but should be the modus operandi for all clinicians who through their work will ultimately influence the management and treatment of the sexually offending individual.

By virtue of their disorder and severity of presenting symptoms, selected patients may benefit from pharmacological interventions. Given that many of the employed biological therapies have the potential to induce serious adverse medical effects, it is advisable that patients submit themselves to a routine medical and laboratory examination prior to the inception of such treatments. This should include a complete physical and, if indicated, neurological examination. If the neuropsychiatric examination is suggestive of an acute or subacute change in mental status or of gross brain pathology, neuroimaging should be considered. Blood indices for a complete blood count, comprehensive metabolic panel, plasma reagin test (RPR), and endocrine assays should be obtained (Bradford, 2001). If clinically indicated, chromosomal karyotyping and analysis, electrocardiography and/or electroencephalography (EEG) should also be obtained.

The Role of the Limbic-Hypothalamic-Pituitary-Gonadal Axis

An extensive body of laboratory research provides evidence in support of gonadal hormones' modulatory effects on neuronal activity. Studies have shown that, probably due to the dimorphic characteristics of the preoptic nucleus of the hypothalamus, hormonal manipulations in utero may undo and reverse gender preferences in both male and female rats. In line with the above study, Davidson, Smith, and Damassa (1977) suggested a link between the medial preoptic area of the hypothalamus and sexual behavior. Moreover, the limbic-hypothalamic-pituitary-gonadal axis has been implicated in the biochemical regulation and control of phenomena such as rage and sexual drive. Evidentiary data continue to be relatively scant in humans.

TABLE 4. Differential Diagnosis of Deviant Sexual Behaviors

Psychotic disorders (e.g., schizophrenia)
Affective disorders (e.g., manic episodes in bipolar disorder)
Drug intoxication (e.g., alcohol intoxication)
Cognitive disorders (e.g., dementia)
Personality disorders (e.g., antisocial personality disorder)

Gaffney and Berlin (1984) hypothesized that a dysfunction at the level of the axis may play a contributory role in the etiology of the paraphilias. In order to test this hypothesis, the authors studied the hypothalamic-pituitary-gonadal axis functioning in men who differed from the norm in their sexual arousal patterns. Pedophilic paraphiliacs ($N = 7$), non-pedophilic paraphiliacs ($N = 5$) and normal controls ($N = 5$) were selected and enrolled into the study. All participants were administered 100mcg of luteinizing hormone-releasing hormone (LHRH), Endogenous hypothalamic hormone, which under normal conditions is secreted into the portal circulation, and after reaching the anterior lobe of the pituitary gland induces the secretion of luteinizing hormone (LH), by the pituitary gland. Follicle stimulating hormone (FSH) and LH samples were obtained before and after the administration of LHRH. FSH responses to LHRH were statistically insignificant in all three groups. Interestingly, the response of LH to LHRH was statistically significant in the pedophilic paraphiliacs ($469+/-100$ng/ml for pedophiles versus $229+/-8$ng/ml for non-pedophilic paraphiliacs versus $216+/-31$ng/ml for controls).

These findings suggest a dysfunctional hypothalamic-pituitary- gonadal axis among the examined pedophilic patients. Somewhat in line with these results, Harrison, Strangeway, McCann, and Catalan (1989) reported the case of a patient with hyperprolactineaemia (prolactin levels measured in the patient 2398 mU/l–normal serum levels range between 0-450 mU/l) and non-exclusive pedophilia (DSM-III-R). Treatment with bromocriptine not only normalized the patient's serum prolactin level but diminished deviant sexual thought patterns. According to the authors, a dysfunction at the level of hypothalamic-pituitary-gonadal axis, as evidenced by hyperprolactineaemia, may have played some role in the etiology of the pedophilic proclivities in the examined patient.

Contrary to Harrison's report, other studies, including data from pharmacological investigations, do not provide evidence supporting a link between sexual deviancy and increased serum prolactin levels (Bancroft, 1989; Cooper, Cernosvsky, & Magnus, 1992; Jeffcoate, Matthews, Edwards, Field, & Besser, 1980). Although preliminary and not conclusive, these data suggest a disturbance of the homeostatic regulatory functions of the hypothalamic-pituitary-gonadal axis, and may be conceptualized as the proxy or correlate for sexual deviancy in some patients.

The Role of Genes

As with many other psychiatric disorders, the role of genetic abnormalities has been explored with regard to sexually related disorders. Patients with Klinefelter's syndrome (usually XXY chromosome karyotypes), for instance, have increased rates of sexual disorders (Baker & Stoller, 1968; Hunter, 1969; Nielsen, 1972; Schroder, De La Chapelle, Hakola, & Virrkurnen, 1981). Klinefelter's syndrome patients usually have a phenotype characterized by a male habitus, large extremities, small penis and rudimentary testes. With the onset of puberty, these patients usually do not acquire secondary sexual characteristics. Their endocrinological profile is characterized by abnormally elevated LH and FSH levels and a lower than normal serum testosterone level.

Individuals with Klinefelter's syndrome can present with behavioral and emotional disturbances, including paraphilic disorders (Crowley, 1964; Knecht, 1993; Nielsen, 1970; Pasqualine, Vidal, & Bur, 1957). Berlin (1983) reported several cases of Klinefelter's syndrome patients (mosaic chromosomal patterns [90% 47 XXY, 10% 46 XY] or 47 XXY chromosomal patterns), who in addition to their genetic disorder had co-morbid paraphilias, including homosexual pedophilia, ephebophilia (ephebophilia: men who are sexually aroused by adolescent boys), transsexualism, and transvestism.

A number of other chromosomal abnormalities/patterns, such as mosaic chromosomal patterns (97.5% XY, 2.5% XX and large heterochromatic region at the centromere of autosome number 19), 46 XY, inversion 9 (p+ q−) chromosomal patterns, and the aforementioned 47 XXY chromosomal patterns have been linked to homosexual pedophilia.

Sexually deviant behaviors and syndromes have also been reported in patients with genetically based neuropsychiatric disorders (Comings, 1990; Comings & Comings, 1982; Rich & Ovsiew, 1994; Rosenbaum, 1941). Federoff, Peyser, Franz, and Folstein (1994) reported on a group of 39 patients with Huntington's disease (HD) who not only presented with a paraphilia but also with hypoactive sexual disorders. Interestingly, sexual deviancy appeared to be more frequent in those HD patients who had inhibited orgasm and increased sexual interest. Similarly, patients with Tourette's disorder (TD) may have higher rates of paraphilia-like behaviors. Kerbeshian (1991), for example, reported the case of a 33-year-old man with TD whose repetitive and paraphilic masturbatory fantasies diminished subsequent to the treatment with a serotonin-specific reuptake inhibitor (SSRI).

Although a single chromosome or gene locus has not yet been identified for many of the known psychiatric syndromes, the above data may suggest the existence of a genetic vulnerability or predisposition towards sexual deviancy.

Neuroradiological Findings

Advances in neuroradiology have made it possible to establish links between neuropharmacological, neurophysiological, and neurobiological phenomena. One of the most powerful means available in psychiatric research is functional neuroimaging. Non-invasive brain-mapping techniques allow the indirect and in vivo measurement of brain activity via analysis of regional hemodynamic/metabolic responses following sensory or cognitive stimulation. Through intricate data analysis a broad understanding of the functional organization of the human brain may thus materialize.

Present-day brain neuroimaging methods can be subdivided based on the predominant feature, into four categories. The first is computed tomography (CT) and magnetic resonance imaging (MRI) techniques that primarily visualize static macroscopic anatomic structures. The second category comprises single-photon emission tomography (SPECT) and positron emission tomography (PET). These functional imaging techniques are used for the in vivo measurement of neurophysiological processes, as well as the in vivo identification of neurotransmitter receptors. The third category encompasses functional magnetic resonance imaging techniques (fMRI). fMRI measures changes in blood volume, blood flow and blood oxygenation during the performance of sensory and cognitive tasks. The fourth category includes the non-invasive methods of electroencephalography (EEG) and magnetoelectroencephalography (MEG). These latter methods are employed in the study and mapping of brain electrical activity (for a brief review on fMRI, SPECT, and PET, see Appendix).

In line with the above, EEG techniques were used to examine electrical brain activity in paraphilic patients. A group of Canadian researchers, for instance (Flor-Henry, Lang, Koles, & Frenzel, 1991), employed quantitative EEG techniques in an attempt to study neural electrical activity in 96 pedophiles (ascertained by PPG) and matched controls. A pattern of increased frontal delta, theta, and alpha power and a pattern of decreased interhemispheric and increased intrahemispheric-interhemispheric coherence, right and left (demonstrable only during verbal processing) was found. Interestingly, these findings were limited to those individuals who showed maximal erotic arousal to prepubescent children.

Dressing and colleagues (2001) examined neuronal activity in a homosexual pedophile using fMRI. During the imaging session the subject was asked to view images of semi-nude young boys (the patient had rated the images as sexually not stimulating and not arousing prior to the session). Activation of the attention network and of the right orbitofrontal cortex was demonstrated following data analysis. Left hemispheric regions germane for speech were not activated.

Schober and colleagues (2001) recently presented PET data on five pedophilic patients (mean age 50). All five subjects were started and maintained for 16 months on leuprolide acetate, a luteinizing hormone-releasing-hormone agonist. For the ensuing nine months, subjects received placebo injections of normal saline (saline/Q3months) instead of the active formulation. All subjects were imaged at baseline and at 13 months in a non-aroused state. Interestingly and somewhat in contrast to the below mentioned study, PET data analysis did not show significant changes in brain activity at 13 months.

PET Scanning and the Role of Opiates in Human Sexuality

A substantial body of research has linked endogenous opiate peptides and their receptors to sexual drive and sexual motivation. Opiate receptors appear to be particularly abundant in certain brain regions such as those associated with the limbic system (Pert, 1981). Sexual arousal is decreased by LH and exogenous opiates (Cushman, 1972). Naloxone, an opiate antagonist, blocks the effects of exogenous opiates on the pituitary gland (Sirinathsinghji, Whittington, Andslay, & Fraser, 1983). Furthermore, β-endorphin and morphine decrease copulatory behaviors in rats, an effect which once again can be blocked by Naloxone (McIntosh, Vallano, & Barfield, 1980).

On the other hand, Naloxone given to laboratory animals (i.e., male rats), without the concomitant administration of opiates, kindles copulatory behaviors and lessens the latency period to ejaculation (Cessa, Paglietti, & Quarantotti, 1979). These data suggest, as reported in the substance abuse literature, that exogenous opiates may indeed decrease sexual drive and general sexual functioning (Mirin, Meyer, Mendelson, & Ellinboe, 1980). Additionally, protracted copulatory behavior in laboratory animals can lead to a virtual depletion of the endogenous opiate, metencephalon, in mid-brain structures (Szechtman et al., 1981). Carfentanil, a mild opiate with high affinity for kappa and mu-opiate receptors, can be radioactively labeled (C11-Carfentanil). C11-Carfentanil can thus serve as a ligand in neuroradiological studies. Due to its receptor binding qualities, C11-Carfentanil can be used for the identification and localization of those neuroanatomical structures that are rich in opiate receptors.

Given that endogenous opiates bind to opiate receptors, Frost and Berlin (1985) hypothesized that C11-Carfentanil binding (ergo radioactive count) should be attenuated following sexual arousal. In order to test this hypothesis, C11-Carfentanil activity was measured during a control resting state and during a state of sexual arousal. Subjects were instructed to fantasize about sexual arousing activities prior, during, and up to 15 minutes after the injection of C11-Carfentanil. The degree of penile erection was used as a proxy for sexual arousal. If erection was full and sustained, arousal was assessed as being adequate.

Though preliminary, this study illustrated that in some individuals sexual arousal resulted in a broad release, and subsequent occupancy, of opiate receptors. Furthermore, sexual arousal seemed to induce a global rather than a slow and incremental change in the opiate system. Interestingly, the amygdala and thalamus, two neuroanatomical structures thought to be important in sexual drive and motivation, did not show statistically significant changes in opiate activities during sexual arousal (Berlin et al., 1988; Frost et al., 1985).

The Role of Brain Pathology

Anecdotal case reports and scientific studies have linked idiopathic or secondary brain abnormalities to hypersexual behaviors or frank paraphilias. Hendricks and colleagues (1988) examined and computed the head CT scans and regional cerebral blood flow (rCBF) estimates of 16 criminally committed and sexually abusive men. In contrast to normal controls, radiological findings in the sexually offending group were significant for the thinner and less dense skulls as well as lower regional blood flow values.

Other types of brain pathology, such as frontotemporal dementia or bilateral hippocampal sclerosis, have been seen in patients with late onset homosexual pedophilia. Mendez, Chow, Ringman, Twitchell, and Hinkin (2000) reported the cases of two professional elderly men who in addition to the above described conditions showed, using 18-fluorodeoxyglucose PET scans, right temporal lobe hypometabolism. Huws,

Shubsachs, and Taylor (1991) reported the case of a man with multiple sclerosis who developed a foot fetish in addition to hypersexuality and disinhibition. An MRI image of this patient's brain showed lesions in the temporal and frontal lobes. Anomalies of the temporal lobes and temporal lobe epilepsy have also been linked to paraphilic disorders, such as fetishism and exhibitionism (Epstein, 1961; Hooshmand & Brawley, 1969; Langevin, 1990; Langevin et al., 1988).

Mitchell and Falconer (1954) reported the case of a patient with epilepsy, cross-dressing behaviors and fetishism, whose paraphilic behaviors abated following temporal lobectomy. Interestingly, bilateral temporal lobe ablation in monkeys results in a syndrome called Klüver-Bucy, that is characterized by hyperorality, placidity, hypermetamorphosis (compulsive exploration of surrounding stimuli) and hypersexuality. In contrast to this experimental animal model, the human variant of the Klüver-Bucy syndrome has been more frequently associated with changes in sexual preference rather than with hypersexuality (Lilly, Cunnings, Benson, & Frankel, 1983).

Early or late onset cognitive disorders have also been associated with sexually offending behaviors or even paraphilas (Cooper, 1987, 1988; Myers, 1991; Regestein & Reich, 1978). Miller, Cummings, McIntyre, Ebers, and Grode (1986), for example, reported the cases of several patients, who subsequent to brain pathology (i.e., traumatic brain injury [TBI]), developed de-novo, and uncharacteristic sexual arousal and behavior patterns. A 39-year-old man, for instance, started to engage in public masturbatory behaviors following the rupture of an anterior communicating artery aneurysm. A 50-year-old man's sexual drive substantially increased subsequent to surgical resection of a subfrontal meningoma. A 31-year-old woman became hypersexual after suffering a right-sided stroke. A 50-year-old man had an increase in his pedophilic proclivities and his sexual drive following the development of a progressing brainstem neoplasm (astrocytoma) with involvement of adjacent thalamic and hypothalamic structures.

In line with the findings of Miller's report, Simpson, Blaszczynski, and Hodgkinson (1999) reviewed in a five-year retrospective study the cases of 445 patients who had suffered a TBI. Subsequent to the TBI, 29 patients (6.5%) engaged in sexually offending behaviors. Only two had a prior history of sexually offending behaviors. Three patients (2.3%) were intoxicated from alcohol at the time of the index offense. Staff members were predominantly the target of the "touching offenses."

Although a distinct neurobiological substrate or correlate of sexual deviancy has not yet been identified, the incidence of deviant sexual behaviors in humans with brain pathology appears to be greater than one expects to find by chance alone. Though very pertinent to this general discussion, the analysis and examination of the role of serotonin, catecholamines, and testosterone is undertaken in some detail in our other article that centers around neurotransmitters, sex hormones, and psychopharmacology.

The pendulum has clearly swung away from the 40s and early 50s when psychoanalysis and a plethora of interrelated theories dominated the field of psychiatry. Dubious concepts and terms, such as castration anxiety, oedipal crisis, and libido cathexis were commonly used to "explain" and to "treat" sexual deviancy (Freud, 1953). Though we certainly do not disagree with the notion that certain types of adverse childhood experiences may unfavorably influence normative psychosexual development, we continue to be troubled by those clinical opinions that attempt to validate and explain the paraphilias on the basis of mere child rearing practices and/or other traumatic early life occurrences.

Despite many years of scientific research, paraphilias continue to evoke numerous questions within the mental health community. The enigma of why some men crave intimacy with children, animals, or corpses remains unanswered. Though the etiology and pathophysiology of paraphilic disorders remains under investigation, the data presented here illustrate and provide evidence suggestive of an abnormality at a biological level. It is, however, imperative to bear in mind that, whatever the organic predisposition or vulnerability towards sexually aggressive or deviant behaviors, biological abnormalities account for only a part of the variance. Indeed, behaviors, motivated or socially learned, are intricate phenomena in that they are influenced by a myriad of environmental and individual factors, which may encompass genetic endowments, intrinsic drive states, as well as cognitive and temperamental dispositions. In our opinion, only critical interpretation and analysis of clinical and scientific data will eventually lead to new and innovative methods that will help to elucidate, and maybe one day explain, the phenomenon of sexual deviancy.

REFERENCES

Abel, G. G., Becker, J. V., Cunningham-Rathner, J., Mittelman, M., & Roul, J. L. (1988). Multiple paraphilic diagnoses among sex offenders. *Bulletin of the Academy of Psychiatry and the Law, 16*(2), 153-168.

Abel, G. G., Becker, J. V., & Mittelman, M. (1987). Self-reported sex crimes of non-incarcerated paraphiliacs. *Journal of Interpersonal Violence, 2,* 3-25.

Abel, G. G., Huffman, J., Warberg, B., & Holland, C. L. (1998). Visual reaction time and plethysmography as measures of sexual interest in child molesters. *Sexual Abuse: A Journal of Research and Treatment, 10*(2), 81-95.

Abel, G. G., & Rouleau, J. L. (1990). The nature and extent of sexual assault. In W. L. Marshall, D. R. Laws, & H. E. Barabree (Eds.), *Handbook of sexual assault* (pp. 9-20). New York: Plenum Press.

Aine, C. J. (1995). A conceptual overview and critique of functional neuroimaging techniques in humans: I. MRI/fMRI and PET. *Critical Reviews in Neurobiology, 9*(2/3), 29-109.

Allnutt, S. H., Bradford, J. M., Greenberg, D. M., & Curry, S. (1996). Co-morbidty of alcoholism and the paraphilias. *Journal of Forensic Sciences, 41*(2), 234-239.

American Psychiatric Association. (1980). *Diagnostic and statistical manual of mental disorders* (3rd ed.). Washington, DC: Author.

American Psychiatric Association. (2000). *Diagnostic and statistical manual of mental disorders* (text revision). Washington, DC: Author.

Anderson, P. B. (1996). Correlates of college's self-reports of heterosexual aggression. *Sex Abuse, 8*(2), 121-133.

Baker, H. J., & Stoller, J. (1968). Can a biological force contribute to gender identity? *American Journal of Psychiatry, 124*(12),1653-1658.

Balon, R. (1998). Pharmacological treatment of paraphilias with a focus on antidepressants. *Journal of Sex and Marital Therapy, 24*(4), 241-254.

Bancroft, J. (1989). The biological basis of human sexuality. In J. Bancroft (Ed.), *Human sexuality and its problems* (pp. 12-145). Edinburgh: Churchill Livingstone.

Berlin, F. S. (1983). Sex offenders: A biomedical perspective and a status report on biomedical treatment. In J. B. Greer, & I. R. Stuart (Eds.), *The sexual aggressor: Current perspectives on treatment* (pp. 83-123). New York: Van NOSTRAND Reinhold Co.

Berlin, F. S., Frost, J. J., Mayberg, H. S., Behal, R., Daniels, R. F., Links, J. M. et al. (1988). *Endogenous opiate secretion in the brain during sexual arousal detectible by PET scanning.* Unpublished Data.

Berlin, F. S., Lehne, G. K., Martin, H. M., Wayne, H. P., Thomas, K., & Fuhrmaneck, J. (1997). The eroticized violent crime: A psychiatric perspective with six clinical examples. *Sexual Addiction & Compulsivity, 4*(1), 9-31.

Berlin, F. S., & Schaerf, F. W. (1985). Laboratory assessment of the paraphilias and their treatment with antiandrogenic medication. In R. C. W. Hall, & T. P. Beresford (Eds.), *Handbook of psychiatric diagnostic procedures* (pp. 273-305). New York: Spectrum Publications.

Blanchard, R., Klassen, P., Dickey, R., Kuban, M. E., & Blak, T. (2001). Sensitivity and specificity of the phallometric test for pedophilia in nonadmitting sex offenders. *Psychological Assessment, 13*(1), 118-126.

Bradford, J. M. W. (1993). The pharmacological treatment of the adolescent sex offender. In H. E. Barbaree (Ed.), *The juvenile sex offender* (pp. 278-288). New York: Guilford Publications.

Bradford, J. M. W. (1998). Treatment of men with paraphilia. *New England Journal of Medicine, 338*, 464-465.

Bradford, J. M. W. (2001). The neurobiology, neuropharmacology, and pharamcological treatment of the paraphilias and compulsive sexual behaviour. *Canadian Journal of Psychiatry, 46*(1), 26-34.

Bradford, J. M. W., Boulet, J., & Pawlak, A. (1992). The paraphilias a multiplicity of deviant behaviours. *Canadian Journal of Psychiatry, 37,* 104-108.

Bradford, J. M. W., Greenberg, D., Gojer, J., Martindale, J. J., & Goldberg, M. (1995, May). *Sertraline in the treatment of pedophilia: An open label study.* Paper presented at the meeting of the American Psychiatric Association, Miami, FL.

Brown, M., Amoroso, D., Ware, E., Puresse, M., & Pilkey, D. (1973). Factors affecting viewing time of pornography. *Journal of Social Psychology, 90,* 125-135.

Cessa, G. L., Paglietti, E., & Quarantotti, B. P. (1979). Induction to copulatory behavior in sexually inactive rats by naloxone. *Science, 204*(13), 203-204.

Comings, D. E. (1990). *Tourette's syndrome and human behavior.* Durate, CA: Hope Press.

Comings, D. E., & Comings, B. G. (1982). A case of familial exhibitionism in Tourette's syndrome successfully treated with haloperidol. *American Journal of Psychiatry, 139*(7), 913-915.

Cooper, A. J. (1987). Medroxyprogesterone acetate (MPA) treatment of sexual acting out men suffering from dementia. *Journal of Clinical Psychiatry, 48,* 368-70.

Cooper, A. J. (1988). Medroxyprogesterone acetate as a treatment for sexual acting out in organic brain syndrome. *American Journal of Psychiatry, 145*(9), 1179-1180.

Cooper, A. J., Cernosvsky, Z., & Magnus, R. V. (1992). The long-term use of cyproterone acetate in pedophilia: A case study. *Journal of Sex and Marital Therapy, 18*(4), 292-302.

Crowley, J. T. (1964). Klinefelter's syndrome and abnormal behavior: A case report. *International Journal of Neuropsychiatry, 5,* 359-363.

Cushman, P. (1972). Sexual behavior in heroin addiction and methadone maintenance: Correlation with plasma luteinizing hormone. *New York State Journal of Medicine, 72,* 1261-1265.

Davidson, J. M., Smith, E. R., & Damassa, D. A. (1977). Comparative analysis of the roles of androgen in the feedback mechanism and sexual behavior. In L. Martini & M. Motta, *Androgens and antiandrogens* (pp. 137-149). New York: Raven Press.

Dressing, H., Obergriesser, T., Tost, H., Kaumeier, S., Ruf, M., & Braus, D. F. (2001). Homosexual pedophilia and functional networks–An fMRI case report and literature review. *Fortgeschrittene Neurologie und Psychiatrie, 69*(11), 539-544.

Epstein, A. (1961). Relationship of fetishism and transvestism to brain and particularly to temporal lobe dysfunction. *Journal of Nervous and Mental Disease, 133,* 247-253.

Evans, P. R. (1968). Masturbatory fantasy and sexual deviation. *Behaviour Research & Therapy, 6,* 17-49.

Fedoroff, J. P., Peyser, C., Franz, M. L., & Folstein, S. E. (1994). Sexual disorders in Huntington's disease. *Journal of Neuropsychiatry and Clinical Neurosciences, 6*(2), 147-153.

Fischer, L., & Smith, G. (1999). Statistical adequacy of the Abel assessment for interest in paraphilias. *Sex Abuse, 11*(3), 195-205.

Flor-Henry, P., Lang, R., Koles, Z. J., & Frenzel, R. R. (1991). Quantitative EEG studies of pedophilia. *International Journal of Psychophysiology, 10*(3), 253-258.

Freud, S. (1953). Three essays on sexuality. In J. Strachey (Ed.), *The standard edition of the complete psychological works of Sigmund Freud, Vol. 7* (pp. 123-246). London: Hogarth Press.

Frosch, J., & Bromberg, W. (1939). The sex offender: A psychiatric study. *American Journal of Orthopsychiatry, 9*, 761-776.

Frost, J. J., Mayberg, H. S., Berlin, F. S., Behal, R., Dannals, R. F., Links, J. M. et al. (1986). Alteration in brain opiate receptor binding in man following sexual arousal using C_{11}-carfentanil and positron emission tomography. *Journal of Computer Assisted Tomography, 9*, 231-236.

Gaffney, G. R., & Berlin, F. S. (1984). Is there hypothalamic-pituitary-gonadal dysfunction in pedophilia? A pilot study. *British Journal of Psychiatry, 145*, 657-660.

Harrison, P., Strangeway, P., McCann. J., & Catalan, J. (1989). Pedophilia and hyperprolactinaemia. *British Journal of Psychiatry, 155*, 847-848.

Hendricks, S. E., Fitzpatrick, D. F., Hartman, K., Quaife, M. A., Stratbucker, R. A., & Graber, B. (1988). Brain structure and function in sexual molesters of children and adolescents. *Journal of Clinical Psychiatry, 49*(3), 108-112.

Hooshmand, H., & Brawley, B. W. (1969). Temporal lobe seizures and exhibitionism. *Neurology, 11*, 1119-1124.

Hunter, H. (1969). A controlled study of the psychopathology and physical measurements of Klinefelter's syndrome. *British Journal of Psychiatry, 115*, 443-448.

Huws, R., Shubsachs, A. P., & Taylor, P. J. (1991). Hypersexuality, fetishism and multiple sclerosis. *British Journal of Psychiatry, 158*, 280-281.

Jeffcoate, J. W., Matthews, R. W., Edwards, C. R., Field, L. H., & Besser, G. M. (1980). The effect of cyproterone acetate on serum testosterone, LH, FSH, and prolactin in male sex offenders. *Clinical Endocrinology, 2*, 189-195.

Kafka, M. P. (1994). Paraphilia-related disorders: Common, neglected, and misunderstood. *Harvard Review of Psychiatry, 2*(1), 39-42.

Kafka, M. P., & Hennen, J. (2002). A DSM-IV axis I comorbidity study of males (n = 120) with paraphilias and paraphilia-related disorders. *Sex Abuse, 14*(4), 349-366.

Kafka, M. P., & Prentky, R. (1992). A comparative study of nonparaphilic sexual addictions and paraphilias in men. *Journal of Clinical Psychiatry, 53*(10), 345-350.

Kaplan, I. H., & Sadock, B. J. (1998). *Kaplan and Sadock's synopsis of psychiatry: Behavioral sciences/clinical psychiatry* (8th ed.). Maryland: Williams & Wilkins.

Kelly, J. R., & Cavanaugh, J. L. (1982). Treatment of the sexually dangerous patient. *Current Psychiatric Therapies, 21*, 101-113.

Kerbeshian, J., & Burd L. (1991). Tourette's syndrome and recurrent paraphilic masturbatory fantasy. *Canadian Journal of Psychiatry, 36*(2), 155-157.

Knecht, T. (1993). Pedophilia and diaper fetishism in a man with Klinefelter syndrome. *Psychiatrische Praxis, 20*(5), 191-192.

Langevin, R. (1990). Sexual anomalies and the brain. In W. L. Marshall, D. R. Laws, & H. E. Barbaree (Eds.), *Handbook of sexual assault: Issues, theories and treatment of the offender* (pp. 103-114). New York: Plenum.

Langevin, R., Bain, J., Wortzman, G., Hucker, S., Dickey, R., & Wright, P. (1988). Sexual sadism: Brain, blood and behavior. *Annals of the New York Academy of Sciences, 528*, 163-171.

Lilly, R., Cunnings, J. L., Benson, D. F., & Frankel, M. (1983). The human Klüver-Bucy syndrome. *Neurology, 33*, 1141-1145.

Marshall, W. L., & Fernandez, Y. M. (2000). Phallometric testing with sexual offenders: Limits to its value. *Clinical Psychology Review, 20*(7), 807-822.

McIntosh, T. K., Vallano, M. L., & Barfield, R. J. (1980). Effects of morphine, beta-endorphin and naloxone on catecholamine levels and sexual behavior in the male rat. *Pharmacology Biochemistry and Behavior, 13*, 435-441.

Mendez, M. F., Chow, T., Ringman, J., Twitchell, G., & Hinkin, C. H. (2000). Pedophilia and temporal disturbances. *Journal of Neuropsychiatry and Clinical Neurosciences, 12*(1), 76-86.

Meyer, J. K. (1995). Paraphilias. In H. I. Kaplan, & B. J. Sadock (Eds.), *Comprehensive textbook of Psychiatry, volume 1* (6th ed.) (pp. 1334-1347). Baltimore, MD: Williams & Wilkins.

Miller, B. L., Cummings, J. L., McIntyre, H., Ebers, G., & Grode, M. (1986). Hypersexuality or altered sexual preference following brain injury. *Journal of Neurology, Neurosurgery, and Psychiatry, 49*, 867-873.

Mirin, S. M., Meyer, R. E., Mendelson, J. H., & Ellinboe, J. (1980). Opiate use and sexual function. *American Journal of Psychiatry, 137*, 909-915.

Mitchell, W., & Falconer, M. A. (1954). Epilepsy with fetishism relieved by temporal lobectomy. *Lancet, 2*, 626-630.

Money, J. (1984). Paraphilias: Phenomenology and classification. *American Journal of Psychotherapy, 38*(2), 164-179.

Myers, B. A. (1991). Treatment of sexual offenses by persons with developmental disabilities. *American Journal on Mental Retardation, 95*(5), 563-569.

Nielsen, J. (1970). Criminality among patients with Klinefelter's syndrome and the XXY syndrome. *British Journal of Psychiatry, 117*, 365-369.

Nielsen, J. (1972). Gender role identity and sexual behavior in persons with sex chromosome aberrations. *Danish Medical Bulletin, 17*(8), 269-275.

O'Donohue, W., Regev, L. G., & Hagstrom, A. (2000). Problems with the DSM-IV diagnosis of pedophilia. *Sex Abuse, 12*(2), 95-105.

Packard, W. S., & Rosner, R. (1985). Psychiatric evaluation of sexual offenders. *Journal of Forensic Sciences, 30*, 715-720.

Pasqualine, R. Q., Vidal, G., & Bur, G. E. (1957). Psychopathology of Klinefelter's syndrome: A review of thirty-one cases. *Lancet, 2*, 164-167.

Pert, C. B. (1981). Type I and Type II opiate receptor distribution in brain: What does it tell us? In J. B. Martin, S. Reichlin, & K. L. Biche (Eds.), *Neurosecretion and brain peptides* (pp. 117-131). New York: Raven.

Raymond, N. C., Coleman, E., Ohlerking, F., Christenson, G. A., & Miner, M. (1999). Psychiatric comorbidity in pedophilic sex offenders. *American Journal of Psychiatry, 156*(5), 786-788.

Regestein, Q. R., & Reich, P. (1978). Pedophilia occurring after the onset of cognitive impairment. *Journal of Nervous and Mental Disease, 166*(11), 794-798.

Rich, S. S., & Ovsiew, F. (1994). Leuprolide acetate for exhibitionism in Huntington's disease. *Movement Disorders, 9*(3), 353-357.

Rosenbaum, D. (1941). Psychosis with Huntington's chorea. *Psychiatry Q, 15*, 93-99.

Rosler, A., & Witztum, E. (2000). Pharmacotherapy of paraphilias in the next millennium. *Behavioral Sciences and the Law, 18*(1), 43-56.

Schober, J. M., Kuhn, P., Kovacs, P., Earle, J., Byrne, P., & Fries, R. (2001, November). *A comparison of standard psychotherapy versus leuprolide acetate with standard psychotherapy for suppression of aberrant sexual arousal*. Paper presented at the 20th Annual Research and Treatment Conference of the Association for the Treatment of Sexual Abusers (ATSA), San Antonio, TX.

Schroder, J., De La Chapelle, A., Hakola, P., & Virrkurnen, M. (1981). The frequency of XYY and XXY men among criminal offenders. *Acta Psychiatrica Scandinavica, 63*, 272-276.

Seligman, L., & Hardenburg, S. A. (2000). Assessment and treatment of paraphilias. *Journal of Counseling & Development, 78* (1), 107-116.

Seto, M. C., Lalumiere, M. L., & Blanchard, R. (2000). The discriminative validity of a phallometric test for pedophilic interests among adolescent sex offenders against children. *Psychological Assessment, 3*, 319-327.

Simpson, G., Blaszczynski, A., & Hodgkinson, A. (1999). Sex offending as a psychological sequela of traumatic brain injury. *Journal of Head Trauma Rehabilitation, 6*, 567-580.

Sirinathsinghji, D. J. S., Whittington, P. E., Andslay, A., & Fraser, H. M. (1983). Beta-Endorphin regulates lordosis in female rats by modulating LH-Rh release. *Nature, 301*(6), 62-64.

Smith, A. D., & Taylor, P. J. (1999). Serious sex offending against women by men with schizophrenia: Relationship of illness and psychiatric symptoms to offending. *British Journal of Psychiatry, 174*, 233-237.

Smith, G., & Fischer, L. (1999). Assessment of juvenile sexual offenders: Reliability and validity of the Abel assessment for interest in paraphilias. *Sex Abuse, 3*, 207-216.

Suppe, F. (1984). Classifying sexual disorders: The diagnostic and statistical manual of the American psychiatric association. *Journal of Homosexuality, 4*, 9-28.

Szechtman, H., Hershkowitz, M., & Simantov, R. (1981). Sexual behavior decreases pain sensitivity and stimulates endogenous opiods in male rats. *European Journal of Pharmacology, 70*, 279-285.

Ward, N. G. (1975). Successful lithium treatment of transvestism associated with manic depression. *Journal of Nervous and Mental Disease, 161*(3), 204-206.

APPENDIX

Neuroradiological Concepts

In this subsection we will briefly review some of the concepts and principles germane to SPECT, PET, MRI, and fMRI. In contrast to CT, which relies on measurement of X-ray absorption and X-ray attenuation, MRI uses the technology of nuclear magnetic resonance (NMR). NMR is based on the principle that nuclei of all atoms spin about a randomly in space orientated axis. When a person, ergo atoms, are placed in a magnetic field, the axis of all odd-numbered nuclei (nucleus with an odd number of either protons or neutrons–for example, hydrogen in the brain) align with the magnetic field. Exposure to non-ionizing high pulse radio frequency (RF) electromagnetic signals upsets this alignment, deviating thereby the axes of nuclei from the magnetic field. As soon as the radio frequency ceases, the axes realign with the magnetic field and produce their own MR signals. The electrical energy released is measured by the MRI scanner. High-resolution, multiplanar images of varied brain structures are generated (e.g., axial, coronal and sagittal images) as a result of this process.

Variations in either duration of the RF pulse sequence and/or the duration of the time collection of data influences image acquisitions. We distinguish T1-weighted scans (spin echo, inversion recovery, short return time [TR] and short TE [Echo Time]) with high anatomic resolution permit superior delineations of gray-white matter structures. T1 scans can be enhanced with gadolinium-diethylenetriamine pentaacetic acid (contrast material). T2-weighted scans (spin echo, long TR and long TE) are optimal for the visualization of brain pathology. Partial T2 scans (proton density, long TR, short TE) permit the discrimination of diseased tissue and fluid. Flair scans (inversion recovery, very long TR and long TE) are even more sensitive and discriminative than T2 scans.

Functional magnetic resonance imaging (fMRI) was first used in the early 1990s. It can provide both individual and group-averaged imaging data with good spatial and temporal resolution. Since non-radioactive tracers are used, fMRI allows longitudinal studies of brain function in individual subjects. For fMRI, several techniques are presently available. The most widely used family of methods exploits the effects of deoxyhemoglobin on MRI signals. This is called the blood oxygen level-dependent (BOLD) signal change. Functional MRI acquires BOLD pulse sequences in one of two ways. In echo planar imaging (EPI), 2D spiral imaging or fast low-angle shot imaging (FLASH), information is acquired in a per-slice manner and data from each slice is combined to constitute a volume. The technique of principles of echo-shifting with a train of observations (PRESTO), however, allows fMRI scanning to directly acquire information in a 3D fashion. PRESTO, which is essentially a modification of the EPI 2D imaging method, provides greater image stability in that there is less signal fluctuation across repeated acquisitions.

Due to greater spatial integrity, there is greater correspondence of shape between the brain and the image, and a lesser degree of imaged tissue lost near cranial cavities. However, PRESTO fMRI does have the problem of greater sensitivity to motion of the scanned subject. This is controlled with vigilant quality control examination of time series data sets as well as both active head restraint (bite bar and restrictive padding) and post-processing image realignment software.

Furthermore, the latest version of PRESTO pulse sequence incorporates a "navigator echo" which enables correction of motion, while also reducing scan time by a factor of 3 to 4. SPECT permits the three-dimensional assessment of regional cerebral blood flow. SPECT requires the use of radiotracers, e.g., technetium-99m (half-life of approximately 6 hours). A small bolus of a tracer is injected into a peripheral vein. This compound circulates through the blood stream, and after crossing the blood-brain barrier it enters the brain cells. Within the cells the ligands are transformed to charged ions. Single gamma photons are emitted and registered by detectors, and two-dimensional images of small sections of the brain (axial, coronal and sagittal planes) are thus produced. PET also requires the use of radioactive compounds, and subsequent to recording processes generates detailed maps of brain activity. One advantage over SPECT is its relatively high level of spatial and temporal resolution. Moreover, PET scanning may provide data about neuronal metabolism. One of its main disadvantages is that it requires an actual imaging camera and a cyclotron, an apparatus where charged particles are accelerated to high energies, making it therefore a relatively costly procedure (Aine, 1995; Kaplan & Sadock, 1998).

The Role of Theory in the Assessment of Sex Offenders

Ray E. Quackenbush

SUMMARY. No generally accepted theory of sex offender behavior exists at this point. As clinical experience and research findings interact within an evolving theoretical framework, the picture of what is important, as well as what is possible to know about a sex offender, is rapidly changing. It is vital that mental health professionals, the legal system, social service agencies, and other consumers and providers of sex offender assessments be aware of both what is possible to learn about an offender as well as the limitations on that knowledge and its application. Prominent theories that influence the assessment of offenders in North America and Europe are presented and examined. Uses and limitations of each theory are discussed. Several trends emerge which could influence the future of sex offender assessment, treatment, management, and policy. *[Article copies available for a fee from The Haworth Document Delivery Service: 1-800-HAWORTH. E-mail address: <docdelivery@haworthpress.com> Website: <http://www.HaworthPress.com> © 2003 by The Haworth Press, Inc. All rights reserved.]*

Address correspondence to: Ray E. Quackenbush, PsyD, Affiliated Psychologists, Ltd., 4801 West Peterson Avenue, Suite 525, Chicago, IL 60646 (E-mail: quaq@earthlink.net).

[Haworth co-indexing entry note]: "The Role of Theory in the Assessment of Sex Offenders." Quackenbush, Ray E. Co-published simultaneously in *Journal of Child Sexual Abuse* (The Haworth Maltreatment & Trauma Press, an imprint of The Haworth Press, Inc.) Vol. 12, No. 3/4, 2003, pp. 77-102; and: *Identifying and Treating Sex Offenders: Current Approaches, Research, and Techniques* (ed: Robert Geffner et al.) The Haworth Maltreatment & Trauma Press, an imprint of The Haworth Press, Inc., 2003, pp. 77-102. Single or multiple copies of this article are available for a fee from The Haworth Document Delivery Service [1-800-HAWORTH, 9:00 a.m. - 5:00 p.m. (EST). E-mail address: docdelivery@haworthpress.com].

KEYWORDS. Sex offender assessment, theory in sex offender assessment, psychological theory, psychological assessment

Assessment in a correctional context can go a long way if the assessment tools are grounded in a theory of criminal behavior (Bonta, 2002). At the present time there is no generally accepted theory of sex offender behavior. While there is a growing amount of published data, there is little discussion that could be described as theoretical contained in the literature dealing with sexual violence. Nevertheless, it may be possible to partially infer a theory or theories from the more commonly used assessment techniques. While few researchers in sex offender behavior would be expected to have an awareness of the major trends in science in general, much of the more recent research supporting sex offender assessment fits well with an emerging meta-theory of science that is concerned with the dynamics of all types of behavior, both physical and psychological.

The effort to understand the theoretical underpinnings of sex offender assessment is worth undertaking because there cannot be a truly atheoretical approach to assessment. In making an assessment, hopefully we do not randomly accumulate bits and pieces of information about a subject and then present them in a haphazard fashion. The methods chosen to collect and analyze the information are dependent not only upon what seems important, but also upon what it seems possible to learn. Whether we are aware of it or not, we look at the subject through a theoretical lens which determines what information we will collect and what information will be ignored. What we do not see may be vitally important, but it goes undiscovered (Holland, 1995). As Einstein (in Johnson, 1995) said, "It is the theory that allows us to see the facts."

There exists a certain amount of misunderstanding in both the popular mind and the minds of some scientists as to the nature of science and its limits. Many people think of science as a subject, but it is not. It is a method (Sulloway, 1996). It is an attempt to understand the universe and humanity's relationship to nature (Bohm & Peat, 1987). The essence of science lies in explanation, in laying bare the fundamental mechanisms of nature (Butz & McCowen, 1997). In science, the so-called facts do not speak for themselves, but assume their meaning based on theoretical and ideological commitments (Sulloway, 1996).

Some sort of structure or theory is essential if we are to effectively inter-relate and interpret observations in any field of knowledge (Forrester, 1990). As it is taught in courses in the philosophy of science, the scientific answer to a question is a set of rules, or as more commonly termed, a model, which is often expressed in the compact language of mathematics (Casti, 1994).

Models of human behavior are often expressed in statistical terms. Statistical models have proven very useful, but they have serious limitations when complex behaviors are studied, and where alternative explanations are possible for the same pattern of data (Cohen & Stewart, 1994). There is a long-honored tradition in science that holds that when several theories appear to account for the same phenomenon, then only one of them can be correct (Bohm & Peat, 1987). This is called the Law of Parsimony. It is a respectable ideal, but one that does not make sense on its own. In thought as in life, a false economy is possible (Midgely, 1995). One theory may not be enough to explain a particular data pattern. Behavioral researchers are well acquainted with situations in which different or even contradictory events produce the same behavior in their subjects. Conversely, subjects can respond differently from one trial to the next even when presented with apparently identical circumstances. Would a more elegant order emerge if the data were graphed in a different way (Johnson, 1995; Quackenbush, 1998)? Simple and complicated behaviors have both been shown to emerge from the same system (Kelso, 1995). Holism is an entirely respectable, perfectly clear concept within modern mathematics (Penrose, 1995). Understanding of the component parts of a composite system is impossible without an understanding of the behavior of the system as a whole (Dyson, 1995).

DIFFICULTIES IN THE FIELD

Illegal behaviors such as sexual offending are difficult or sometimes impossible to study in the psychological laboratory. There are obvious ethical dilemmas, and even when experimental studies are possible, psychologists are often unsure whether their findings will generalize to real life behavior (Sulloway, 1996). Naturalistic studies of some behaviors face serious methodological problems. For example, most sexual assaults are never officially reported. Also, such research does not clearly fall within the domain of one particular discipline. There are communication problems between workers in various, widely differing disciplines. Few researchers can keep up with the diversity (Finkelhor, 1986; Quackenbush, 1998).

Slife and Williams (1997) have presented a critique of theory as used in psychology. Koch (1959-1963), in his influential history of the development of psychology, observed that psychology settled on its methods before it developed its questions. The natural sciences on the other hand developed their methods as a specific response to particular theoretical problems. There has never been a lack of theoretical activity in psychology. But this activity is fragmented, and fails to take into account the theoretical themes and problems that motivate the enterprise of psychology as a whole. Slife and Williams feel that the result is a general disaffection with theory in psychology. The recent trend toward eclecticism in clinical psychology is seen as evidence of this disaffection with theory (Slife & Williams, 1997).

Theories of sexual offending are hampered by a lack of knowledge. Despite recent advances in sex offender assessment (Borum & Otto, 2000), particularly in risk estimation and assessment of psychopathy, there are still serious problems with what is known about sex offenders (Hanson & Harris, 2001). For example, no one knows what the actual occurrence rate of sexual offenses is, even though there is widespread agreement among workers in the field that most occurrences go unreported (Bradford, 2001). Even when sexual offenses result in criminal charges, they may not be counted as sex-related crimes for a variety of reasons (Quinsey, Harris, Rice, & Cormier, 1998).

Most research has dealt with adult male offenders, while there has been less research dealing with juvenile sexual offenders (Brown & Forth, 1997), and even less known about female offenders (Adkerson, 2001; Lewis & Stanley, 2000; Wood, Grossman, & Fichtner, 2000). The present chapter also deals only with adult male offenders. For legal as well as psychological reasons, sex offenders are usually highly reluctant to disclose their offenses (Ahlmeyer, Heil, McKee, & English, 2000). For this and other reasons, there are virtually insurmountable problems in securing samples of sex offenders for research purposes. Researchers are forced to rely upon samples of convenience (Quinsey et al., 1998) usually drawn from populations of convicted offenders, who may not be at all representative of sex offenders in general (Wood et al., 2000). Sexual offenders are actually a highly heterogeneous population (Brown & Forth, 1997; Gruben, 1999). The reliance on convenient samples of convicted offenders means that almost nothing is known about the characteristics of those who are not reported to authorities.

Studies of sex offender recidivism all are biased toward underestimating the true rate of occurrence (Hanson & Bussiere, 1998; Quackenbush, 1998, 2000a, 2000b, 2000c; Quinsey et al., 1998). There are also serious problems in the methodology used to study reoffense. Investigators usually use "rap sheet" information rather than relying on police reports of the offenses. Few studies of reoffense cover a period of more than five years (Hanson & Bussiere, 1998), but research suggests that some offenders have different rates of reoffense over shorter as compared to longer periods of time (Hanson & Harris, 2001). It is likely that offenders with the fewest social ties are undercounted in determining reoffense rates (Quinsey et al., 1998), despite the fact that they may be more at risk to commit a reoffense (Hanson & Harris, 2001). Due to uneven methods of reporting in the United States, it is impossible to accurately follow the criminal career of an offender who moves between legal jurisdictions. This is less of a problem in countries such as Canada, where crime reporting is more centralized. Not surprisingly, much reoffense research comes from Canada. In all populations studied to date, sexual reoffense rates have been lower than the rates of reoffense for most other crimes. The low base rate is a source of difficulty in making actuarial estimates of the risk of reoffense (Doran & Epperson, 2001; Gruben, 1999; Quinsey et al., 1998; Rice & Harris, 1995).

The literature contains many inconsistencies. For example, one of the earliest and seemingly most robust findings in the literature is that both the frequency of offending and the likelihood of reoffense are highly related to the type of victim chosen by the offender, as well as the relationship between the offender and victim (Fitch, 1962 as cited in Quinsey et al., 1998; Frisbie, 1969; Frisbie & Dondis, 1965; Hanson & Bussiere, 1998; Mohr, Turner, & Jerry, 1964). Father-daughter incest offenders with no other victims are seen as lowest risk, opposite sex, extrafamilial child molesters are seen as intermediate risk, and same sex child molesters are the highest risk. Some research seems to support the tendency for offenders to recommit the same type of offense again rather than to switch to other types (Hanson, 2001; Quinsey et al., 1998). This view is based primarily on studies of sex offenders who have reoffended, and continues to be widely held today.

A different line of research is now emerging based upon offender studies using the polygraph (Colorado Department of Public Safety, 2000), as well as on studies of victims (English, 1998, 2001). This research seems to reveal that a significant amount of crossover occurs where a sex offender deviates from targeting a single type of victim and targets victims in other age, gender, or relationship categories, or exhibits multiple types of offending behavior (Ahlmeyer et al., 2000; Colorado Department of Public Safety, 2000). The fundamental separation between those who target children and those who target adults is being brought into question. It may be that sex offenders do not fit neatly into any typological scheme at all. Individual experience appears to be highly variable (English, 2001; Peugh & Belenko, 2001), and less predictable than was previously thought. Substance abuse may play a mediating role in sexual offending. It is not at all clear how alcohol and drugs impact sexual violence (Peugh & Belenko, 2001).

We do not have comprehensive theories concerning sexual offenses or sexual offenders. This may explain the broad-based approach that is often taken in assessing sex offenders (Wood et al., 2000). Schwartz (1997) presented a summary of prominent theories regarding sex offenders. She noted that despite 90 years of work in the field, there remains a hot debate as to whether or not sex offenders suffer from some form of mental illness. She cataloged 21 theoretical approaches to understanding sexual violence ranging from single dimensions such as the biological to several integrative approaches. She pointed out that while each discipline tends to view the problem through its own lens, nevertheless, the emerging trend is moving towards integrative approaches and acknowledges that each discipline holds a piece of the puzzle (Schwartz, 1997).

Integrative Approaches to Understanding Sex Offending

One of the early integrative approaches mentioned by Schwartz is that of Murphy, Coleman, Haynes, and Stalgartis's (1979) Integrative Theory of Rape. The model divides men into four groups with numerous gradations between the groups. The first group includes highly psychopathic individuals who demonstrate hostility toward women as well as a variety of emotional conflicts. The second group is similar in all dimensions, but less psychopathic. The third features little psychopathy and limited antisocial tendencies, while the fourth consists of men who are neither sexually assaultive nor coercive (Schwartz, 1997). This theory combines several dynamics and seems to have the advantage of explaining why some men are not rapists. It suffers from a relatively narrow focus that does not account for much of what is known about sexual violence.

David Finkelhor (1984) developed a four-factor theory of child sexual abuse that accounts for the individual psychology of the offender, as well as victim characteristics and environmental influences. Finkelhor's model has been influential in understanding child maltreatment in general, not just child sexual abuse (Schwartz, 1997). While it integrates knowledge in several fields, it is limited in that it does not account for sexual violence against adults.

Marshall and Barbaree (1990) have presented an Integrated Theory of Sexual Deviancy that includes hormonal influences, the effects of poor parenting, sociocultural attitudes and limited environmental influences. The authors emphasize that all of these factors must be taken into account in treatment planning (Schwartz, 1997). Somewhat resembling Finkelhor's (1984) model, Marshall and Barbaree's approach is not limited to child sexual abuse.

Prentky and Burgess (1993) have developed a model that integrates caretaker instability during development, developmental history of abuse, and biological factors. The result is an individual with multiple problems experiencing empathy and expressing anger, and who demonstrates deviant sexual arousal and repetitive or compulsive assaultive behavior (Schwartz, 1997). An advantage of this model is that each offender is treated as an individual with unique needs.

Schwartz and Masters (1993) combined psychodynamic, trauma-based theories of sexual addiction together with cognitive-behavioral models to develop a theory of sexual deviance and therapeutic response. The use of relapse prevention techniques originating in the addictions field flows naturally from this model. The model allows for a blending of various therapeutic approaches (Schwartz, 1997).

Testing Procedures

A variety of psychometric measures have been employed in researching sex offenders (Hanson, Cox, & Woszcyna, 1991). Most frequently, investigators have attempted to discriminate sex offenders from others with personality measures or with measures of general psychopathology. Unfortunately, these attempts have achieved only limited success (Quinsey et al., 1998). Measures of psychological instability are largely irrelevant to the risk of future reoffense (Bonta, 2002). Few studies of predictive validity have been attempted with offender populations (Bonta, 2002). Empathy has figured prominently in psychometric research of sex offenders. Recent research has shown that the issues surrounding models of empathy, as well as the measures used to evaluate empathy among sex offenders, are in need of clarification (Marshall, Hamilton, & Fernandez, 2001; McKibben, Proulx, & Lusier, 2001). At the present time, there seems to be no individual test or recognized battery of psychological tests that successfully discriminates between sex offenders and others (Bonta, 2002; Wood et al., 2000). Despite this, a standardized battery of psychometric tests is routinely employed in England and to a lesser extent in Ireland (Beech, Fisher, Beckett, & Scott-Fordham, 1998; Quakenbush, 2000a, 2000b) to assess sexual offenders, while in Canada and the United States, the psychometric batteries used are less standardized (Gutheil & Stein, 2000).

Accepted professional standards for the assessment of violence risk have not yet been established (Slovic, Monahan, & McGregor, 2000) despite the recognition of the importance of assessment in sex offender management (Association for the Treatment of Sexual Abusers [ATSA], 1999). A detailed model for the forensic assessment of sex offender risk has been proposed by Otto (2001), but it still reflects a broad-based, atheoretical approach. Clinicians often rely on uninformed, intuitive beliefs regarding factors associated with recidivism, with the result that predictive accuracy is lessened (Wood, Grosman, Kulkarni, & Fichtner, 1999). There is extensive documentation in the literature that unaided clinical judgement is the least accurate method to estimate the risk of reoffense or to arrive at a diagnosis (Quinsey et al., 1998; Rice & Harris, 1997), often being no better than chance (Gardner, Lidz, Mulvey, & Shaw, 1996).

Psychological testing has found wide acceptance in the assessment of sex offenders. Nevertheless, there is no agreement in the field as to what should be included in a battery of tests (Pithers, 1999). Psychological tests provide empirically quantified information which allows a more precise measurement of offender characteristics than can be obtained from an interview alone (Meyer et al., 2001). The sophisticated integration of information derived from a battery of psychological tests hopefully optimizes the knowledge gained in an assessment (Grove, Zald, Lebow, Snits, & Nelson, 2000; Meyer et al., 2001).

Most psychological tests used in the assessment of sex offenders reflect personality characteristics. Some, such as the Minnesota Multiphasic Personality Inventory-2 (Hathaway & McKinley, 1989) and the Millon Clinical Multiaxial Inventory-III (Dyer & McCann, 2000; Retzlaff, 2000; Rogers, Salekin, & Sewell, 2000a, 2000b; Wiener, 2000) are widely used in forensic assessment in general. Major personality tests, such as the MMPI-2, MCMI-III, Neo Personality Inventory, and 16-PF, incorporate well-developed, empirically derived theories of personality. Despite their widespread usage, the particular personality traits measured are somewhat controversial when applied to this population (Marshall et al., 2001).

Despite the lack of agreement about the particular psychometric tests that would be most appropriate for the assessment of sexual offenders, the tests themselves are firmly rooted in the rich theoretical tradition of personality theory. Elaborate statistical procedures are routinely employed to ensure that a psychological test is both reliable and valid, consistently and accurately measuring what it purports to measure. Generalization of the test to other populations is a serious issue and depends upon the similarity of the other populations to the developmental sample, as well as the situation in which the test is employed (Groth-Marnat, 1990). Relatively few psychological tests have been developed and validated specifically for the assessment of sexual offenders. The few that have been developed and validated for sexual offender populations such as the Multiphasic Sex Inventory II (Nichols & Molinder, 2000) and the Abel Screening (Abel, 1995) compare subjects to a sample of known sexual offenders for various characteristics believed to be significant in offense etiology. They do not represent a comprehensive theory of sexual offending.

The assessment literature, when it does deal with offenders, focuses almost exclusively on measuring factors related to risk of reoffense with only modest focus on factors which might be used to reduce the risk of future offenses (Borum & Otto, 2000). Psychometric tests in general are not sensitive to recidivism by sex offenders (Firestone et al., 1999). Nevertheless, two broad areas associated with the risk of sexual reoffense have emerged from the literature: (a) deviant sexual interest as shown by history and often validated by use of the polygraph or the penile pelthysmograph, and (b) psychopathy (Hanson & Harris, 1998; Seto & Lalumiere, 2001; Witt, DelRusso, Oppenheim, & Ferguson, 1996).

The Role of Psychopathy

Psychopathy is a clinical construct defined by a constellation of interpersonal, affective, and lifestyle traits (Hare, 1999). It is viewed as a serious personality disorder that manifests early in life and persists throughout the life span (Brown & Forth, 1997). Psychopathy is similar to, but not the same as, antisocial personality disorder (American Psychiatric Association, 2000). There is already a well developed and rapidly evolving body of theory concerning psychopathy. Although several instruments exist to evaluate it, the accepted standard is the Psychopathy Checklist-Revised (PCL-R) (Hare, 1991; Witt et al., 1996). Violence and future criminal behavior appears to be predicted by the PCL-R as well as or better than other existing measures (Rice, 1997; Rogers, Salekin, & Sewell, 1996). The PCL-R is widely used in Europe and North America (R. Hare, personal communication, March 3, 2002). Sexual recidivism is strongly predicted by the combination of phallometric evidence of deviant sexual arousal and a high PCL-R score (Hare, 1999).

Psychopathy appears to this author to be the single most important personality construct in understanding sexual violence. Criminal behavior may be related to different factors in psychopaths and non-psychopaths. The mixture of the two in studies of sexual recidivism may mask relationships that are important in only one subgroup. For example, both age and a history of alcohol abuse are strongly related to recidivism among non-psychopathic sexual offenders, but not among psychopaths (Harris, Rice, & Quinsey, 1994). At the same time, both psychopaths and non-psychopaths are quite similar in terms of prior sexual offending and age at onset of sexual offending (Brown & Forth, 1997). Psychopaths may not be so much specialized sexual offenders as they are more general, highly versatile offenders (Hare, 1999).

The etiology of psychopathy is complex and is beginning to be explored (Lalumiere & Quinsey, 1996; Rice, 2001). Harris, Rice, and Lalumiere (2001) have begun to explore the independent contributions of three constructs associated with male criminal violence: (a) neuro-developmental insults, (b) antisocial parenting, and (c) psychopathy using structural equation modeling. They have developed a complex, two-path model for criminal violence that shows promise for understanding general criminal behavior and not just sexual offending. The model helps explain why violence by psychopaths is predicted differently than violence by non-psychopaths. It also accounts for the disparate role played by alcohol abuse in psychopaths and non-psychopaths, as well as the age-related decline in violence in non-psychopaths but not in psychopaths. In short, it accounts for inconsistencies. They also posit an adaptive role for psychopathy, pointing out that psychopaths engage more in goal-directed violence than non-psychopaths, and seem to target victims for sexual offenses who are at an age to reproduce. This model provides a start toward a comprehensive theoretical model of sexual violence. It also has some elements in common with the theoretical implications of actuarial risk assessment.

The Role of Actuarial Risk Assessment

One of the most important areas in the assessment of sex offenders is actuarial risk assessment. It involves assigning statistical weights to previously identified risk factors and then using an algorithm to compute an estimate of the likelihood of an event occurring. The technique is widely used in business, particularly insurance. When applied to the risk of sexual reoffense, it may be used by any one of a variety of professionals and does not require any particular training or expertise other than learning how to use the scoring rules and algorithm. It results in an estimate of what category of risk an offender may fit into. Actuarial risk assessment does not provide a probabilistic prediction of someone reoffending, although there exists a common misconception that it does. The actuarial risk estimate always includes the possibility of not reoffending as well as the risk of reoffense (Rice & Harris, 1997).

Actuarial risk assessment has a number of advantages that have earned it a prominent place in sex offender assessment. It is relatively easy to use, not requiring the cooperation or even the presence of the person whose risk is being assessed. The instruments are scored from archival information. The scoring rules are written so as to minimize the use of personal judgement in scoring the answers to questions (Pithers, 1999; Quackenbush, 2000b). The most important advantage of actuarial risk assessment is that at present, it is the most accurate means available to estimate the likelihood of an offender committing a sexual reoffense (Bonta, 2002; Gardner et al., 1996; Harris, Rice, & Quinsey, 1993; Rice & Harris, 1997). Clinical assessments of the risk of sexual recidivism yielded an r of .10 while actuarial assessments produced an r of .46 (Hanson & Bussiere, 1998). While it is not yet fully accepted without challenge in every United States legal jurisdiction, actuarial risk assessment has been mandated by the European Parliament for sex offender assessment in all 15 European Union member countries.

Multivariate statistical techniques are employed to determine the factors that seem to predict sexual violence (Harris et al., 1993; Quinsey et al., 1998). The predictor factors chosen are predictors of convenience (Doran & Epperson, 2001; Quinsey et al., 1998). They have been gleaned from studies of convicted sex offenders whose records are otherwise available for study. No studies have so far been able to examine sex offenders who have not been found out and officially reported. The meta-analysis by Hanson and Bussiere (1996, 1998) provides a comprehensive survey of the research on predictors of sexual offending. Since they were derived from studies of convicted offenders, they do not reflect characteristics that might differentiate sex offenders from the general population. Relatively little research has been done to identify factors which predict a lowered risk of reoffense. It is necessary to combine several factors in order to achieve a satisfactory level of accuracy (Hanson & Harris, 1998). On the other hand, the risk predictors so far identified appear to be culturally invariant. Instruments based upon them have been cross-validated in several countries (Barbaree, Seto, Langdon, & Peacock, 2001; Quackenbush, 2000b; Quinsey et al., 1998).

A convicted sex offender is actually more likely to be convicted of a new non-sexual offense than another sex offense (Quinsey et al., 1998). Sex offenses appear to occur at a lower base rate than other crimes. This leads to a problem in predicting their occurrence. Low base rate behaviors are inherently difficult to predict. Actuarial instruments do not predict the occurrence of a sex offense. Rather, they produce an estimate that includes both the possibility of reoffending and the possibility of not reoffending. Determining that someone is at high risk to reoffend is not the same thing as predicting that they will reoffend. In practice, sex offender assessments rarely, if ever, use actuarial instruments as stand alone devices. The actuarial risk assessment is only one piece, albeit an important piece, of the information in a sex offender assessment. Actuarial risk assessments are properly used to inform decisions, not to make the decisions themselves. There is a lively debate within the field as to how much one can or ought to attempt to adjust the risk estimate due to non-actuarial factors (Gruben, 1999; Steadman et al., 2000).

In the United States, the STATIC-99 (Hanson & Thornton, 1999), MnSOST-R (Epperson, Kaul, & Huot, 1997), and the RRASOR (Hanson, 1997) are probably the most commonly utilized actuarials. Steadman et al. (2000) have pointed out that while they are clearly superior to unstructured violence risk assessments, many clinicians have yet to accept their use. This may be due to two interrelated problems. First, virtually all the existing risk assessment tools are derived from main effects linear regression models that imply that a single solution fits all subjects. Second, while they represent a significant statistical improvement over unaided clinical judgement, the magnitude of the improvement is not always understood as clinically significant to the others in predictive capability. Potential research on proximal antecedents of reoffending, including noncompliance with supervision, substance abuse, access to potential victims, and acute psychiatric symptoms, would likely improve predictive accuracy (Barbaree et al., 2001; Gruben, 1999).

Unfortunately, most of the psychological and criminological literature does not differentiate between static and dynamic predictors of recidivism risk. It can be difficult to detect dynamic predictors. They can be subdivided into stable factors that can be expected to persist for months or even years, such as personality disorders or substance abuse, and acute predictors that may last from minutes to days, such as intoxication or acute anger (Hanson & Harris, 2001). Much of the difficulty researchers face in studying predictors of sexual recidivism is inherent in the methodology used to study them. An inherent weakness of statistics is that as the number of variables being studied increases, so does the difficulty in identifying significant relationships between them. Another weakness lies in the inability of statistics to deal with events that rarely occur and are treated by the methodology as noise to be disregarded or screened out (Mandelbrodt, 1983). In other words, it is difficult to deal with complex behavior using a statistical methodology. Complex behaviors can be modeled more easily using nonlinear methods, among others.

While there is a justifiably strong interest in the assessment of sex offenders who initially present to the judicial or mental health systems, it is also vitally important to reassess those offenders who have received a period of treatment intended to reduce their risk of reoffense. Just as with the initial assessment, reassessment can be approached with psychometric tests and, to a limited extent, with actuarial risk assessment. One can administer a battery of psychological tests before treatment and compare the results to those obtained when the same battery is administered following a period of treatment. To the extent that the traits measured are believed to relate to reduction in the risk of reoffense, one can gauge progress in treatment. At present, there is not a consensus as to what tests to use and what traits to measure.

One can also attempt to determine if there has been any change in actuarially determined risk. Since most actuarial risk assessment instruments rely upon static predictors, the same instruments cannot be used to reassess risk following treatment. Hanson and Harris (2001) have developed the Sex Offender Need Assessment Rating (SONAR) to attempt to provide an actuarial measure that can be used to modify the actuarial estimates made initially using other instruments. The SONAR utilizes a combination of stable and acute dynamic variables to allow the adjustment of long-term actuarial predictions provided by other instruments. The SONAR represents an ongoing research project that holds promise for refining sex offender assessment and reassessment.

The Theory Behind Sex Offender Assessment

Psychological assessment of sex offenders may seem to be nearly free of theory. We rely upon a multimethod assessment battery in an attempt to efficiently maximize the validity of our assessments of sex offenders (Meyer et al., 1994). The clinician takes test scores and combines them with history, other records provided, information obtained from interviewing the offender, the results of physiological measures, and the estimate of risk from one or more actuarial instruments, and attempts to answer the referral question(s) and communicate the results. The process is heavily influenced by the theories embodied in the tests used as well as by the theoretical model of sexual violence in the mind of the examiner. Lacking a comprehensive theory of sexual violence, we must rely on idiosyncratic combinations of data to develop what hopefully, and sometimes is, a meaningful portrait of the subject, his proclivities, weaknesses, strengths, and potential for future reoffense.

It is a daunting task to identify the meaningful elements that should be the building blocks of a theory of sexual violence. The biological, social, and psychological systems involved are highly complex. It is not uncommon for contradictory or inconsistent results to emerge in the research. Almost without exception, all efforts to date have relied on linear, statistical reasoning. For researchers who are not specifically trained to work with the dynamics inherent in complex systems, the contradictory findings may seem "unscientific." The law of parsimony is not absolute, but when should an investigator disregard it? There is an increasing awareness in psychology that bottom-up (reductionist) and top-down (holistic) approaches to theory building cannot be researched independently because they are intimately linked to one another (Ochsner & Lieberman, 2001). At the same time, practice is moved by theory (Morawski, 2001). Psychology is closely akin to the physical and biological sciences in some ways, but it also has much in common with the humanities (Smith, 2001). The various methods employed in psychological assessment are relatively independent of each other. As a result of this independence, investigators should be able to harness the unique qualities of each method to develop an understanding of the complex phenomena involved in sexual violence. The resulting understanding hopefully will have higher validity than would otherwise be possible (Meyer et al., 1994).

When evaluators attempt to utilize psychological tests to evaluate a sex offender, the hope is that the various measures of concepts like depression will be close enough to each other to provide a meaningful metric. Despite many personality tests being cross validated for construct validity, it is common that two different personality tests will reveal differing results for the same subject measured on the same occasion. At the same time, whatever personality trait is being measured is modified in its effect on the subject by a host of other variables. There are a wide variety of theories that the evaluator could potentially draw upon to explain the interaction of personality traits for a given subject. Some of these have received little or no empirical verification. There are very few theoretical guideposts that the evaluator can use as a guide when making a personality assessment of a sex offender (Dolan, Millington, & Park, 2002). For some offenders depression plays a prominent role in their sexual violence, but for others, it does not. The variety of micro-theories involved with the psychometric assessment of sex offenders is tentative, inconsistent and difficult to apply. There is a need for much more research to identify what personality traits are important to understanding sexual violence. The need is just as great to identify how these traits operate together under different circumstances to produce sexual violence.

Personality theory is rich and varied. Despite over one hundred years of theory building and research, there is no single, generally accepted theory of personality in psychology. Psychopathy represents a promising theoretical development at a higher level of integration. By combining elements of interpersonal, affective, and lifestyle traits to produce a model of behavior that encompasses the entire life span, Cleckly (1976), Hare (1991), and others have produced a theory that shows genuine promise in understanding criminal behavior in general and sexual violence in particular. The theory of psychopathy has been incorporated into more holistic models to achieve more comprehensive theories of both criminal violence generally, and sexual violence in particular (Harris et al., 2001). It is a promising line of research that should lead to new insights.

Actuarial risk estimation is based more on a mathematical technique than on a theory of human behavior. Predictors of risk are identified by examining studies that identify traits or dynamics that have been shown to have some correlation with reoffense. To date, no one has developed an actuarial instrument that can differentiate between sex offenders and the general population. The putative predictors may have been chosen originally for investigation based upon some theoretical model, but inclusion in an actuarial instrument is based solely upon correlation with sexual reoffense. Actuarial risk assessment may appear to be free of theory. However, since most actuarial tools are based on a main effects regression approach (a linear process), they may not adequately reflect the contingent nature of the assessment process (Steadman et al., 2000).

The assessment of sex offenders may not seem to rely heavily on any theory, but that is not the case. Assessment is heavily dependent on statistics. All psychological tests and every actuarial instrument have been developed using the theoretical models embodied by statistics. Psychology is not alone. All of the social sciences have adopted statistics as their lingua franca. In so doing, they have adopted a theoretical lens that allows only a linear view of reality. Mathematically, a function is linear if its value, for any set of values assigned to it, is simply a weighted sum of those values (Holland, 1995). It is possible in the abstract world of mathematics for something to be purely linear or nonlinear. The real world is different. In reality, linearity is always an idealization. In reality, nonlinearity dominates (Johnson, 1995). An essential feature of any nonlinear system is that many different states can exist under the same operating conditions. The one obtained in a given set of circumstances depends on the history of its creation. The result is that it is often impossible to control an experiment and to interpret the outcome (Hall, 1991). It also follows that there must be inexactness in psychological assessment.

Lacking comprehensive theories of sexual violence, assessment of sexual offenders has become highly reductionist. Researchers in the social sciences, like most of their hard science cousins, have been trained to think linearly rather than comprehensively. This deep cultural undercurrent structures life and guides professional careers in subtle but highly consistent ways that are not consciously formulated (Hall, 1981; Kuhn as cited in Gleick, 1987). Unpredictability in sex offender behavior stems not only from randomness, but also from deterministic, nonlinear components that are at work within all the complex systems involved. It is now understood that unpredictable data, once thought to be random, may instead be the result of deterministic uncertainty, or chaos in the mathematical sense (Meyer et al., 1994). For modern science, the main goal is prediction. This means that only those aspects of a system are deemed to be relevant that make it suitable for manipulation or control (Kellert, 1993). There is no logical reason why several theories may not offer alternative, but equally valid and important accounts of a particular aspect of nature (Bohm & Peat, 1987). Psychologists cannot always predict what a person will do. Sometimes the outcome cannot be known until the behavior happens (Bodin, 1981).

The scientific worldview was built up over centuries by explaining complicated puzzles in terms of internal simplicities. Looking one level down may be humanity's greatest construction. It reduces complicated questions to internal simplicities, and it has given us enormous power to understand and manipulate our world (Cohen & Stewart, 1994). Peitgan, Hartmut, and Dietmar (1992) caution us that the magnificent successes of the natural sciences have fed the illusion that the development of natural systems could be ever more accurately predicted. They remind us that it is exactly those persons at the active core of modern science who proclaim that the ability to see ever more accurately into future developments is unattainable. Stricter determinism and apparently accidental development are not mutually exclusive. Their coexistence is more the rule than the exception in nature (Peitgan, Hartmut, & Dietmar, 1992). We may never be able to predict sexual violence with great precision. The present author would suggest, however, that if future research begins to incorporate nonlinear models along with the linear, statistical ones now employed, then a more complete and useful understanding of sexual violence could emerge.

What the Future Might Hold

In mathematically linear systems, small changes produce small effects, and large effects are due to large changes or to a sum of many small changes. In nonlinear systems, by contrast, small changes may have dramatic effects because they might be amplified by self-reinforcing feedback (Capra, 1996). A small change in one variable, at the right place and time, can produce a large effect elsewhere in the system. Alternatively, a large change in one variable could produce no impact on another variable (Lorenz, 1993). The practical impossibility of predicting long-term behavior in detail for the contingent systems of psychology is overwhelming (Bak, 1996; Lorenz, 1993).

There is growing evidence of nonlinear dynamics in the fields of psychology and psychiatry. If forecasting methods utilizing dynamic properties were to be combined with statistical hypothesis testing, it would be difficult for mainstream psychology to ignore (Tschacher & Scheier, 1997). This may seem a novel idea, but the earliest documented mathematical model of human behavior is the Verlust model of population growth, a nonlinear model that dates from 1837. It models the behavior of populations limited by finite resources (Abraham, 1994; Briggs & Peat, 1989; Schroeder, 1991). Today, the Verlust equation is widely used in such scientific disciplines as biology, ecology, demographics, sociology, and to a limited degree, psychology. There are many other examples of such models. In 1998, a nonlinear model of incest was developed that allows simulations to test the effects of changes in the dynamic variables on the likelihood of occurrence of sexual abuse in a family (Quackenbush, 1998).

Gendreau, Goggin, and Smith (2002) caution that the number of predictor variables typically employed in reaching conclusions about criminal behavior are miniscule compared to the standards of other human performance literature, which relies on up to a thousand predictors. What is urgently needed is a holistic approach that would combine the bits of data and micro-theories that characterize sex offender assessment today into a comprehensive theory of sexual violence. In this author's opinion, we do not have all of the data yet to allow such a grand model of human behavior to be constructed. However, two current lines of research show promise in this direction. Both are mathematically linear, but they are comprehensive enough to allow a nonlinear theory to be developed based upon them.

The first is the SONAR project of Karl Hanson and Andrew Harris (2001). Hanson and Harris (2001) examined how well the dynamic risk factors identified in an earlier study could be organized into a structured risk assessment. Their work combined social cognitive theory with the results of earlier research into proximal dynamics of recidivism. The dynamics identified were divided into five stable factors: (a) intimacy deficits, (b) negative social influences, (c) attitudes tolerant of sexual offending, (d) sexual self-regulation, and (e) general self-regulation; and four acute factors: (a) substance abuse, (b) negative mood, (c) anger, and (d) victim access. A structured risk assessment instrument, the Sex Offender Need Assessment Rating (SONAR) was constructed.

Hanson and Harris (2001) note that while all SONAR items were intended to be dynamic, the possibility exists that they serve as proxy variables for enduring propensities. They also caution that short-term recidivism risk factors may not be the same as long-term risk factors. This could result in their study being better at determining the timing of reoffending than for determining which offenders will recidivate over long follow-up periods. The authors are continuing with their line of research and are gathering data to determine the predictive validity of the SONAR. If Hanson and Harris' linear model were to be developed concurrently as a nonlinear model, it would be possible to conduct computerized simulations utilizing all the possible combinations of dynamic variables. This would allow important additional information to be gained that could be used to modify the original model and improve its predictive power.

Human behavior is frequently inconsistent and paradoxical. A linear model can estimate the overall likelihood of reoffense, but it is less able to describe how reoffense occurs. A nonlinear model can produce a portrait of how reoffense occurs. In doing so, it can provide indications of when and how the variables involved interact with each other at differing strengths to produce or not produce reoffense. It can gracefully accommodate inconsistencies. It can also point out unanticipated behaviors that would become outliers in statistical data, but can represent actual routes to relapse in real life. It can even determine with great precision the limits of accuracy possible for the model.

If a nonlinear model were used to inform Hanson and Harris' SONAR research, other significant risk or protective factors not anticipated by the authors might be identified. The particular circumstances in which relapse was most likely to occur or not could also be stated. The resulting risk assessment instrument would be potentially much more useful. This combination of models would also serve to provide a basis for the development of a more comprehensive theoretical model of relapse than is presently available.

The second line of research comes from the work of Harris, Rice, and Lalumiere (2001) regarding psychopathy and criminal violence. The authors complain that there are so many factors shown to be empirically related to violence that it seems to be impossible to interpret them in a theoretically sensible fashion. This problem is inherent in linear models with their inability to deal with large numbers of variables. They focused their research on three classes of variables: neurodevelopmental insults, antisocial parenting, and psychopathy. Using linear, statistical methodology, the authors developed a two-path model of the origins of criminal violence. One path involves pathological damage from neurodevelopmental insult, while the other involves a nonpathological evolved life strategy. The model explains why violence by psychopaths is predicted differently from that of nonpsychopaths. It also accounts for a number of inconsistent findings.

The model utilizes a number of bidirectional relationships between variables. Without deviating from linear mathematics, the authors have come very close to a nonlinear model. In fact, a two-path model strongly suggests bifurcation of the system. Bifurcation is the most thoroughly researched route to unpredictability in deterministic systems (Kellert, 1993). A mathematician should have little difficulty in transforming Harris, Rice, and Lalumiere's (2001) linear model into a nonlinear one. The resulting model would have the potential to reveal relationships and outcomes that are unforeseen in the present line of research. The theory of sexual violence could either become even more complex than what the authors complained of, or a new unifying principle could be revealed. Either way, we would move closer to a comprehensive theoretical model of sexual violence.

It is exciting to think about what could be done with other integrative theories of sexual violence such as that of Finkelhor (1984), Murphy and associates (1979), Marshall and Barbaree (1990), Prentky and Burgess (1993), and Schwartz and Masters (1993), if the theories were restated in the mathematical terms of a nonlinear model. There is no upper limit to the number of dynamic variables that can be gracefully handled at one time in a nonlinear model. At the present time, much of the knowledge of sexual violence appears incomplete, paradoxical and inconsistent. While they offer an explanation of highly complex, multiplely determined behaviors, nonlinear models are themselves often relatively simple. Quackenbush's (1998) model of incest describes the phenomena in terms of only four dynamic systems that include the complexities of all the other dynamics which impact on this form of sexual violence (although it does take 286 pages to describe and explain). Other models could account for a broader range of sexual violence. If such a model seems farfetched, one need look no further than widely used models of the atmosphere, which regularly employ several million dynamic variables at a time (Lorenz, 1993).

Will sex offender assessment remain dependant upon micro-theories and idiosyncratically organized bits of data, or will the field move toward a comprehensive theory of sexual violence? Very few social scientists are trained to use nonlinear methodologies, but many mathematicians and biological scientists are. If a few psychologists were to join forces with nonlinear dyanamicists, a new theoretical understanding of sexual violence might be the outcome.

REFERENCES

Abel, G. (1995). *Abel assessment for sexual interest.* Atlanta, GA: Abel Screening, Inc.

Abraham, R. (1994). *Chaos, gaia, eros.* San Francisco: Harper.

Adkerson, D. (2001, Spring). *Female sexual offenders: Gender specific considerations.* Paper presented to Illinois Association for the Treatment of Sexual Abusers Meeting, Chicago, IL.

Ahlmeyer, S., Heil, P., McKee, B., & English, K. (2000). The impact of polygraphy on admissions of victims and offenses in adult sexual offenders. *Sexual Abuse: A Journal of Research and Treatment, 12*(2), 123-138.

American Psychiatric Association. (2000). *Diagnostic and statistical manual* (4th ed. rev.). Washington, DC: Author.

Association for the Treatment of Sexual Abusers. (1999). *Risk assessment.* Beaverton, OR: Author.

Bak, P. (1996). *How nature works: The science of self-organized criticality.* New York: Copernicus.

Barbaree, H. E., Seto, M. C, Langdon, C. M., & Peacock, E. J. (2001). Evaluating the predictive accuracy of six risk assessment instruments for adult sex offenders. *Criminal Justice and Behavior, 28*(4), 490-521.

Beech, A., Fisher, D., Beckett, R., & Scott-Fordham, A. (1998). *Research findings no. 79: An evaluation of the prison sex offender treatment programme.* London: Home Office Research, Development, and Statistics Directorate.

Bodin, A. M. (1981). The interactional view: Family therapy approaches of the mental research institute. In D. A. Gurman, & D. Kniskern (Eds.), *Handbook of family therapy, Volume I* (pp. 267-309). New York: Brunner/Mazel.

Bohm, D., & Peat, D. (1987). *Science, order and creativity.* New York: Bantam.

Bonta, J. (2002). Offender risk assessment: Guidelines for selection and use. *Criminal Justice and Behavior, 29,* 4, 355-379.

Borum, R., & Otto, R. (2000). Advances in forensic assessment and treatment: An overview and introduction to the special issue. *Law and Human Behavior, 24*(1), 1-7.

Bradford, M. W. (2001). The neurobiology, neuropharmacology, and pharmacological treatment of the paraphilias and compulsive sexual behaviour. *Canadian Journal of Psychiatry, 46,* 26-34.

Briggs, J., & Peat, F. D. (1989). *The turbulent mirror.* New York: Harper & Row.

Brown, S., & Forth, A. D. (1997). Psychopathy and sexual assault: Static risk factors, emotional precursors, and rapist subtypes. *Journal of Consulting and Clinical Psychology, 65*(5), 848-857.

Butz, M. R., & McCowen, W. (1997). *Strange attractors: Chaos, complexity and the art of family therapy.* New York: John Wiley & Sons, Inc.

Capra, F. (1996). *The web of life.* New York: Anchor Books.

Casti, J. L. (1994). *Complexification.* New York: Harper Collins.

Cleckley, H. (1976). *The mask of sanity* (5th ed.). St. Louis, MO: Mosby.

Cohen, J., & Stewart, I. (1994). *The collapse of chaos.* New York: Penguin.

Colorado Department of Public Safety. (2000). Combo of polygraph & treatment reveals many sex offenders offend across multiple relationship, age gender, & crime type categories. *Elements of Change, 5*(1), 1-8.

Dolan, M., Millington, J., & Park, I. (2002). Personality and neuropsychological function in violent, sexual and arson offenders. *Medicine Science and Law, 42*(1), 34-43.

Doran, M., & Epperson, D. L. (2001). Great analysis, but problematic assumptions: A critique of Janus and Meehl (1997). *Sexual Abuse: A Journal of Research and Treatment, 13*(1), 45-52.

Dyer, F., & McCann, J. T. (2000). The millon clinical inventories, research critical of their forensic application, and daubert criteria. *Law and Human Behavior, 24*(4), 487-497.

Dyson, F. (1995). The scientist as rebel. In J. Cornwell (Ed.), *Nature's imagination* (pp. 1-11). New York: Oxford University Press.

English, K. (1998). The containment approach: An aggressive strategy for the community management of adult sex offenders. *Psychology, Public Policy, and Law, 4*(1/2), 218-235.

English, K. (2001, Spring). *A different look at who reoffends.* Paper presented to Illinois Association for the Treatment of Sexual Abusers Meeting, Chicago, IL.

Epperson, D. L., Kaul, J. D., & Huot, S. J. (1997). *Minnesota sex offender screening tool-revised (mnsost-r): Development, performance, and recommended risk level cut scores.* St. Paul, MN: Minnesota Department of Corrections.

Finkelhor, D. (1984). *Child sexual abuse: New theory and research.* New York: The Free Press.

Finkelhor, D. (1986). *A sourcebook on child sexual abuse.* Beverly Hills, CA: Beverly Hills Sage Publications.

Firestone, P., Bradford, J. M., McCoy, M., Greenberg, D. M., Larose, M. R., & Curry, S. (1999). Prediction of recidivism in incest offenders. *Journal of Interpersonal Violence, 14*(5), 511-531.

Forrester, J. (1990). *Principles of systems.* Portland, OR: Productivity Press.

Frisbie, L. V. (1969). *Another look at sex offenders in California* (California Mental Health Research Monograph, No. 12). Sacramento: State of California Department of Mental Hygiene.

Frisbie, L. V., & Dondis, E. H. (1965). *Recidivism among treated sex offenders* (California Mental Health Research Monograph, No. 5). Sacramento: State of California Department of Mental Health.

Gardner, W., Lidz, C. W., Mulvey, E. P., & Shaw, E. C. (1996). Clinical versus actuarial predictions of violence in patients with mental illnesses. *Journal of Consulting and Clinical Psychology, 64*(3), 602-609.

Gendreau, P., Goggin, C., & Smith, P. (2002). Is the PCL-R really the "unparalleled" measure of offender risk? *Criminal Justice and Behavior, 29*(4), 380-396.

Gleick, J. (1987). *Chaos: The making of a new science.* New York: Grossett/Putnam.

Groth-Marnat, G. (1990). *Handbook of psychological assessment* (2nd ed.). New York: John Wiley, & Sons.

Grove, W., Zald, D. H., Lebow, B. S., Snits, B. E., & Nelson, C. (2000). Clinical versus mechanical prediction: A meta-analysis. *Psychological Assessment, 12*(1), 19-30.

Gruben, D. (1999). Actuarial and clinical assessment of risk in sex offenders. *Journal of Interpersonal Violence, 14*(3), 331-343.

Gutheil, T., & Stein, M. D. (2000). Daubert-based gatekeeping and psychiatric/psychological testimony in court: Review and proposal. *Journal of Psychiatry and Law, 28*, 235-252.

Hall, E. (1981). *Beyond culture.* New York: Anchor.

Hall, N. (1991). *Exploring chaos.* New York: W.W. Norton & Co.

Hanson, R. K. (1997). *The development of a brief actuarial risk scale for sexual offense recidivism.* Ottawa, Canada: Department of the Solicitor General of Canada.

Hanson, R. K. (2001). *Age and sexual recidivism: A comparison of rapists and child molesters.* Ottawa, Canada: Department of the Solicitor General of Canada.

Hanson, R. K., & Bussiere, M. T. (1996). *Predictors of sexual offender recidivism: A meta-analysis.* Ottawa, Canada: Ministry of the Solicitor General of Canada.

Hanson, R. K., & Bussiere, M. T. (1998). Predicting relapse: A meta-analysis of sexual offender recidivism studies. *Journal of Consulting and Clinical Psychology, 66*(2), 348-362.

Hanson, R., Cox, B. J., & Woszcyna, C. (1991). *Sexuality, personality and attitude: Questionnaires for sexual offenders: A review.* Ottawa, Canada: Corrections Branch, Ministry of the Solicitor General of Canada.

Hanson, R., & Harris, A. (1998). *Dynamic predictors of recidivism.* Ottawa, Canada: Public Works and Government Services Canada.

Hanson, R., & Harris, A. J. R. (2001). A structured approach to evaluating change among sex offenders. *Sexual Abuse: A Journal of Research and Treatment, 13*(2), 105-122.

Hanson, R., & Thornton, D. (1999). *Static-99: Improving actuarial risk assessment for sex offenders.* Ottawa, Canada: Solicitor General of Canada.

Hare, R. (1991). *The hare psychopathy checklist-revised.* Toronto, ON: Multi-Health Systems, Inc.

Hare, R. (1999). Psychopathy as a risk factor for violence. *Psychiatric Quarterly, 70*(3), 181-197.

Harris, G., Rice, M. E., & Lalumiere, M. (2001). Criminal violence: The roles of psychopathy, neurodevelopmental insults, and antisocial parenting. *Criminal Justice and Behavior, 28*(4), 402-426.

Harris, G., Rice, M. E., & Quinsey, V. L. (1993). Violent recidivism of mentally disordered offenders. *Criminal Justice and Behavior, 20*(4), 315-335.

Harris, G., Rice, M. E., & Quinsey, V. L. (1994). Psychopathy as a taxon: Evidence that psychopaths are a discrete class. *Journal of Consulting and Clinical Psychology, 62*(2), 387-397.

Hathaway, S., & McKinley, J. C. (1989). *MMPI-2: Manual for administration and scoring.* Minneapolis, MN: University of Minnesota Press.

Holland, J. (1995). *Hidden order.* Reading, MA: Addison-Wesley Publishing Co.

Johnson, G. (1995). *Fire in the mind.* New York: Knopf.

Kellert, S. (1993). *In the wake of chaos.* Chicago: University of Chicago Press.

Kelso, J. (1995). *Dynamic patterns.* Cambridge, MA: MIT Press.

Koch, S. (1959-1963). *Psychology: A study of a science* (Vols. 1-6). New York: McGraw-Hill.

Lalumiere, M., & Quinsey, V. L. (1996). Sexual deviance, antisociality, mating effort, and the use of sexually coercive behaviors. *Personal and Individual Differences, 21*(1), 33-48.

Lewis, C., & Stanley, C. R. (2000). Women accused of sexual offenses. *Behavioral Sciences and the Law, 18*, 73-81.

Lorenz, E. (1993). *The essence of chaos.* Seattle, WA: University of Washington Press.

Mandelbrodt, B. (1983). *The fractal geometry of nature.* New York: W.H. Freeman & Co.

Marshall, W., Hamilton, K., & Fernandez, Y. (2001). Empathy deficits and cognitive distortions in child molesters. *Sexual Abuse: A Journal of Research and Treatment, 13*(2), 105-122.

Marshall, W. L., & Barbaree, H. E. (1990). An integrated theory of the etiology of sexual offending. In W. L. Marshall, D. R. Laws, & H. E. Barbaree (Eds.), *Handbook of sexual assault: Issues, theories, and the treatment of the offender* (pp. 257-275). New York: Julian Press.

McKibben, A., Proulx, J., & Lusier, P. (2001). Sexual aggressors' perceptions of effectiveness of strategies to cope with negative emotions and deviant sexual fantasies. *Sexual Abuse: A Journal of Research and Treatment, 13*(4), 257-274.

Meyer, G., Finn, S. E., Eyde, L. D., Kay, G. G., Moreland, K. L., Dies, R. R. et al. (1994). *Proceedings of the 3rd annual chaos network conference.* Urbana, IL: People Technologies.

Midgley, M. (1995). Reductive megalomania. In J. Cornwell (Ed.), *Nature's imagination* (pp. 133-147). New York: Oxford University Press.

Mohr, J. W., Turner, R. E., & Jerry, M. B. (1964). *Pedophilia and exhibitionism.* Toronto, Canada: University of Toronto Press.

Morawski, J. (2001). Gifts bestowed, gifts withheld: Assessing psychological theory with a kochian attitude. *American Psychologist, 56*(5), 433-440.

Murphy, W. D., Coleman, E. M., Haynes, M. R., & Stalgartis, S. (1979). *Etiological theories of coercive sexual behavior and their relationship to prevention.* Unpublished manuscript.

Nichols, H., & Molinder, I. (2000). *Multiphasic sex inventory.* Tacoma, WA: Nichols and Molinder Assessments.

Ochsner, K., & Lieberman, M. D. (2001). The emergence of social cognitive neuroscience. *American Psychologist, 56*(9), 717-734.

Otto, R. (2001, April). *Sex offender risk assessment.* Presentation to the American Academy of Forensic Psychology, St. Louis, MO.

Peitgan, H., Harmut, J., & Dietmar, S. (1992). *Chaos and fractals: New frontiers of science.* New York: Springer-Verlag.

Penrose, R. (1995). Must mathematical physics be reductionist? In J. Cornwell (Ed.), *Nature's imagination* (pp. 12-27). New York: Oxford University Press.

Peugh, J., & Belenko, S. (2001). Examining the substance abuse patterns and treatment needs of incarcerated sex offenders. *Sexual Abuse: A Journal of Research and Treatment, 13*(3), 179-196.

Pithers, W. (1999). Definition, enhancement, and relevance to the treatment of sexual abusers. *Journal of Interpersonal Violence, 14*(3), 257-284.

Prentky, R. A., & Burgess, A. W. (1993). Hypothetical biological substrates of a fantasy-based drive mechanism for repetitive sexual aggression. In A. W. Burgess (Ed.), *Rape and sexual assault III* (pp. 235-256). New York: Garland.

Quackenbush, R. (1998). *A nonlinear dynamical model of the family dynamics of incest.* [diss], San Franciso: California Institute of Integral Studies.

Quackenbush, R. (2000a, September). *Actuarial assessment of sex offenders in Ireland.* Millennium Conference of the National Organization for the Treatment of Abusers. Dublin, Ireland.

Quackenbush, R. (2000b). *The assessment of sex offenders in Ireland and the Irish sex offender risk tool.* Dublin, Ireland: Granada Institute.

Quackenbush, R. (2000c, October). *The chances of doing it again: Actuarial assessment of the risk of sexual reoffense in Ireland.* Presented at the 31st Annual Conference of the Psychological Society of Ireland. Ireland.

Quinsey, V., Harris, G. T., Rice, M. E., & Cormier, C. A. (1998). *Violent offenders: Appraising and managing risk.* Washington, DC: American Psychological Association.

Retzlaff, P. (2000). Comment on the validity of the mcmi-iii. *Law and Human Behavior, 24*(4), 499-450.

Rice, M. (1997). Violent offender research and implications for the criminal justice system. *American Psychologist, 2*(4), 414-423.

Rice, M. (2001, May). *Psychopathy, sex offenders, and treatment.* Paper presented to the National SVP Summit, Chicago, IL.

Rice, M., & Harris, G. T. (1995). Violent recidivism: Assessing predictive validity. *Journal of Consulting and Clinical Psychology, 63*(5), 737-748.

Rice, M., & Harris, G. T. (1997). Cross-validation and extension of the violence risk appraisal guide for child molesters and rapists. *Law and Human Behavior, 21*(2), 231-241.

Rogers, R., Salekin, R. T., & Sewell, K. W. (2000a). The MCMI-II and the Daubert standard: Separating rhetoric from reality. *Law and Human Behavior, 24*(4), 501-505.

Rogers, R., Salekin, R. T., & Sewell, K. W. (2000b). Validation of the Millon Clinical Multiaxial Inventory for axis II disorders: Does it meet the Daubert standard? *Law and Human Behavior, 24*(4), 425-443.

Salekin, R., Rogers, R., & Sewell, K. W. (1996). A review and meta-analysis of the psychopathy checklist and psychopathy checklist-revised: Predictive validity of dangerousness. *Clinical Psychology Science Practice, 3*, 203-215.

Schroeder, M. (1991). *Fractal, chaos, power laws.* New York: W.H. Freeman & Co.

Schwartz, B. (1997). Theories of sex offenders. In B. Schwartz, & H. Cellini (Eds.), *The sex offender: New insights, treatment innovations and legal developments* (pp. 2-32). Kingston, NJ: Civic Research Institute.

Schwartz, M. F., & Masters, W. H. (1993). Integration of trauma-based, cognitive behavioral, systemic and addiction approaches for treatment of hypersexual pair-bonding disorder. In P. J. Carnes (Ed.), *Sexual addiction and compulsivity, Vol. I* (pp. 57-76). New York: Brunner Mazel.

Seto, M., & Lalumiere, M. L. (2001). A brief screening scale to identify pedophilic interests. *Sexual Abuse: A Journal of Research and Treatment, 13*(1), 15-26.

Slife, B., & Williams, R. N. (1997). Toward a theoretical psychology. *American Psychologist, 52*(2), 117-129.

Slovic, P., Monahan, J., & McGregor, D. G. (2000). Violence risk assessment and risk communication: The effects of using actual cases, providing instruction, and employing probability versus frequency formats. *Law and Human Behavior, 24*(3), 271-296.

Smith, M. (2001). Sigmund Koch as critical humanist. *American Psychologist, 56*(5), 441-444.

Steadman, H., Silver, E., Monahan, J., Applebaum, P. S., Robbins, P. C., Mulvey, E. P. et al. (2000). A classification tree approach to the development of actuarial violence risk assessment tools. *Law and Human Behavior, 24*(1), 83-100.

Sulloway, F. (1996). *Born to rebel: Birth order, family dynamics, and creative lives.* New York: Pantheon.

Tschacher, W., & Scheier, C. (1997). Complex psychological systems: Synergetics and chaos. In F. Masterpasqua, & P. Perna (Eds.), *The psychological meaning of chaos: Translating theory into practice* (pp. 273-298). Washington, DC: American Psychological Association.

Wiener, R. (2000). Point and counterpoint: Forensic use of the millon inventories. *Law and Human Behavior, 24*(4), 485.

Witt, P. H., DelRusso, J., Oppenheim, J., & Ferguson, G. (1996). Sex offender risk assessment and the law. *Journal of Psychiatry and Law*, Fall, 343-377.

Wood, R., Grossman, L. S., & Fitchner, C. G. (2000). Psychological assessment, treatment and outcome with sex offenders. *Behavioral Science and the Law, 18*(1), 23-41.

Wood, R., Grossman, L. S., Kulkarni, R., & Fichtner, C. G. (1999). Sexual offenders in custody for control, care and treatment. *Current Opinion in Psychiatry, 12,* 659-663.

ASSESSMENT AND FORENSIC ISSUES

Boundaries and Family Practices: Implications for Assessing Child Abuse

Toni Cavanagh Johnson
Richard I. Hooper

SUMMARY. Family practices related to hygiene, affection behavior, and privacy were studied using a sample of mental health and child welfare professionals. The professionals were asked to use their own experience to state up to what age it was acceptable for parents and children of the same gender and mixed gender to engage in certain family practices. For virtually all family practices, respondents reported lower appropriate ages for mixed gender pairs. Family practices were acceptable for mothers with their daughters up to older ages than fathers with their sons. Results indicate high variability in the responses regarding appropriate ages, as well as whether the behavior was ever acceptable. The implications of these sub-

---

Address correspondence via e-mail to Toni Cavanagh Johnson, PhD, at Toni@TCavJohn.com

[Haworth co-indexing entry note]: "Boundaries and Family Practices: Implications for Assessing Child Abuse." Johnson, Toni Cavanagh, and Richard I. Hooper. Co-published simultaneously in *Journal of Child Sexual Abuse* (The Haworth Maltreatment & Trauma Press, an imprint of The Haworth Press, Inc.) Vol. 12, No. 3/4, 2003, pp. 103-125; and: *Identifying and Treating Sex Offenders: Current Approaches, Research, and Techniques* (ed: Robert Geffner et al.)The Haworth Maltreatment & Trauma Press, an imprint of The Haworth Press, Inc., 2003, pp. 103-125. Single or multiple copies of this article are available for a fee from The Haworth Document Delivery Service [1-800-HAWORTH, 9:00 a.m. - 5:00 p.m. (EST). E-mail address: docdelivery@haworthpress.com].

stantial differences among professionals who often assess these practices as "soft signs" related to abuse are discussed. *[Article copies available for a fee from The Haworth Document Delivery Service: 1-800-HAWORTH. E-mail address: <docdelivery@haworthpress.com> Website: <http://www.HaworthPress.com> © 2003 by The Haworth Press, Inc. All rights reserved.]*

KEYWORDS. Child abuse, age boundaries, clinician responses, family practices, hygiene, affection, privacy, appropriate touch, sex abuse assessment

BOUNDARY CONCERNS

"Boundaries" is a term that can refer to the often unspoken conventions that people follow regarding interpersonal behaviors. There are emotional, physical, sexual, role, and other boundaries that are set, sometimes unconsciously, between people. Many factors such as age, culture, religion and upbringing can influence boundaries. Obvious boundary violations occur when a child's genitals are penetrated or fondled. Yet, there are more subtle, personal boundary violations that may be a part of or a prelude to sexual abuse, or intrusive behaviors that are not illegal but inappropriate and confusing to children.

Child welfare workers and mental health providers are frequently presented with children who engage in worrisome sexual behaviors, either touching their own bodies excessively or touching other children, adolescents, or adults in a way that is considered beyond what is natural and healthy. Often the first issue that is addressed is whether the child has been touched on his or her private parts in an abusive manner. When the child does not acknowledge having been sexually abused, the worker is frequently at a loss as to how to proceed.

An area of research more recently explored is the intersection between certain family practices and increased sexual behaviors in children. Friedrich, Fisher, Broughton, Houston, and Shafran (1998) indicate that some family practices are related to an increased variety of sexual behaviors in children. A factor they label "family sexuality" which they describe as a more relaxed approach to co-sleeping, co-bathing, family nudity, opportunities to see adult movies, and to witness sexual intercourse accounts for 5.7% of the variance when looking at sexual behaviors in children. Friedrich and colleagues do not say that more relaxed family practices necessarily increase disturbed sexual behaviors, only the number and types of sexual behaviors in which children engage. Because these family practices can increase sexual behaviors and confusion about boundaries and sexuality, Friedrich et al. created a Safety Checklist (Friedrich, 2002). The Safety Checklist asks parents about many issues related to boundaries including questions on co-sleeping, co-bathing, and family nudity in the home.

Gil and Johnson (1993) found that when children are experiencing difficulty with their sexual behaviors, information on the family practices related to co-sleeping, co-bathing, nudity, kissing, and privacy are valuable to explore. In some cases the child is being exposed to an increase in adult behavior, talk, sexual innuendo, and sexual behaviors, and boundaries in the home need to be tightened (Gil & Johnson, 1993).

Johnson (1999) describes extensive boundary violations that may occur in the homes of young children who engage in problematic sexual behaviors. Behaviors include those that decrease an individual's emotional and physical privacy, increase intrusive interpersonal practices, and sexualize the atmosphere in the home. The boundary confusion in children's homes may be as potent as direct hands-on sexual abuse in creating sexual confusion, anxiety and disturbed sexual behaviors in young children. Johnson (1999) describes "sexually-reactive" children whose worrisome sexual behaviors are a product of the confusion and anxiety that can be generated by living in these environments. A series of questionnaires to assess boundaries and family practices in homes has been developed by Johnson (1998a, 1998b).

Academic researchers and clinicians have suggested that crossing certain boundaries may be a subtle form of sexual abuse (Lewis & Janda, 1988; Srouf & Fleeson, 1986). Terms such as "emotional incest" (Bolton, Morris, & MacEachron, 1989) and "sexualized attention" (Haynes- Seman & Krugman, 1989) have been used to describe behaviors that overstep the boundaries of acceptable family interactions. The abuse of sexuality model (Bolton, Morris, & MacEachron, 1989) provides descriptions of family environments that may be sexually abusive or sexually overwhelming. In the permissive environments described by the authors, a child may be exposed to nudity or adult sexual behaviors without the adult recognizing that these behaviors may be over-stimulating to the child.

Defining Boundaries

In their study entitled *Defining Sexual Boundaries Between Children and Adults: A Potential New Approach to Child Sexual Abuse Prevention*, Disimone-Weiss (2000) surveyed the opinions of professionals including child psychologists, child psychiatrists, and pediatricians regarding when selected behaviors between parents and children related to nudity, co-sleeping, and kissing on the lips become inappropriate. An interaction between child and parent gender was found for all investigated behaviors. The age at which behaviors related to nudity and co-sleeping were said to become inappropriate was younger for different-gender parent and child than for same-gender parent and child. The opposite was found for kissing. Psychologists and psychiatrists were not found to differ significantly in their responses, yet pediatricians generally responded with significantly older age cut-offs.

Dr. Spock (1976), whose advice did not come from a concern about sexual abuse but from a developmental perspective, wrote:

> I don't want to claim that all children are bothered by parental nudity. No study has been made of normal children. But since we know that it's a possibility, I think it's a little wiser for parents to give their children the benefit of the doubt, and as a general rule . . . keep the child out of the bathroom while a parent is bathing. (p. 45)

Due to his belief that it is important to know what is normative sexual socialization to contrast it with possible sexual abuse, Rosenfeld, Seigal, and Bailey (1987) surveyed parents about sexually related home behaviors. An anonymous questionnaire was used to survey parents' affectionate and sexual patterns. Open and closed ended questions were asked concerning bathing practices. The closed ended questions used a five-point rating scale with three responses: never, sometimes, and always. No significant differences were found, and thus data reported by mothers and fathers were aggregated. Mothers were rated as bathing more frequently with their daughters and fathers more frequently with their sons. It was uncommon for mothers to bathe or shower with sons older than 8 years of age or for fathers to bathe or shower with daughters older than 9 years of age. When assessing why parents stopped bathing with their children, 12.3% mentioned a rule the parents made, usually because the child had behaved in a way that, at least to the parent's eye, was sexual. For instance, the mother of a 4-year-old girl remarked that her daughter "bathed once with father (when she was 2 years of age). She wanted to play with his penis and he decided not to bathe with her." The mother of a 6-year-old boy stated that she had felt uncomfortable about bathing with her son in the past six months because of his open curiosity about her body. In a few cases, the parents had not yet decided to stop bathing with their child when the child decided to no longer bathe or shower with the parent. For instance, the mother of a 6-year-old girl said that within the last few months the child decided she did not want to shower with her father anymore.

Harrison-Speake and Willis (1995) studied parents' perceptions of the appropriateness of different kinds of touch including parents kissing children on the lips, sleeping with them, and giving them a bath. Approval of the various practices was lower for older children. Higher approval ratings were obtained for mothers than for fathers for kissing and bathing. African-Americans gave consistently lower approval ratings for ever engaging in the behaviors than Caucasians.

Atteberry-Bennett (1987) attempted to determine the point at which various behaviors were considered by respondents to be abusive and when intervention was warranted. This study used a sample from Virginia of 255 psychotherapists (psychologists, social workers, and counselors), protective service workers employed by the Department of Social Services, legal professionals (lawyers and judges), law enforcement agents (probation and parole officers), and parents. Using a vignette format, the investigators varied the gender of the parent, gender of child, age of child, and the type of behavior. Some behaviors that were studied were (a) parent often hugs child, (b) parent often kisses child on the lips as he/she goes to work in the morning, (c) parent often enters the bathroom without knocking while the child is bathing, (d) parent is often nude in front of child, (e) parent often sleeps in same bed as child, (f) parent often photographs child nude, (g) parent often touches child's genitals, and (h) parent often has sexual intercourse with child (Atteberry-Bennett, 1987, p. 40). Respondents were asked whether outside intervention would be required in response to these behaviors and what sorts of interventions would be most appropriate.

Results indicated that significant numbers of professionals of all types considered intervention required for behaviors such as frequent hugging of a child, kissing a child on the lips (as when leaving for work in the morning), entering the bathroom without knocking while the child is bathing, co-sleeping, and exposure to parental nudity. There were some differences between the opinions of the respondents with psychotherapists consistently rating the vignettes more abusive than all other groups of professionals or parents.

Seventy-five percent of respondents considered intervention required in cases in which a mother "often" appeared nude in front of her 5-year-old son, and 80% thought intervention required in cases in which a father "often" slept in the same bed as his five-year-old daughter. Approximately 47% of respondents favored intervention in cases in which a mother "often" kissed her 10-year-old son on the lips when leaving for work, and 51% where a father "often" entered the bathroom while his five-year-old daughter was bathing. Virtually 100% of respondents believed intervention was required in cases of a parent photographing a small child nude.

Caution Regarding Overreactions to Parent/Child Interactions

While there is literature in the child abuse field warning of excesses and potential problems with little privacy and loose boundaries between family members, there are others who are concerned with pathologizing certain family practices. Okami (1995) voices considerable concern over what he describes as an overreaction to family practices such as co-sleeping, co-bathing, kissing children on the lips, or being nude in front of children. He points out that experiences such as exposure to parental nudity or sexuality may be constructed of very different "meanings" within a family whose values include beliefs in the "naturalness" of nudity and sexuality than within the context of family whose values include endorsement of "conservative" attitudes toward nudity and sexuality. He cites anthropological and ethnographic data showing that child exposure to parental nudity and parent-child co-sleeping is very common cross-culturally.

Research into childhood exposure to parental and other adult nudity has provided neutral or mixed results, or results open to interpretation, but have not indicated that it has dire aftereffects on children (Lewis & Janda, 1988; Okami, Olmstead, Abramson, & Pendleton, 1998; Story, 1979). In a study of college undergraduates that asked about early childhood experiences, a positive outcome for boys who observed their parents nude when they were between the ages of 0-5 was self-reported comfort with physical affection. For girls at this age it was related to an increased frequency of sexual behavior (Lewis & Janda, 1988). Witnessing parental nudity during ages 6-11 for boys and girls was positively related to a tendency to engage in casual sexual relationships (Lewis & Janda, 1988). A more positive "body self-concept" was found in boys 3 to 5 years old who were the sons of social nudists (Story, 1979). Male undergraduate students indicated that sleeping in their parents' bed when younger than 12 was related to increased self-esteem and less guilt and anxiety about sex. For females, it was modestly related to increased comfort with physical contact as well as increased sexuality (Lewis & Janda, 1988).

There are advocates for more closeness between family members. In her book *The Family Bed*, Thevenin (1987) advocates that children and parents sleep together in the same bed. She argues that it is the most natural and practical way to soothe children and increase their feelings of security. She does not give an age for the children to leave the family bed but indicates it could be over 10 years old (Thevenin, 1987).

Placing a Marker in the Sand

In this era of sexual abuse allegations, family practices related to behaviors between parents and children have come under increased scrutiny. In divorce custody cases where there are allegations of sexual abuse, questions frequently arise about the family practices of the parent with his or her child if hands-on sexual abuse is not acknowledged by the child (Faller, 1991b). In some cases one parent accuses the other of inappropriate sleeping, bathing, kissing, hugging, or nudity with the child, suggesting this may be a grooming behavior or abusive in its own right. Should the father be bathing with his 5-year-old daughter? Should the mother be sleeping with her 8-year-old son?

Are there family practices related to physical boundaries in homes in the United States that we can measure? Although there may be a wide range of what is considered acceptable, are there some limits? Is sleeping in bed with a child of the opposite sex acceptable? Up to what age is this acceptable? Is this different for mothers and daughters, mothers and sons, fathers and sons, and fathers and daughters?

While there are certainly differences in family practices in the United States, it is the intent of this research to place a marker in the sand regarding physical boundaries in families. This will provide some gauge of family practices currently considered acceptable in the United States between parents and children in relation to their age for: (a) bathing together, (b) showering together, (c) sleeping in the same bed with a single parent, (d) hugging between parents and their children, (e) kissing on the mouth, (f) changing clothes together (including underwear), (g) giving back rubs, (h) parents' washing their children's bodies, (i) applying medicine to private parts, and (j) cleaning children after they use the toilet.

METHOD

Design and Procedures

This study used data collected from mental health and child welfare professionals attending trainings provided by the first author during

1999 and 2000 on the subject of children with sexual behavior problems. The trainings were held in Missouri, Illinois, Nebraska, Maine, Florida, Georgia, and New York. It is estimated that 70% of the participants returned the questionnaire (based on attendance and survey returns). The questionnaires were handed out prior to the training, and time was allowed for them to be filled out before the training started. A box was provided in which the completed questionnaires could be deposited during the first break. Completing and turning in questionnaires was on a voluntary basis. Anonymity of participants was assured since no names were included on the forms. The only identifying information was type of current work, gender, race, and level of education.

Population and Sample

A nonrandom, purposive sample was used to maximize the number of clinicians and practitioners participating in this project. The sample of 717 participants was taken from trainings held at in Missouri, Illinois, Nebraska, Maine, Florida, Georgia, and New York in 1999 and 2000. Participants ranged in age from 20 to 84, with a mean age of 39 years of age.

Demographics

This sample of seminar participants was predominately female (77%), Caucasian (79%), and middle aged (mean age of 39.2 years, $SD =$ 11.5). Nine percent of the sample was African-American, 7% Hispanic, 4% Asian, and 1% Other. Over 27% were college graduates with a bachelors of science. An additional 69.6% of participants held graduate degrees of either a masters or PhD. Some participants had experienced emotional abuse (29.3%), physical abuse (14.6%), sexual abuse (19%), were emotionally neglected (25.8%), observed violence in their family (26.4%), or had been physically neglected (5.1%) as a child or teenager.

Variables and Instruments

The Family Practices Questionnaire (Johnson, 1998c) versions 5 and 6 were used to measure all variables in this study. Both versions contain demographic information about the practitioners, followed by 13 questions regarding appropriate ages for mothers and fathers to be involved with their sons and daughters in a variety of physical contact, such as taking baths, washing their children's bodies, or cleaning their children after they have used the toilet.

All items common to both versions were included in this study. Additionally, one question, new to version 6, "What ages are suitable for parents and children changing clothes (including underwear) in the same room?," was included in this study. The independent variables in this study were distinguishing characteristics of the participants, while the dependent variables were their responses to appropriate ages for situational physical contact between mothers and fathers and their sons and daughters.

Variables

The variables analyzed in this study were three areas of intimate behaviors: (a) hygiene, (b) affection, and (c) privacy. The Hygiene category included five "suitable age" questions regarding taking baths, showers, washing children in the bath, cleaning after toilet use, and placing medicine on children's private parts. The Affection variable included three "suitable age" questions regarding parents kissing children on the mouth, giving back and neck rubs, and hugs with body contact. The final category, Privacy, included four questions addressing "suitable ages" where parents were naked with children, children seeing their parents on the toilet, parents and children changing clothes, and parents engaged in sex while children are sleeping in the same room.

Statistical Procedures

Descriptive statistics were used to explore the individual independent and dependent variables by parent/child gender combinations. ANOVA and t-tests were used to identify significant gender pair differences of mean appropriate ages regarding physical boundaries.

RESULTS

Hygiene Scores

The five hygiene indicators of this study were questions regarding taking baths, showers, washing children in the bath, cleaning after toilet use, and placing medicine on children's private parts. Table 1 shows participants' responses to suitability for parents and children to be together while engaging in hygiene activities.

The data are reported by ages for mother/son (M/S), mother/daughter (M/D), father/son (F/S) and father/daughter (F/D) in Table 2. ANOVA was used to determine if ages given for mother/son, mother/daughter, father/son, and father/daughter were significantly different, setting alpha to .001. As shown in Table 2, there were significant age differences, at the 0.001 level, in 4 of the 5 family hygiene behaviors. Only suitable ages for parents cleaning their children after using the toilet were not significantly different. Additionally, suitable ages for hygiene behaviors did not vary significantly ($p < .001$) by race or by respondent history of prior abuse or neglect.

T-tests were calculated for the hygiene activities where significant differences between gender pairs were found. Results are found in Table 3. It is noteworthy that all mother/father gender pairs were significantly different, except when considering mother/son and father/son gender pairs for washing children's bodies while giving them a bath.

Affection Scores

The three affection indicators of this study were questions regarding appropriate ages to kiss children on the mouth, give back, neck, or shoulder rubs, and hugs with body contact. Table 4 shows participants' responses as to what ages it is suitable for parents and children to be engaged in intimate physical contact while engaged in affection activities.

The data are reported by ages for mother/son (M/S), mother/daughter (M/D), father/son (F/S) and father/daughter (F/D) in Table 5. Results of ANOVA for suitable ages for affection are also found in Table 5. None of the three behaviors were significantly different when considering the mother/father/son/daughter ages. Furthermore, suitable ages for affection behaviors did not vary significantly ($p < .001$) by race or by respondent history of prior abuse or neglect.

TABLE. 1 Percent Indicated for Suitable Ages for Hygiene Activities

	Taking baths together (%)	Taking showers (%)	Washing children (%)	Cleaning post toilet (%)	Medicine on private parts (%)
No age	23.8	27.0	1.0	1.8	4.2
Some ages	75.9	72.7	98.2	97.2	91.0
All ages	0.3	0.3	0.8	1.0	4.8

TABLE 2. Suitable Ages, in Years, for Hygiene Care of Children

	Taking baths together				Taking showers				Washing children				Cleaning post toilet				Medicine on private parts			
Group Mean	3.3				3.3				4.7				4.0				6.1			
	M/S	M/D	F/S	F/D	M/S	M/D	F/S	F/D	M/S	M/D	F/S	F/D	M/S	M/D	F/S	F/D	M/S	M/D	F/S	F/D
Mean	3.0	3.7	3.7	2.67	3.2	4.3	2.9	2.9	4.7	5.0	4.9	4.3	4.0	4.1	4.1	3.9	6.1	6.6	6.3	5.1
Median	3.0	3.0	3.0	2.0	3.0	4.0	3.0	3.0	5.0	5.0	5.0	4.00	4.0	4.0	4.00	4.00	5.0	6.0	5.0	5.0
Mode	2.0	2.0	2.0	2.0	3.0	3.0	2.0	2.00	5.0	5.0	5.0	4.00	3.0	3.0	3.00	3.00	5.0	5.0	5.0	5.0
Std.Dev.	2.0	2.3	2.3	1.96	2.1	2.3	2.1	2.13	1.8	2.0	1.9	1.86	1.4	1.4	1.47	1.428	3.2	3.5	3.6	3.0
	***F = 12.69				***F = 27.39				***F = 15.26				F = 2.82				***F = 10.94			

M/S = Mother/son
M/D = Mother/daughter
F/S = Father/son
F/D = Father/daughter
*** $p < .001$

113

Privacy Scores

The five privacy indicators of this study were questions regarding ages of children when/if it is appropriate for adults to be naked around their children (yes/no response), children being present while parents are using the toilet, parents and children changing clothes (including underwear) in the same room, parents engaged in prolonged sexual interactions with children asleep in the same room (yes/no response), and sleeping with a single parent. Table 6 shows participants' responses as to what ages it is suitable for parents and children to be together while privacy activities are occurring.

The data are reported by ages for mother/son (M/S), mother/daughter (M/D), father/son (F/S) and father/daughter (F/D) in Table 7. Results of the ANOVAs for Privacy behaviors are found in Table 8. All three privacy behaviors that measured gender of parent/child were found to be significantly different by gender combinations. However, suitable ages for hygiene behaviors did not vary significantly ($p < .001$) by race or by respondent history of prior abuse or neglect. It should be noted that two privacy behaviors were not measured by gender combinations, so are not listed in Table 8. These two questions include: (a) age after which parents should try not to be naked around their children, and (b) age that

TABLE 3. Results of Hygiene T-Tests by Mother/Son-Father/Son and Mother/ Daughter-Father/Daughter Gender Pairs

	Taking baths together		Taking showers		Washing children		Medicine on private parts	
	F/S	F/D	F/S	F/D	F/S	F/D	F/S	F/D
M/S	7.71***		3.25**		1.87 (n.s.)		2.06*	
M/D		51.85***		12.12***		8.72*		9.86***

*** $p < .001$, ** $p < .01$, * $p < .05$

TABLE 4. Percent Indicated for Suitable Ages for Affection Behaviors

	Kissing on mouth (%)	Back & neck rubs (%)	Hugs (%)
No age	19.6	4.4	4.8
Some ages	40.1	23.5	10.7
All ages	40.3	72.1	84.5

it is alright for parents to engage in prolonged sexual interactions with children asleep in the same room.

T-tests were calculated for the privacy behaviors where significant differences between gender pairs were found. Results are found in Table 9. Significant differences were found between all mother/son-father/son and mother/daughter-father/daughter gender pairs.

DISCUSSION

Hygiene Behaviors

Most respondents agree that it is appropriate for parents and caretakers to be involved in hygiene activities such as taking baths and showers together, washing their children in the bathtub, cleaning them after they use the toilet, and putting medicine on their private parts. Overall, re-

TABLE 5. ANOVAs of Suitable Ages for Affection by Gender Combinations

	Kissing on mouth				Back & neck rubs				Hugs			
Group Mean	5.0				8.0				8.6			
	M/S	M/D	F/S	F/D	M/S	M/D	F/S	F/D	M/S	M/D	F/S	F/D
Mean	5.5	4.5	4.9	5.2	7.8	8.4	8.2	7.5	8.1	9.1	9.0	8.1
Median	5.0	5.0	5.0	5.0	8.0	8.0	8.0	8.0	8.0	10.0	9.5	8.0
Mode	5.0	5.0	5.0	3.0	10.0	10.0	10.0	10.0	10.0	10.0	10.0	10.0
Std.Dev.	3.3	3.3	3.2	3.2	3.8	4.0	3.8	3.7	5.0	5.0	4.8	3.9
	F = 1.10, n.s.				F = 1.26, n.s.				F = 0.76, n.s.			

TABLE 6. Percent Indicated for Suitable Ages for Privacy Activities

	Adults naked w/ children	Children see parents using toilet	Changing clothes together	Sexual interactions in same room	Sleeping w/ single parent
No age	10.8% (no)	17.3%	11.0%	79.9% (no)	15.6%
Some ages	89.2 (yes)	73.3	78	20.1 (yes)	78.9
All ages		9.4	11.0		5.5

spondents consistently report lower appropriate hygiene behavior ages for mother/son and father/daughter. This lower age for opposite gender pairs likely stems from social norms and concerns regarding sexual abuse.

While four of the five hygiene behaviors (taking baths and showers, washing children, and putting medicine on private parts) were significantly different by parent/child gender pairs, the differences were small. For example, while the differences in appropriate ages for taking baths together were statistically significant ($p < .001$), the practical age differences were actually quite small. The differences in appropriate ages for taking baths together ranged from 2.67 years (father/daughter) to 3.7 years (father/son), only about a 1-year difference. There was a 1.4 year age range difference for taking showers together (mother/daughter 4.3

TABLE 7. Suitable Ages for Privacy Behaviors

	Adults naked w/ children	Children see parents using toilet				Changing clothes together				Sexual interactions in same room	Sleeping w/ single parent			
Group Mean		4.8				5.6					5.4			
	Age if yes	M/S	M/D	F/S	F/D	M/S	M/D	F/S	F/D	Age if yes	M/S	M/D	F/S	F/D
Mean	4.6	3.7	6.2	6.0	3.4	4.9	6.6	6.5	4.4	2.3	5.2	5.7	5.6	4.9
Median	4.0	3.0	4.0	4.0	3.00	5.0	5.0	5.0	4.00	2.0	5.0	5.0	5.0	5.0
Mode	5.0	3.0	3.0	3.0	2.00	5.0	5.0	5.0	4.00	1.0	5.0	5.0	5.0	5.0
Std.Dev.	2.5	2.0	6.0	5.7	2.1	2.5	5.9	5.2	2.4	1.6	2.8	3.1	3.0	2.8

TABLE 8. ANOVAs of Suitable Ages for Privacy Behaviors by Gender Combinations

	Children see parents using toilet				Changing clothes together				Sleeping w/ single parent			
	M/S	M/D	F/S	F/D	M/S	M/D	F/S	F/D	M/S	M/D	F/S	F/D
Mean	3.7	6.2	6.0	3.4	4.9	6.6	6.5	4.4	5.2	5.7	5.6	4.9
Median	3.0	4.0	4.0	3.00	5.0	5.0	5.0	4.00	5.0	5.0	5.0	5.0
Mode	3.0	3.0	3.0	2.00	5.0	5.0	5.0	4.00	5.0	5.0	5.0	5.0
Std.Dev.	2.0	6.0	5.7	2.1	2.5	5.9	5.2	2.4	2.8	3.1	3.0	2.8
	***F = 46.0				***F = 14.9				***F = 6.8			

*** $p < .001$

TABLE 9. Results of Privacy T-Tests by Mother/Son-Father/Son and Mother/Daughter-Father/Daughter Gender Pairs

	Children see parents using toilet		Changing clothes together		Sleeping w/ single parent	
	F/S	F/D	F/S	F/D	F/S	F/D
M/S	13.38***		7.34***		3.42***	
M/D		16.30***		10.52***		7.08***

*** $t < .001$

to father/daughter 2.9), a 0.7 year age difference for washing children in a bathtub (mother/daughter 5.0 to father/son 4.3), and a 1.5 year age range difference for putting medicine on private parts (mother/daughter 6.6 to father/daughter 5.1). Overall, the reported age differences were between 0.7 and 1.5 years.

While the age differences were not great, the differences were statistically significant by t-tests on the mother/father gender pairs. There appears to be a strong tendency for respondents to find it acceptable for the same gender parent and child to engage in hygiene behaviors together rather than mixed gender parents and children. This held true except when the parent was purposely bathing the child and cleaning the child after the child used the toilet. Then there was no statistical difference regarding mothers or fathers engaging with the other gender child. It is hypothesized that these behaviors are considered child-care responsibilities of parents and thus less prone to sexualization. Also the genitals of the parent are not involved in these cases. Interestingly, the age for parents to apply medicine to the genitals is considerably older, yet still with the acceptable ages younger for mixed gender parents.

Affection Behaviors

As was found for hygiene behaviors, most participants agreed that affection behaviors such as kissing on the mouth, giving back and neck rubs, and hugs were appropriate at some ages or all ages (84.4%-95.6%). Similarly, lower appropriate ages were reported for opposite gender parent/child pairs, except for kissing on the mouth. Disimone-Weiss (2000) also found the ages were higher for kissing for opposite gender parent/child pairs. However, these age differences, when tested using ANOVA, were not found to be significantly different.

Privacy Behaviors

The pattern of lower reported ages for opposite gender parent/child pairs continued for privacy behaviors, as reported in Table 8. The highest reported ages were for same gender parent/child pairs, with the highest ages reported for mother/daughter pairs. The age range for children seeing parents using the toilet was 3.4 years (father/daughter) to 6.2 years (mother/daughter). For changing clothes together the ages ranged from 4.4 years (father/daughter) to 6.6 (mother/daughter). For sleeping with a single parent the ages ranged from 4.9 years (father/daughter) to 5.7 years (mother/daughter). These ages differed by between 0.8 to 2.8 years. This age difference is greater than the age range for hygiene behaviors (0.7-1.5 years). The narrower age range for hygiene may be related to the respondents' discomfort with parents and children being in close physical proximity when both their genitals are exposed as in bathing and showering. Eighty-nine percent of the respondents agreed with adults being naked around children up to 4.6 years, thus the lower ages for bathing and showering appear to be the physical proximity and, perhaps, the amount of time together naked in this close proximity.

Race and Past History of Abuse

It was anticipated that there would be differences in respondents' answers regarding the ages at which family practices related to hygiene, privacy, and affection behaviors would occur based on the race or ethnicity of the respondent. No significant differences were found. It is possible that the high level of education of the respondents may have washed out differences that may occur in other populations. Since the respondents were all mental health and child welfare workers, their training and observation of many families may have influenced their answers.

Secondly, it was of interest that respondents reporting childhood emotional, physical, and sexual abuse or neglect, or witnessing domestic violence did not report significantly different appropriate ages for hygiene, privacy, and affection behaviors when compared to respondents who reported no abuse history. It is possible that any diffusion of boundaries learned from their homes of origin may have been mitigated by their education, training, and their work helping people who have suffered child abuse and neglect.

General Guidelines

Child Protective Services, therapists, pediatricians, school-teachers, day-care providers, and others who work closely with children remain alert to potential "soft signs" in the child's life that may indicate abuse or neglect. When suspicion arises about sexual abuse, the family's child-care practices may come under scrutiny. The data discussed in this article show what a large group of professionals believe about the suitable ages for parents and children to interact in certain standard family situations related to hygiene, affection and privacy.

An important feature of the data gathered in this study is the wide variation between respondents regarding whether certain family practices are ever acceptable, and at what ages they are acceptable. These great differences may account for some of the significant variability in practice when cases are evaluated and decisions regarding possible abuse are made.

For instance, the data in Table 4 show that 40.3% of the sample of mental health and child welfare workers indicated that it is acceptable at all ages for parents and children to kiss on the mouth while 40.1% said it is only acceptable at some ages, and 19.6% said it is not acceptable at any age. For the group who think kissing on the mouth is acceptable, the average acceptable age is 5 years old. That means that 84% of these professionals who said it was appropriate find it acceptable for parents and children to kiss on the mouth up to 8.2 years old. Another 13.6% (the second standard deviation above the mean) believe it is acceptable for parents and children to kiss on the mouth up to 11.4 years of age.

With these data in mind, what could happen when a child protective services (CPS) worker is asked to respond to a school principal's call who says an 8-year-old boy has tried to kiss his teachers and class-mates, both male and female, on the mouth? The CPS worker questions the boy about sexual contact and gets a negative response. The CPS worker suggests that the school counselor see the boy. The school counselor makes no progress and sends the boy to a therapist who determines that this boy's mother and father and all of his relatives kiss him on the mouth. The therapist does not think parents should ever kiss children on the mouth and certainly not kissing eight-year-old boys, and calls CPS. The CPS worker finds parents kissing their children an acceptable practice at any age and cannot see how this concern of the therapist is relevant. It is possible that the issue of the boy kissing the adults and children on the mouth could become obscured by the focus on the professionals' focus on the acceptability of parents kissing their children, which may or may not be relevant to the boy's issues.

This study found similar results as Rosenfeld et al. (1987) and Harrison-Speake and Willis (1995) regarding the ages for family practices. The data indicate that only young ages are considered suitable for showering, bathing, children seeing parents using the toilet, and parents being nude around their children. As there is a significant difference between the ages found suitable for same gender versus mixed gender parents and children for these activities, this may reflect a concern with young children seeing the genitals of the other gender parent. According to Okami and colleagues (1998), this may reflect a rather puritanical tradition in the United States regarding showing our unclothed bodies.

With the data on showering in mind, consider the case of a 4-year-old girl whose mother and father have been separated for a year. The 4-year-old tells her mother that she likes showering with her father and wants to shower with her mother also. The mother who has been suspicious because her daughter has started openly masturbating and being interested in seeing her mother naked calls Child Protective Services (CPS), who interviews the child and father who both acknowledge they shower together. The child responds negatively to questions regarding any form of sexual abuse. The CPS worker says since it is not a secret, there is no contact between the father's penis and the child, the little girl likes it, and it is a fast way to wash the child, there is no problem, although the worker recommends the showering stop. The father does not stop. The mother divorces the father the following year and asks for only monitored visits alleging very intrusive and possibly sexually abusive behavior during the divorce proceeding. The judge, who does not see anything wrong with showering, believes the mother is trying to alienate the affection of the child and is guilty of making repeated false allegations of sexual abuse. The judge admonishes the mother to stop this or removal of the child from her custody will be considered.

The data in this survey indicate that the average age found acceptable for father-daughter showering is 2.9 with a standard deviation of 2.13 years. Hence, 84% of the sample population would accept this practice up to about 5 years of age, and an additional 13.6% would accept father/daughter showering up to approximately 7 years of age. The data also indicate that almost 27% of the professionals sampled felt the practice was never acceptable. If the mother had spoken to a CPS worker when the child was 4, who felt that fathers and daughter showering together was never acceptable, or gone before a judge in the family law matter, who believed fathers showering with daughters was only acceptable up until 3 and was aware that the father had been told to stop the practice, would the outcome of the case be different?

The cases demonstrate that if a limited sampling of a child's or parent's behavior is considered when there is suspicion of abuse, the individual worker's opinion on certain family practices can have a substantial impact on case decision-making. It is hoped that the data in this article can help establish some markers to assist workers when they are confronted with such cases. Being aware of the wide range of opinions will encourage the workers to consult with colleagues and look at a wide range of the family's practices and all other aspects of the case when making decisions. While workers always try to look at the entire case, some workers zero in on certain aspects of a case, such as family practices, and this can color the worker's judgment. The attitudes of the mother, father and children regarding the behaviors and the pre-separation history of the concerning family practices (if there has been a separation or divorce) need also be considered.

Like Disimone-Weiss (2000) this study found that women are always allowed an older age or a longer time in a child's life than men to engage in the family practices studied. We found that the ages found suitable for fathers and daughters to engage in baths, showers or nudity are the youngest ages found suitable for any combination of same or mixed gender parents and children for any behavior. Is this a societal assumption about the role of women as mothers and the primary caretakers of children? Or are these results perhaps based on an assumption these behaviors may be possible precursors to sexual abuse and that women do not sexually abuse children? In a recent study Burton (2000) found that in an anonymous survey of incarcerated adolescent sexual offenders ($N =$ 122), 20% of the sample said that a woman or women had committed sexual offenses against them when they were children (Burton, 1999). In addition several researchers and writers have found mounting evidence regarding adult and adolescent female perpetrators (Faller, 1991a; Higgs, Canavan, & Meyer, 1992; Kaufman, Wallace, Johnson, & Reeder, 1995; Rosencrans, 1997; Travin, Cullen, & Protter, 1989; Worling, 1995) and sexually aggressive female children (Burton, Nesmith, & Badten, 1997; Johnson, 1989).

The limited age range during which fathers are "allowed" to interact in certain family practices with their own children may be supported by concern in the United States about the potential sexual deviance of men if they are given too much access to children, particularly when nude. In this era of focus on sexual abuse, this concern about men may be subtly eroding their comfort with their young children and may be decreasing the amount of physical contact men have with their children. This could have a negative effect on father-child attachments, particularly for father-daughter relationships.

Nudity in and of itself may have little or no effect on young children if it is in the service of changing clothes, bathing, showering or other natural behaviors. Sleeping with children at any age is likely not to have negative effects if the reasons are clear and the physical contact between the persons does not intrude into their sense of privacy and body boundaries. The problems with these behaviors most likely happen when they co-occur with other boundary violations, when the atmosphere is sexualized, and when people are trying to meet their emotional needs through the children (Johnson, 1998b).

When men and women who were sexually abused as children have children of their own, sometimes they are uncertain when to discontinue certain family practices related to hygiene, affection, and privacy, especially if this was part of their own victimization. Perhaps the information included in this article can be helpful to those abuse victims who are unsure. It has been found that in families with children who have sexual behavior problems, a large number of the parents have been abused (Burton et al., 1997; Johnson, 1988, 1989; Johnson & Berry, 1989). This may account for some of the boundary violations which occur in their homes and which appear to contribute to the premature sexualization of the child's behavior (Johnson, 1999).

A Marker in the Sand

The mean age differences between mother/son, mother/daughter, father/son and father/daughter pairs for the family practices were fairly small, although generally significantly different. Thus, it is suggested that the overall group means for all parent/child pairs are the most helpful for Child Protective Services, therapists, counselors, teachers, and others to use when consulting with parents who want to know an age at which to consider discontinuing certain family practices. As noted in Tables 1, 5, and 6, the group means are:

1. Hygiene Behaviors: parents and children bathing and showering together until 3.3 years, 4.7 years for washing children's bodies, 4.0 for parents wiping children after they toilet, and 6.1 years old for applying medicine to their private parts.
2. Affection Behavior: parents kissing children on the mouth until 5 years of age, giving back and neck rubs until 8 years of age, giving hugs until 8.6 years of age.

3. Privacy Behaviors: adults naked with children until 4.6 years old, children seeing parents using toilet until 4.8 years, parents and children changing together including underwear until 5.6 years of age, sexual interactions with a child in the same room until child is 2.3 years old, and children sleeping with a single parent until 5.4 years of age.

Limitation and Asset

A limitation of this study is that the educational level of the respondents is high compared to the general population, and all of the participants are child protective service workers and mental health professionals. Their educational level and professional status may affect their judgment regarding family practices. While educational level is a limitation, it is also a strength in the context of abuse and neglect work, as the participants are all people who work with children and are mandated reporters. Since family practices are frequently used as a "soft sign" of possible abuse, the opinions of these professionals are currently used for decision-making. Rather than professionals basing judgments on their own opinions garnered from their upbringing, these data inform practitioners about the opinions of 717 fellow professionals.

REFERENCES

Atteberry-Bennett, J. (1987). *Child sexual abuse: Definitions and interventions of parents and professionals.* Unpublished doctoral dissertation, University of Virginia.

Bolton, F., Morris, L., & MacEachron, A. (1989). *Males at risk.* Newbury Park, CA: Sage.

Burton, D. (1999). *Victimization by females among adolescent sexual offenders.* Unpublished paper.

Burton, D. (2000). Were adolescent sexual offenders children with sexual behavior problems? *Sexual Abuse: A Journal of Research and Treatment, 12*(1), 37-48.

Burton, D., Nesmith, A., & Badten, L. (1997). Clinician's views of sexually aggressive children: A theoretical exploration. *Child Abuse & Neglect, 21,* 157-170.

Disimone-Weiss, R. (2000). Defining sexual boundaries between children and adults: A potential new approach to child abuse prevention. *Sciences and Engineering,* Allegheny University, 60.

Faller, K. C. (1991a). Polyincestuous families: An exploratory study. *Journal of Interpersonal Violence, 6,* 310-322.

Faller, K. (1991b). Possible explanations for child sexual abuse allegations in divorce. *American Journal of Orthopsychiatry, 61*(1), 86-91.

Friedrich, W. N. (2002). *Psychological assessment of sexually abused children and their families.* Thousand Oaks, CA: Sage Publications.

Friedrich, W., Fisher, J., Broughton, D., Houston, M., & Shafran, C. (1998). Normative sexual behavior in children: A contemporary sample. *Pediatrics, 101*(4), 693-696.

Gil, E., & Johnson, T. C. (Eds.). (1993). *Clinical evaluation. Sexualized children: Assessment and treatment of sexualized children and children who molest.* Rockville, MD: Launch Press.

Harrison-Speake, K., & Willis, F. (1995). Ratings of the appropriateness of touch among family members. *Journal of Nonverbal Behavior, 19*(2), 85-100.

Haynes-Seman, C., &. Krugman, R. (1989). Sexualized attention: Normal interaction or precursor to sexual abuse? *American Journal of Orthopsychiatry, 59,* 238-245.

Higgs, D. C., Canavan, M. M., & Meyer, W. J. (1992). Moving from defense to offense: The development of an adolescent female sex offender. *Journal of Sex Research, 29,* 131-139.

Johnson, T. C. (1988). Child perpetrators–children who molest other children: Preliminary findings. *Child Abuse & Neglect, 12,* 219-229.

Johnson, T. C. (1989). Female child perpetrators: Children who molest other children. *Child Abuse & Neglect, 13,* 571-584.

Johnson, T. C. (1998a). *Sexuality curriculum for children and young adolescents, and their parents.* South Pasadena, CA: Author.

Johnson, T. C. (1998b). *Treatment exercises for abused children and children with sexual behavior problems.* South Pasadena, CA: Author.

Johnson, T. C. (1998c). *The Family Practices Questionnaire versions 5 and 6.* (Available from T. C. Johnson, 1101 Fremont Avenue, Suite 101, South Pasadena, CA 91030).

Johnson, T. C. (1999). *Understanding your child's sexual behavior.* Oakland, CA: New Harbinger Publications.

Johnson, T. C., & Berry, C. (1989). Children who molest other children: A treatment program. *Journal of Interpersonal Violence, 4*(2), 185-203.

Kaufman, K. L., Wallace, A. M., Johnson, C. F., & Reeder, M. L. (1995). Comparing female and male perpetrators' modus operandi. *Journal of Interpersonal Violence, 10,* 322-333.

Lewis, R. J., & Janda, L. H. (1988). The relationship between adult sexual adjustment and childhood experiences regarding exposure to nudity, sleeping in the parental bed, and parental attitudes toward sexuality. *Archives of Sexual Behavior, 17,* 349-362.

Okami, P. (1995). Childhood exposure to parental nudity, parent-child co-sleeping, and "primal scenes": A review of clinical opinion and empirical evidence. *Journal of Sex Research, 32*(1), 51-63.

Okami, P. R., Olmstead, R., Abramson, P., & Pendleton, L. (1998). Early childhood exposure to parental nudity and scenes of parental sexuality ("Primal Scenes"): An 18-year longitudinal study of outcome. *Archives of Sexual Behavior, 27*(4), 361-384.

Rosencrans, B. (1997). *The last secret: Daughters sexually abused by mothers.* Brandon, VT: Safer Society.

Rosenfeld, A. A., Seigal, B., & Bailey, R. (1987). Familial bathing patterns: Implications for cases of alleged molestation and for pediatric practice. *Pediatrics, 79,* 224-229.

Spock, B. (1976). *Baby and child care.* New York: Pocket Books.

Sroufe, A., & Fleeson, J. (1986). *Attachment and the construction of relationships: Relationships and development.* Hillsdale, NJ: Erlbaum.

Story, M. (1979). Factors associated with more positive body self-concepts in preschool children. *Journal of Social Psychology, 108,* 49-56.

Thevenin, T. (1987). *The family bed.* Wayne, NJ: Avery Publishing Group, Inc.

Travin, S., Cullen, K., & Protter, B. (1989). Female sex offenders: Severe victims and victimizers. *Journal of Forensic Sciences, 35,* 140-150.

Worling, J. R. (1995). Sexual abuse histories of adolescent male sex offenders: Differences on the basis of the age and gender of their victims. *Journal of Abnormal Psychology, 104,* 610-613.

Practical Considerations in the Interview and Evaluation of Sexual Offenders

Clark R. Clipson

SUMMARY. The evaluation and assessment of sexual offenders is different than any other type of evaluation, and most clinicians are not properly trained to interview this population. This article addresses the clinical and ethical issues particular to the interview, assessment, and evaluation of these types of offenders. It offers both practical information regarding the interview itself, along with an overview of classification systems, paraphilias, and assessment techniques used with this population. In addition, issues related to risk assessment and risk management are also addressed, and an introduction to the use of actuarial risk assessment instruments is provided. *[Article copies available for a fee from The Haworth Document Delivery Service: 1-800-HAWORTH. E-mail address: <docdelivery@haworthpress.com> Website: <http://www.HaworthPress.com> © 2003 by The Haworth Press, Inc. All rights reserved.]*

KEYWORDS. Sex offender, interview, evaluation, risk assessment

---

Address correspondence to: Clark R. Clipson, PhD, 3921 Goldfinch Street, San Diego, CA 92103.

[Haworth co-indexing entry note]: "Practical Considerations in the Interview and Evaluation of Sexual Offenders." Clipson, Clark, R. Co-published simultaneously in *Journal of Child Sexual Abuse* (The Haworth Maltreatment & Trauma Press, an imprint of The Haworth Press, Inc.) Vol. 12, No. 3/4, 2003, pp. 127-173; and: *Identifying and Treating Sex Offenders: Current Approaches, Research, and Techniques* (ed: Robert Geffner et al.) The Haworth Maltreatment & Trauma Press, an imprint of The Haworth Press, Inc., 2003, pp. 127-173. Single or multiple copies of this article are available for a fee from The Haworth Document Delivery Service [1-800-HAWORTH, 9:00 a.m. - 5:00 p.m. (EST). E-mail address: docdelivery@haworthpress.com].

Digital Object Identifier: 10.1300/J070v12n03_06

The evaluation of sexual offenders offers a challenge unlike that found in either a general clinical practice or even in a forensic setting. All forensic assessments must address the possibility that the person being interviewed may minimize, deny, exaggerate, or feign a psychiatric disorder to obtain a desired outcome. The sexual offender in particular is prone to be dishonest about his behavior for several reasons. Obviously, he may wish to avoid the consequences of his illegal sexual behavior. He may also have learned over the years that it is not permissible to be open about his sexual deviance. On another level, he may not even be willing to admit his sexual interests and behaviors to himself, much less acknowledge them to a professional. Adding yet another layer of complexity to the issue is the vast, often confusing research literature related to sexual offenders.

With the recent advent in several states of the new sexually violent predator laws, there has been an explosion of information regarding the typology, risk assessment, and treatment of sex offenders (Hanson, Morton, & Harris, 2002). In contrast, there has been relatively little information published regarding how to conduct an effective interview with this population, and even less that attempts to bridge the gap between research and practice in a manner that provides concise, meaningful (and practical) information to the clinician who is asked to evaluate someone who has committed a sexual offense. This article is designed to provide clinicians with an overall framework in which to conduct an evaluation that identifies the information necessary for an adequate assessment, even if the sexual offender is denying or minimizing his involvement in a sexual offense.

Obviously, any evaluation with a sexual offender will be most useful if the offender is willing to discuss his sexual interests and admit to the commission of any sexual offenses. Under such circumstances, the assessment will provide information not only relevant to risk assessment, but will also lead to classification of the dynamics of the offense(s), and the most meaningful types of intervention required for treatment. However, an evaluation is also quite useful in cases where the individual has been convicted of a sexual offense, yet continues to deny responsibility for the crime. This is not an uncommon situation. Under such circumstances, the offender will often reveal information about himself and the offense that he did not intend to, as a comprehensive evaluation provides several ways of getting at the desired information–if one approach does not work, either persistence or a different way of asking the same question will. In addition, the interview of a sexual offender requires more time than the typical clinical interview, so that the very length of the evaluation serves to reveal efforts to conceal or deny information.

CONCEPTUAL ISSUES IN THE EVALUATION OF SEXUAL OFFENDERS

Before an effective assessment of sexual offenders can be conducted, the interviewer must have a clear understanding of some of basic issues: sexual deviance, the difference between a sexual offense and sexual deviance, and paraphilias.

Sexual Deviance

People differ sexually in four ways (Berlin, 1999). First, there are the kinds of sexual behaviors they find enjoyable. Second are the kinds of partners they are attracted to. Third, they vary in the intensity of their sexual desire, both temperamentally and situationally (for example, because of stress or a medical condition). Finally, they vary in attitudes regarding their sexual preferences along a continuum from ego-syntonic to ego-dystonic. It is useful to keep these dimensions of human sexuality in mind throughout the discussion of sexual deviance and sex offenses.

It is recognized that distinguishing sexual behavior that is "normal" from that which is deviant can be very difficult. For one thing, deviance is culturally defined, as some sexual practices that would be deviant in American society may be accepted and even encouraged in other cultures. For example, in some South Pacific cultures such as the Kaingang tribe, it is common for children to receive a great deal of sexual stimulation from adults (Mead, 1949). In addition, there is a temporal component to defining deviant behavior within the same culture. Some behaviors that were once considered deviant in our culture are now considered normal, such as masturbation and having premarital intercourse. Homosexuality was once included in the American Psychiatric Association's (1968) *Diagnostic and Statistical Manual of Mental Disorders* as a sexual deviation. Finally, the definition of what behaviors constitute sexual deviance can vary within a given culture at the same time depending on the subculture within which one lives.

So how can sexual deviance be reliably defined? For the purpose of this discussion, there are four components that are relied upon in defining sexual deviance (see Table 1). The first is statistical. That is, does a significant percentage of the population in question (herein defined as

TABLE 1. Defining Sexual Deviance

Sexual deviance can be defined by:

    (1) the prevalence of the sexual interest or behavior;

    (2) the potential effect on the recipient of the sexual interest or behavior;

    (3) the impact of the sexual interest or behavior on a person's adaptive functioning; and

    (4) the persistence or chronicity of a sexual interest or behavior.

modern American society) engage in a given behavior? By this definition, masturbation, premarital sexual behavior, homosexuality, having casual sex, visiting a prostitute, engaging in sexual fantasies, having an extramarital affair, and viewing adult pornography with non-violent themes would be considered normal (Hunt, 1974; Kinsey, Pomeroy, & Martin, 1948; Kinsey, Pomeroy, Martin, & Gebhard, 1953; Mott & Haum, 1988; Zelnik & Kanter, 1980). In addition, by this definition it is normal for an adult heterosexual male to be sexually attracted to post-pubescent adolescent females without necessarily acting on that attraction (Abel, Lawry, Karlstrom, Osborn, & Gillespie, 1994).

The second defining criterion for sexual deviance pertains to the recipient of a given sexual behavior. At the heart of the issue are the questions of consent and potential harm. That is, a sexual behavior may be gratifying for the person engaging in it, but it may cause harm to the person who is on the receiving end of that behavior. Our society believes that another person should freely give consent before they are engaged in a sexual behavior. For example, it is easy to imagine that a woman who is raped or who discovers a "peeping tom" outside her window will be traumatized by this experience, both because she did not give her consent for this behavior to occur, and because she is the victim of an aggressive act. Similarly, although not all children's sexual experiences with adults have been shown to be harmful (Rind, Tromovitch, & Bauserman, 1998), so many children and adolescents are traumatized by their sexual contact with adults that the prohibition against molestation is quite warranted (Haugaard & Reppucci, 1988). In addition, the issue of whether children and adolescents are capable of providing consent for sexual behaviors with adults is also highly debatable, and no doubt varies given the age, cognitive capacity, and experience of the child or adolescent involved.

The third defining criterion for sexual deviance is related to the impact it has upon the person's adaptive functioning. That is, to what extent does the sexual behavior interfere with a person's social and occupational functioning? While masturbation may be "normal" based upon the statistical frequency of its occurrence in our society, it may be considered deviant if it interferes with a person's marriage or ability to work. For example, if a man preferred to masturbate instead of engage in sexual activities with his wife, and this resulted in problems in the marital relationship, then the man's preference for masturbation might be seen as deviant.

The fourth and final criterion for defining a sexual interest or practice as deviant pertains to the persistence or chronicity of that behavior (Kafka, 1993). Several studies (Crepault & Coulture, 1980; Templeman & Stinnett, 1991) have demonstrated that paraphilic fantasies occur in a normal population. However, in non-offenders these fantasies do not preoccupy the person or interfere with the establishment of romantic and sexual relationships with consensual partners. The DSM-IV (American Psychiatric Association [APA], 1994) criteria for paraphilia prescribes that the deviant sexual interest persist for at least six months. Persistence of the deviant behavior helps distinguish those sex offenders with paraphilias from those without.

At the present time, there is no consensus regarding whether all of these factors (prevalence, consent and harm to another, interference in adaptive functioning, and persistence) are necessary for a particular sexual behavior to be defined as deviant. Some researchers believe that mere prevalence would be insufficient to establish a sexual practice as deviant; they would say that as long as no one is being harmed by the practice, it is not deviant. By this definition, many fetishes would not be considered deviant, as there is typically no victim involved and often no interference in the person's ability to function in society. Precisely because of its relative nature, the question of what constitutes deviant sexual behavior may never be fully resolved.

Sexual Offenses

Sexual deviance and sexual offenses are not the same thing. A sexual offense is determined by legal statute; that is, for a sexual act to be considered a sex offense, it must be considered a crime in a given jurisdiction. The person who is convicted of that crime would then be designated as a sex offender (APA, 1998). Some deviant sexual behaviors (fetishes, cross-dressing, etc.) are not crimes, while some common sexual practices that would not be considered deviant are illegal in some states and provinces. A person can be sexually deviant and not have been apprehended for a sexual offense.

In thinking about sex offenses, it is useful to conceptualize the behavior from three different perspectives: (a) the behavior itself, (b) the consequences of that behavior, and (c) the motivation for the behavior. For a sexual act to be a sexual offense, it must be defined statutorily as illegal. Table 2 lists the most common types of sexual offenses.

The behaviors that are classified as sexual offenses vary widely in terms of their severity, from peeping to sexual homicide. Most of these behaviors are held to be reprehensible by most people, especially those that place others at risk of harm. The more likely someone is to be harmed, the more reprehensible the sexual offense. Gaining an understanding of what happened during the sexual offense, both from the perspective of third parties as well as from the offender himself, helps to classify the offender and will often provide significant clues with regards to addressing the issue of motivation.

The consequences of the sexual offense also vary widely, from benign reactions to severe traumatization and in the extreme, death. Outside of its emotional impact, the consequences of the behavior itself are of relatively little concern to the evaluator of the sexual offender. This is actually a benefit to the person conducting the assessment, as for the most part he or she is able to avoid focusing on the victim's reaction during the assessment. On a personal note, I have observed that for myself and most other evaluators of sex offenders, it is our awareness of the consequences to victims of sexual offenses that serves as a powerful motivator for our work with the perpetrators of these offenses. Far from

TABLE 2. Types of Sexual Offenses

Contact Offenses	Non-Contact Offenses
Rape	Exhibitionism
Child molestation	Voyeurism
Public masturbation	Frottage
Prostitution	
Sexual homicide	

being indifferent to the pain of the victims, we work to understand and treat the offender to prevent others from becoming victims. Some critics have raised the question of whether sexual behavior that is designated as a sexual offense is right or wrong. The answer is simple: It is wrong because the act can, and indeed is likely, to cause harm or damage to the victim.

Finally, of central importance to the evaluator is the question of what motivated the sexual offense. Motivation cannot, in many cases, be determined from the behavior itself. Each case must be examined on an individual basis in order to understand the motivation for the crime. The sexual offense is classified by the motivation that underlies it, which in turn leads to an assessment of how likely the offender is to reoffend, and what kinds of treatment or risk management he is likely to require.

Individuals may commit similar sex offenses for different reasons. A sexual assault may represent an abuse of power that may be largely unrelated to sexual stimulation or satisfaction. It may be the result of antisocial opportunism, it may be the result of diminished capacity as in the case of someone who is psychotic, mentally retarded, manic, intoxicated, brain damaged, or developmentally immature, or it may be the expression of a deviant sexual interest. As Berlin et al. (1997) note, sexual offenses committed by those with deviant sexual interests "are the only type of criminal activity enacted in response to a powerful, albeit at times pathological, biological drive. A paraphiliac disorder cannot be punished or legislated away" (p. 1). For the most part, deviant sexual interests are most prevalent among those who victimize strangers, who use force, who select male victims, or who select victims much younger (or much older) than themselves (Barbaree & Marshall, 1988; Freund & Watson, 1991; Quinsey, 1984, 1986). In other words, some sexual offenses are motivated by paraphilias, but many are not.

Paraphilias

A paraphilia (literally "beyond usual love") is defined in the 4th edition of the *Diagnostic and Statistical Manual of Mental Disorders* (APA, 1994) as "recurring, intense sexually arousing fantasies, sexual urges, or behaviors generally involving (1) nonhuman objects, (2) the suffering or humiliation of oneself or one's partner, or (3) children or other nonconsenting persons, that occur over a period of at least 6 months" (pp. 522-523). Some people with paraphilias assert that their disorder causes them no distress and that their only problem is the reaction they receive from society, while others report extreme guilt, shame, and depression at the feeling of being compelled to perform sexual activities that they regard as immoral or socially unacceptable. By this definition, a person can have a paraphilia even if they do not act on their urges but are only disturbed by them. This definition also notes that a person who has the sexual fantasies or urges but is not troubled by them and does not act them out does not have the disorder. Thus, it is recognized that paraphilias occur on a continuum, and that it may be normal for a person to have "sexually deviant" thoughts or persistent mild, non-clinical sexual fantasies and urges (Kendall & Hammen, 1995). Indeed, some studies have found that it is quite common for non-clinical populations of males to have the same types of paraphiliac interests as those who are being treated for having committed sex offenses (Crepault & Coulture, 1980; Templeman & Stinnett, 1991).

It is also recognized that for some people with paraphilias, the deviant fantasies or stimuli are obligatory for sexual arousal, while for others, the paraphiliac preference occurs only episodically, such as during times of stress. At other times the individual may be able to function sexually without the paraphiliac fantasies or other stimuli. Many paraphiliac fantasies and behaviors begin in childhood or early adolescence, becoming better defined and elaborated in the late teens and in early adulthood. Indeed, Abel and Rouleau (1990a) found that the majority of those who commit sexual offenses develop their deviant sexual interest prior to the age of 18. By definition, paraphilias are recurrent and the disorders tend to be chronic and lifelong. Paraphiliac behaviors may increase in response to stress, in relation to other psychiatric disorders, or with increased opportunity (APA, 1994).

There are no reliable estimates of the number of people who have one or more of these disorders, as many of them never come to professional attention unless they are convicted of a sexual offense. Interestingly, paraphilias are almost never diagnosed in females, and approximately half of the people with paraphilias that do come to clinical attention are married (APA, 1994). Kafka (1993) notes that approximately 5% of the patients in clinics that specialize in the treatment of paraphiliac disorders are women, and that most of these women are diagnosed either with sexual masochism or sexual promiscuity. There is some evidence that sex offenders as a group are relatively well educated, and that most of them are employed (Abel, Becker, Cunningham-Rathner, Rouleau, & Murphy, 1987). All socioeconomic levels and ethnic groups are represented in this population. For reasons that are unclear, Catholics and Protestants are overrepresented among those with paraphilias, while there are relatively few Jews and Muslims among this population (Abel et al., 1987).

Paraphilias are distinguished on the basis of the object of the person's attraction. The various paraphilias are listed in Table 3.

It is now widely accepted that if a person has one paraphilia, he is likely to have others that occur either consecutively or contiguously, with some offenders displaying as many as 10 different paraphiliac interests over the course of their lifetime (Abel & Rouleau, 1990a). The average number of paraphilias found in a self-report study of 516 self-referred cases was 2.02 per subject (Abel et al., 1987). It would be incorrect, therefore, to assume that someone who was arrested for rape of an adult female would be unlikely to molest a male child. Those who are exhibitionists, voyeurs, and who engage in frottage commit the most offenses, with many such offenders averaging crimes that number in the hundreds. Abel and his colleagues (1987) found that on average, rapists in their sample admitted committing an average of just over seven rapes during the course of their lifetime. In another survey of more severe sex offenders (Weinrott & Saylor, 1991), the mean number of victims reported by rapists was just over 11. The number of offenses committed by child molesters in the Abel sample varied significantly by victim type, with those favoring male stranger victims committing the most offenses (average of 281 offenses) and those who molested female stranger victims committing far fewer (average of 23 offenses). Among incest perpetrators, those who admitted molesting female victims committed more offenses (average 81 offenses) than did those who admitted molesting male victims (average 62 offenses).

In addition to their primary sexual interests, many men who have paraphilias also demonstrate what Kafka (1993) refers to as paraphilia-related disorders. These include compulsive masturbation, periods of protracted promiscuity, dependence upon pornography, and an over-reliance on anonymous sexual outlets such as prostitutes, attendance at sex shows, and having sex over the telephone or Internet. Often times men with paraphilias or paraphilia-related disorders will prefer or engage in these activities even when a consenting sexual partner is available to them. For example, Carter, Prentky, Knight, and Vanderveer (1987) found that child molesters were more likely than rapists to use pornography prior to and during an offense, and to employ pornography to relieve an impulse to act out.

An extensive discussion of what causes paraphilias is beyond the scope of this article. The short answer is that we do not yet completely understand the basis of these disorders. While environmental factors

TABLE 3. Sixteen Types of Paraphilias

Arousal to odors–requiring exposure to certain smells in order to become sexually aroused

Coercive paraphilia–sexual arousal to the use of coercion or force during sex

Coprophilia–sex involving the use of feces

Ephebephilia–attraction to post-pubescent adolescents

Exhibitionism–exposure of one's genitals to an unsuspecting stranger

Fetishism–the use of non-living objects to induce sexual arousal

Frotteurism–touching and rubbing against a nonconsenting person

Hypoxyphilia–a type of sexual masochism that involves sexual arousal by oxygen deprivation

Klismaphilia–sex involving the use of enemas

Lust murder–an extreme form of sexual sadism in which a person acts out sexually violent fantasies, often with a series of victims

Necrophilia–sex with corpses

Obscene mail–sending obscene mail, either through the postal service or over the Internet

Partialism–exclusive focus on part of the body not typically associated with sexuality, such as a limb

Pedophilia–attraction to pre-pubescent children

Public masturbation–becoming sexually aroused by masturbating in a place in which one is likely to be discovered

Sexual masochism–sexual arousal through being humiliated, beaten, bound, or otherwise made to suffer

Sexual sadism–becoming sexually aroused by acts that cause another person to suffer psychologically or physically

Telephone scatologia–obscene telephone calls

Transvestic fetishism–becoming sexually aroused by cross-dressing

Urophilia–sex involving the use of urine

Voyeurism–becoming sexually aroused by observing an unsuspecting person who is naked, in the process of disrobing, or engaging in sexual activity

Zoophilia (bestiality)–sex with animals

have received the most attention (in particular factors such as victimization and precocious exposure to sexual stimulation), it appears quite likely that there is a biological component to most, if not all, cases. For example, reports of deviant sexual behavior in males have been associated with temporal lobe disorders, whether these lesions are the result of traumatic injury or idiopathic epilepsy (Kafka, 1993). In addition, there are reports of elevated testosterone levels in repetitively violent sex offenders, and the effectiveness of anti-androgen therapy has been well documented (Hall, 1995). Finally, it appears that there is an inverse relationship between serotonin levels and sexual behavior, with reduced serotonin related to an increase in deviant sexual behavior as well as other impulse disorders, mood disorders, and obsessive-compulsive disorder (Kafka, 1993). Langevin (1990) has also identified cerebral dysfunction associated with the left hemisphere in a number of sex offenders who are often noted to display various symptoms of dysphasia.

THE GOALS OF THE EVALUATION

Any clinical interview conducted by a mental health professional has the goal of understanding the individual and developing an intervention plan based upon an integration of that understanding with the current state of our professional knowledge. The evaluation of a sex offender is always performed with these and other goals in mind. Most sexual offender evaluations address the following referral questions:

1. Does the offender have a psychiatric condition that predisposes him to the commission of sexual offenses?
2. What is the likelihood that the offender will commit another sexual offense, and/or under what circumstances is he most likely to do so?
3. What are the offender's treatment needs, and what is the optimal treatment setting in which these needs can be met?
4. What level and intensity of community supervision does this offender require in order to prevent the community from being placed at undue risk?

In addition, the evaluator may be asked to address the individual and situational dynamics involved in a particular case. The identification of these intrapersonal, situational, and victim characteristics can be quite useful in answering some of the other questions above, such as the individual's treatment needs and the level of supervision required.

Classification

The first goal of any clinical evaluation is that of coming to some understanding of the person being interviewed. In the case of a sex offender, a general diagnostic impression should of course be reached. As most sex offenders meet the criteria for some type of personality disorder (APA, 1998), this possibility should always be explored, along with the presence of substance abuse or dependence, which is also quite common in this population. In addition, the presence of a thought or mood disorder or other psychopathology should be evaluated, and an assessment of overall cognitive functioning should also be performed. However, beyond reaching a diagnostic impression using the standard professional nomenclature, evaluators should address this question: "Is the sexual offense a manifestation of a psychiatric condition, and if so, is it a paraphilia or something else?" Using this information along with the type(s) of sexual offenses the perpetrator is known to have committed, the classification process may begin.

Understanding of Intrapersonal Dynamics

Placing someone in a diagnostic category or typing him by sexual offense does not tell us much about the underlying motivation of the particular offender being evaluated. In addition to the general categorization of the individual and his behavior, a more sophisticated clinical understanding of that person and his sexual behavior is also necessary. This understanding can be attempted using theories of personality development, although in my own experience, psychodynamic and cognitive-behavioral theories are most commonly used. This type of understanding, although not as strongly related to risk assessment as the factors involved in classification, is relevant to treatment and risk management.

Understanding of Contextual Factors

The sexual offender does not operate in a vacuum, and although most of the research regarding sex offenders has focused on characteristics of the individual perpetrator, it is also important to consider external factors. The two most important variables to consider besides the sexual offender himself are characteristics of the victim(s) chosen by the offender and situational factors related to the offenses. For example, some offenders tend to select victims that share particular traits or characteristics, while others will select a wide variety of victim types. In addition, some offenders will only act out when under stress or after a significant loss, others while intoxicated, and still others only when the opportunity arises, often while they are committing an unrelated antisocial act. Finally, some offenders have established patterns of finding and establishing contact with potential victims. Being aware of these factors for a given sex offender becomes crucial in developing effective risk management plans.

Risk Assessment

In almost every evaluation of a sex offender, the referral source wants to know how "dangerous" the person is, or how likely they are to commit another sexual offense. Consequently, risk assessment is a central part of any sex offender evaluation. A level of risk is generally provided in terms such as low, moderate, or high. Evaluations can be even more useful if they address the question of under what circumstances an offender is likely to commit a sexual reoffense (Korpi, 1998).

Treatment

After completion of the first four goals in the assessment process, an individualized treatment plan should be developed for the offender. While in most cases the perpetrator will be referred to a program that specializes in the treatment of sex offenders, programs should be somewhat flexible in their implementation to accommodate the individual needs of each participant. In some cases, usually those that involve unremitting psychosis or significant cognitive impairment, referrals to other practitioners may be necessary. The evaluation should note any specific needs that the treatment program should address for a particular offender in addition to the usual offense-specific treatment offered by that program.

Placement and Level of Supervision

The final question that should be addressed by any evaluation of a sexual offender is that of placement. Generally speaking, placement should be determined by the likelihood of reoffense along with a consideration of the resources available to the offender. A general rule of thumb is that offenders at low risk can probably be maintained in the community along with treatment and/or supervision, while those at high risk should be incarcerated while being treated. Those at moderate risk levels to reoffend pose a less clear-cut solution to this question, and careful consideration of dynamic and situational factors is required in order to form an opinion regarding placement.

For those offenders who are placed in the community, the level of supervision that is required to prevent further sexual offenses from occurring must also be addressed. Clinicians and legal agents have a wide variety of options at their disposal, although the resources available for community supervision will vary dramatically from jurisdiction to jurisdiction.

ETHICAL ISSUES IN THE EVALUATION OF SEX OFFENDERS

There are three professional ethical issues that are central to conducting evaluations with sex offenders. These will be briefly discussed here. For a more complete discussion of general professional ethics within a forensic context, the reader is referred to Melton, Petrila, Poythress, and Slobogin (1997).

Competence

Both the *Ethical Principles of Psychologists and Code of Conduct* published by the American Psychological Association (1992) and the *Specialty Guidelines for Forensic Psychologists* written by the Committee on Ethical Guidelines for Forensic Psychologists (1991) emphasize the importance of competence in the conduct of our professional duties. The evaluation of sexual offenders requires more than the basic clinical training normally received in a graduate program. It also requires, at a minimum, familiarity with specialized assessment techniques and current knowledge of the research related to this population. Given the context in which the evaluation is conducted, it may also require familiarity with the legal system and relevant legal statutes as well as the demands of serving as an expert witness. This type of expertise is not easily arrived at.

The number of forensic training programs that might offer such instruction remains limited, while the number of facilities specializing in the treatment of sex offenders is also few. As a result, there are not many formal opportunities to acquire the expertise necessary to conduct competent evaluations of sex offenders. For most professionals, competence must be attained through some combination of reading, on-the-job training, clinical experience, consultation, and attendance of professional workshops.

One last note about competence that is often under-appreciated is that knowledge of one's professional competence includes an awareness of what we cannot do or what we do not know. Referral sources will occasionally request that we answer questions that either (a) cannot be answered given our current state of knowledge, or that (b) we as individual practitioners cannot answer. In either case, it is our professional responsibility to inform our referral source of our limitations, and perhaps assist them to frame their questions in such a manner that our services can be of use to them.

Informed Consent

It is our professional obligation to inform those we evaluate about the purpose of the evaluation, how it will be used, and who is likely to see it. As in any issue involving informed consent, three components are necessary in order for the consent to be valid. First, the person should be considered competent to give consent for the evaluation. This is typically not an issue in the conduct of sexual offender evaluations unless the individual is acutely psychotic or mentally retarded. Secondly, the discussion of such topics as the purpose of the evaluation should be conducted in a language that is readily understood by the offender. Finally, the offender should be told if they have a choice whether to participate in the evaluation, and if so, what the likely consequences are should they decline to participate. Informed consent should be obtained in writing as well as discussed at the outset of the assessment process.

In addition to the common elements of any type of informed consent, sex offenders should also be told who has requested that they be evaluated, the purpose for which the evaluation will be used, and the kinds of information that will be asked of them. Any limitations regarding confidentiality should be clearly explained, particularly the requirement in most states that any previously undisclosed sexual offenses must be reported. Some offenders might also question the competence of the person conducting the evaluation. To the extent that this does not represent a manipulation on the part of the offender, the evaluator should answer appropriate questions.

Confidentiality

An important aspect of informed consent is addressing any limitations of confidentiality that might be involved. One important aspect of this limitation that pertains to almost every sex offender evaluation is that of the professional obligation to report any previously unreported cases of child or elder abuse. While this may of course inhibit the offender from being completely forthcoming about undetected offenses, it will not deter the rare offender who has already decided to be open with the examiner. For most offenders, it is doubtful that stating this "duty to report" will have any significant impact on their disclosures.

Other important aspects of the limitations of confidentiality refer to situations in which the offender presents a risk of danger to himself or someone else. In a legal context, informing the offender about who is likely to read the report is also indicated, as well as whether the evaluator is likely to have to testify in the case.

THE CONTEXT OF THE INTERVIEW

Interview styles vary in accordance with the personalities of the clinician, and there is probably no style that is preferred over another. The obvious exception to this is an interviewer who comes across as judgmental, arrogant, or who conveys that they have already reached a conclusion regarding the outcome of the evaluation. Conveying the impression that the interviewer is aware that people have a variety of sexual interests and engage in a variety of sexual behaviors is useful in combating a sense of judgment. In addition, interviewers who are fearful or hostile towards the offender are not likely to obtain the information they need. An overall style that conveys genuine interest in the offender, curiosity about what happened and why, and an acceptance of the offender as a human being with their own needs and feelings will go a long way towards breaking down resistance. Abel (1997) notes that some mention of the availability and effectiveness of treatment can also be helpful in some cases, as the offender is informed that there is a possible solution to their problems. In addition, maintaining a detached response style in relation to the offender's attempts to either intimidate or manipulate the evaluator may also prove beneficial.

The goal of the interview–understanding the offender and his risks and needs–should always be in the forefront of the interviewer's mind. Any temptation to engage the offender in an admission of guilt or an expression of remorse is likely to be counterproductive to this goal. The interviewer should be direct, and willing to point out any inconsistencies between the offender's own statements or self-report and the information obtained from other sources. How one does this again is more a matter of style: some clinicians prefer a soft-pedaled, "Columbo" approach while others are more forceful and assertive. Doing what works with a given individual means the interviewer is doing the right thing.

Interviews of sexual offenders are likely to require anywhere from one to three hours because of the amount of information that needs to be obtained, and because there is often a great deal of resistance that must be dealt with. The length of time involved serves a useful function in terms of detecting efforts at dissimulation, as it is difficult to maintain deceptive behaviors over longer periods of time. The longer the interview, the more likely offenders will make contradictory statements or commit "slips of the tongue" that convey more information than they intended. Anxiety and fatigue are on the side of the evaluator.

Evaluators differ in their preference regarding the timing of when they discuss sexual offenses and/or the sexual history of the offender. Some prefer to wait until after a more general history taking has occurred, hoping that this will aid in creating an alliance with the offender and thereby decrease resistance. My own preference is usually to initiate a discussion of the individual's sexual offenses just after we have reviewed the ethical and legal concerns of the evaluation. I find that doing this often facilitates the emergence of contradictory information later in the interview, which can be explored towards the end. In addition, it is also towards the end of the interview that I will confront the offender with any discrepancies between his self-report and information obtained from other sources. This approach puts time and fatigue on my side (increasing the possibility that the offender will forget what he said previously), and also increases the likelihood that I can obtain as much information as possible in case the offender responds defensively and/or terminates the interview.

Legal Status of the Offender at the Time of Assessment

For the most part, an effective clinical evaluation of a sexual offender is only possible in light of a true finding. The appropriate role of an evaluator is to provide the referral source with answers to the questions that we are best suited by our training and experience to answer: the diagnosis and dynamics of the offender, his risk to reoffend, and his treatment, placement, and supervision needs. It is not our job to discover or question evidence, become fact-finders, or to assume the role of advocate for either the offender or their victim(s). These are roles for which attorneys and the court are far more qualified.

Mental health professionals are unable to establish whether an individual committed a sexual crime or not, even though many sex offenders may attempt to turn their interview into a forum that seeks to establish their innocence. It is their right to assert their lack of guilt, of course, but as evaluators we must operate in accordance with the "truth" as it has been established in a court of law. It is a frequent occurrence that sex offenders of all types will employ deception in the self-report of their offenses and sexual interests, and we must allow other, more appropriate agencies to determine what really happened. The persuasiveness of some offenders is a significant force with which to reckon, especially when they seek to point out flaws in the legal system or their defense that resulted in their conviction. Some of them become convincing "jailhouse lawyers" in their own right, and if psychopathic, can be charismatic and convincing.

Despite the caveats and precautions discussed above, clinicians are occasionally asked to evaluate an individual who has not yet been convicted of a sexual offense, but who has merely been accused or arrested on such charges. This situation most frequently seems to arise in the context of custody disputes, when one parent (usually the mother) claims that the other parent (usually the father) molested a child, whose story may often change over time. At other times the court may simply want to have more information about an individual that can only be gained through a psychological evaluation. Such evaluations should be undertaken with great care, of course, as no interview, psychological test, or battery of tests can establish whether an individual has committed a sex offense or not (APA, 1998; Boer et al., 1997; Nichols & Molinder, 1984; Sewall & Salekin, 1997).

Nonetheless, an evaluation performed prior to the determination of guilt or innocence can provide several useful functions. First, it can evaluate an individual's general cognitive and personality functioning to determine the presence of a severe mental disorder, mental retardation, or cerebral dysfunction. Second, the evaluation can gather useful information regarding the individual's background, specifically in the areas of sexual development, family history, childhood abuse, anger management, social history, and psychiatric history, so the court can incorporate this information as it sees fit during trial. In the event that the individual is convicted, the court can rely on information gained in the evaluation during the penalty phase of trial in order to ensure that the individual receives appropriate treatment, supervision, and/or placement.

Evaluators may also be asked by the court to perform what is generally referred to as a *Stoll* evaluation, referring to the court case of that name (*People v. Stoll*, 1989). In this case, the California Supreme Court upheld expert testimony that relied upon an interview and the use of standardized personality tests in order to determine if a defendant displayed signs of "deviance" or "abnormality." Also referred to as "profiling," this type of evaluation results in an opinion of how closely an individual may fit or fail to fit one of the sex offender typologies. While there is no standardized way of conducting these types of evaluations, DiFrancesca (1999) suggests that the individual undergo the Abel test and a polygraph evaluation along with a psychological evaluation. While the Abel test may provide some additional validity with regards to understanding an individual's sexual preferences, the polygraph evaluation is a more informal screening tool. That is, the individual's reaction to the request that they undergo a lie detector test is often more telling than their actual performance on the instrument, which may be unreliable and is inadmissible in court (APA, 1998).

How competent mental health professionals are at profiling remains unclear. A review of the literature focusing on the use of the MMPI and phallometric assessment found little empirical data to support clinicians' ability to be of much use in profiling (Murphy & Peters, 1992). However, a more recent study found that reliance on crime scene variables was very useful in predicting rapist type (Knight, Warren, Reboussin, & Soley, 1998). More studies using the Abel test of visual reaction time to assess sexual preference in conjunction with a structured clinical interview and personality tests is needed.

Countertransference Reactions

It is emotionally difficult to read police reports describing crime scenes and victim statements regarding their injuries and emotional reactions to being sexually assaulted. Anyone exposed to this material will likely feel a mixture of revulsion, horror, sympathy, and compassion for the victim, and anger at the offender. Similar feelings may also arise during the interview with the offender. It is very difficult for many mental health professionals to imagine themselves in the presence of a convicted (or even accused) sexual offender and being able to maintain any semblance of impartiality or neutrality. It is impossible to do this if the clinician reacts on a personal level, imagining how they would feel if this offense had happened to themselves or their loved ones.

However, this is exactly what is demanded of clinicians who elect to become involved in the evaluation and treatment of sexual offenders. We must find ways to deal with our personal responses to the offenses and the offenders that we encounter, while at the same time being able to establish an alliance with the individual we are evaluating. If we are to perform our professional duties effectively, we must be able to bring to our interviews the attitude of curiosity and a certain amount of empathy that we would bring to any other evaluation.

In speaking with other evaluators, I have found that we have similar styles in how we approach this issue. Many of us deal with our emotional reactions to the crime reports prior to and after the interviews. We share our feelings with others to decrease the sense of isolation and vicarious traumatization that can occur. Sometimes we vent our feelings through an expression of our outrage or horror, while at other times we joke and use humor as a means of distancing ourselves from the tragedy we are confronted with.

By bracketing our emotional reactions in this way, we are able to come to the interview with the offender on a more professional and intellectual level. This attitude is one of genuine interest in coming to an understanding of the offender, his behaviors, and what motivates him. Familiarity with and reliance on the extensive body of research that has accumulated on sex offenders is of great benefit in this regard. It is also an attitude that expects the offender to be defensive and deceitful because of how others typically react to him and his crimes, without taking these manipulative efforts personally. It is an attitude that keeps in mind that the purpose of our evaluation is to benefit the court or other referral source so that this offender receives appropriate placement, treatment, and/or supervision. Finally, we need to keep in mind that our evaluation should also benefit the offender, even though it is the rare offender who sees things in this way.

In addition to our emotional reactions, mental health professionals also bring individual biases into our work. Such biases could include ethnic prejudices or overgeneralizations about a given population. These beliefs might be expressed in statements such as, "All sex offenders are bad people," "All sex offenders should be castrated and locked away forever," or "All sex offenders have something biologically wrong with them, and they can't help what they do." Any prejudice based on our ignorance or unfamiliarity, or any tendency to engage in vague overgeneralizations should be recognized by the clinician and attempts made to avoid these traps. While we cannot (nor should we) eliminate our feelings and our personal opinions, we should be aware of them and be able to put them aside while performing our professional duties.

The Issue of Deception

It is well established that many sex offenders will attempt to deceive or manipulate mental health professionals who are evaluating them

(Langevin, 1988). The likelihood of this occurring may increase when the offender believes that any admission of sexual deviance may result in negative consequences, such as a civil commitment or placement in an inpatient or residential treatment program.

Nichols and Molinder (1984) identify three types of deception typically employed by sex offenders. The first is that of dishonesty, expressed either as outright lies or as omissions. This can be quite startling, as some perpetrators will maintain their innocence in the face of multiple witness statements or DNA evidence. The second is that of distortion, in which the offender justifies and rationalizes his offense, often blaming others for what happened. Finally, sex offenders engage in the frequent use of denial, minimizing the seriousness of what they did, and deceiving themselves (and others) into believing that they do not really have a problem and that it will never happen again. Confirmation of these defensive styles is found in the work of Langevin (1988) and Kennedy and Grubin (1992).

It is worth mentioning that some alleged sex offenders will admit to having committed an offense or to having a sexually deviant interest when they in fact do not. These offenders will typically report that they made the false admission in order to accept a lesser sentence, in order to avoid putting the victim through the stress of a trial, or to put the situation behind them in an attempt to get on with their lives. Of course, such situations are probably quite rare, but they illustrate how difficult it can be to determine what has really happened when individuals are motivated to appear either better or worse than they really are (Sewell & Salekin, 1997).

Many evaluators rely upon the validity indicators of various self-report instruments, such as the Minnesota Multiphasic Personality Inventory-2 (MMPI-2), the Millon Clinical Multiaxial Inventory-III (MCMI-III), or the Multiphasic Sex Inventory (MSI), to aid in the detection of dissimulation. While most studies with the MMPI and MSI tended to find the expected differences in response patterns to these scales between those who admitted committing a sexual offense and those who did not, Sewell and Salekin (1997) conclude from their review that these self-report measures are too obvious to be reliable in helping to distinguish dissimulators. Similarly, studies with phallometric assessment techniques have also proved to be disappointing (APA, 1998). Although there is limited but substantial evidence that the Abel Screening Test is less amenable to faking, these results remain preliminary as of this writing (Abel et al., 1994), and the cost of purchasing and using this instrument prohibits many practitioners from its routine use.

Mental health professionals are left with having to determine whether a sexual offender is dissimulating through a comparison of interview, psychometric, and third party data. Given the population, the possibility of manipulation and deceit should always be considered, and the likelihood of conflicting information being obtained is quite high. A combination of the techniques of confrontation, clarification, and confirmation of self-report data are the clinician's best aids in addressing this thorny problem.

THE ASSESSMENT FORMAT

In the following sections, an overview of the assessment process will be reviewed, along with comments designed to aid in the evaluation of the sexual offender. This discussion assumes a general knowledge of interview techniques and data gathering on the part of the evaluator.

Review All Existing Available Data

As in all forensic evaluations, the routine utilization of third party information is crucial. Indeed, the absence of this type of data could severely compromise the validity of the evaluation. The evaluator should request from the referring party any of the following documents that may exist: (a) victim statements, (b) police reports, (c) probation or parole officer's reports, (d) correctional department records, (e) child protection services investigations, (f) previous psychological evaluations, (g) educational assessments, (h) prior or current mental health records, (i) prior or current medical records, (j) prior neurological or neuropsychological assessments, and (k) any statements regarding the offense(s) made by the offender to other investigators.

These documents should be listed and acknowledged in the written psychological evaluation of the offender. Evaluations that do not include this collateral information should be interpreted with great caution.

Interview the Offender

The clinical interview is the most important part of the sex offender's evaluation (Marshall, 1996). It is through the interview that the clinician is able to best detect personality traits, interpersonal skills, and defensiveness, in addition to assessing the conscious self-presentation that the offender displays.

It is recommended that the interview be highly structured to ensure that it is comprehensive enough to aid in the detection of dissimulation (Abel, 1997; Lanyon, 2001). It is strongly recommended that until such structured interviews are published, evaluators should create their own structured interview tool for use during the evaluation of a sexual offender.

Structured interviews are designed to assist in identifying the presence of paraphilias, types of sexual dysfunction, the behavioral progression, and cognitive distortions that are known to occur with various types of sex offenders. In this manner, it can aid in placing the offender within one or more classification systems. It can also be used to answer common referral questions such as risk of reoffense, danger to the community, and the type of treatment, placement, or level of supervision required to meet the needs of the offender and provide protection for the public. If the offender has already participated in or completed a treatment program, a structured interview can be useful in evaluating the effectiveness of that treatment.

Any interview, despite its primacy in importance, is intended to be used as part of a broader assessment. Conducting an interview with the sexual offender by itself is insufficient in providing adequate information for a comprehensive evaluation. The inclusion of third party information is essential, as is obtaining additional historical information other than that provided in this assessment tool. The referral question and the context in which the evaluation takes place will indicate the use of additional psychological tests or actuarial risk prediction tools.

It is recommended that during the interview, the evaluator attempt to record the offender's responses as close to verbatim as possible. This helps prevent the introduction of interviewer bias through paraphrasing, while also allowing the offender to express himself in his own words by the use of quotes in the written report. Careful documentation of interview material is essential in forensic settings, and the use of a structured interview aids in this documentation. In addition, the interviewer may choose to record the interview, using either an auditory or audiovisual format, to improve accuracy in the reporting of the offender's self-report, and/or to provide a record of the interview for the courts. Some interviewers may even wish to have the offender complete a structured interview in a written format, and then review their answers with them later.

Questions should be posed in non-clinical, everyday language to facilitate the development of a positive relationship with the offender. The interviewer is encouraged to note the sexual vocabulary used by the offender, and to use similar words if able to do so in a natural manner, even if this is not a term the evaluator would normally use. For example, if the offender uses the term "jack off" in reference to masturbation, the examiner might substitute this term when asking questions about masturbation. If this cannot be done in a natural and comfortable manner, however, the evaluator should use a vocabulary with which he or she is comfortable to avoid sounding phony or contrived.

Leading questions should be avoided during the portion of the interview concerned with the sexual offense so that the offender is not led into saying something they do not mean, and so the evaluator does not provide the offender with an answer to a question out of convenience. For example, the offender should be asked how he was feeling just prior to the offense, rather than being asked if he was angry, depressed, etc. However, during the sexual history portion of the interview, leading questions are asked purposely in order to facilitate disclosure of deviant sexual interests. For example, the offender can be asked when the first time he masturbated might be, as opposed to asking if he has ever masturbated.

The following components should be included in any interview of sexual offenders.

1. *Demographic data.* The usual personal information one collects during an evaluation can be noted here, in addition to other information that is directly related to risk assessment. The information gathered will be dictated by the risk assessment method used by the evaluator.

2. *Details of the sexual assault.* The offense (or offenses) should be examined in great detail. Offenders are most likely to evidence denial, minimization, or cognitive distortions in this portion of the interview. It is important to go through the specifics of what transpired, assisting the offender to tell his story in as much detail as possible. It is useful to think of this section like watching a movie–when the interviewer can clearly visualize and follow the story, he or she is probably obtaining as accurate a picture of the crime as the offender will allow. When facts are omitted or discrepant with one another, or the examiner feels confused, it is useful to "rewind the tape," getting the offender to review the story again, carefully and in more detail. The offender should be

asked how he set up the circumstances in which to commit the offense, his thoughts and feelings before, during and after the offense, any accompanying fantasies, and the actual details of the offense itself as well as what happened afterwards and how and when he was apprehended. Particular attention should be paid to any use of manipulation, coercion, threat or violence.

3. *Victim empathy.* Here the goal is to determine something about the relationship between the offender and his victim, or at least how the offender perceives that relationship. Of particular interest is what the offender believes the victim was experiencing during and perhaps after the offense. This is a likely place for cognitive distortions to abound. It is also an opportunity to learn about how secrecy was attempted, and whether any type of coercion, whether subtle or overt, was used.

4. *Insight.* The offender's thoughts about his offense pattern should be explored in this section, along with questions about how others might react to his crimes. Justifications and rationalizations are likely to be expressed here, as well as evidence of progress in treatment, if relevant.

5. *Relapse prevention.* This section addresses any past or current treatment for sexual offending, seeking to determine the content and type of any such treatment. It should also address whether an offender completed treatment and if not, why. The offender should be invited to relate how he plans to keep from reoffending in the future, and whether he has undergone treatment or not. He might also be asked to discuss how he plans to meet his future sexual needs.

6. *Victimization.* The offender's own history of physical, sexual and emotional abuse should be explored, along with whether he was exposed to domestic violence.

7. *Family history.* This should include the composition of the offender's family of origin while growing up, parents' marital status, education, and occupations, religious upbringing, changes, losses, separations, and stresses that affected the family, and the offender's relationship to his parents.

8. *Developmental history.* Here the interview should address any information available regarding the offender's mother during her pregnancy, labor and delivery, as well as the presence of any

developmental delays, emotional problems, or behavioral problems while growing up. Of particular interest might be the presence of delinquent behaviors, such as fighting, arson, stealing, lying, etc.

9. *Academic and occupational history.* In this section, the interview should explore the offender's educational history, particularly the presence of any learning disabilities or special abilities. Relevant occupational history includes military service, specific job skills, types of jobs held, lengths of employment, reasons for termination, periods of unemployment, financial responsibility, and any illegal means of self-support.

10. *Social, relationship, and marital history.* Here the interview should explore the offender's early temperament, childhood and adolescent peer relationships, dating and marital history, current friendships, and social skills. If applicable, the evaluator should ask about the offender's relationship with his own children, reasons for divorce, and the quality of his relationship with a current partner.

11. *Sexual history.* This section should explore the many facets of the offender's sexual development, behaviors, fantasies, and preferences. It should include childhood sexual experiences, parental messages, numbers and types of sexual partners, and the offender's comfort level with his own sexuality. It should also address sexual practices with the offender's most recent sexual partner in some detail, and also address areas of sexual dysfunction. Following the advice of Abel (1997), interviewers are encouraged to ask directly about each of the paraphilias. Whenever the offender indicates that he has engaged in fantasies or behaviors related to a particular deviant sexual interest, the evaluator is encouraged to inquire about the age of onset, frequency of these occurrences, situations in which they might occur, and the degree of comfort the offender feels with these impulses.

12. *Legal history.* This should include both sexual and non-sexual offenses. Each offense should be explored in some detail with the offender, as some offenses may involve violent or sexual impulses that are not readily apparent from the charges or convictions listed.

13. *Medical history.* Here the evaluator should explore the offender's history of significant illness, surgery and injury, particularly any head injuries. The family medical history should also be explored, along with any physical limitations the offender might have. Cur-

rent medical concerns and medications should also be documented.

14. *Substance abuse history.* This portion of the history should include detailed exploration of the offender's history of alcohol and drug abuse, including both illegal and prescription medications. The age of first use, pattern and effects of use, and (if applicable), when the offender last used a particular substance and why he stopped, all merit inquiry. Any history of drug or alcohol treatment should also be documented here.

15. *Psychiatric history.* In this section, the evaluator should address the offender's history of psychiatric symptoms and treatment, including both outpatient and inpatient settings, prescribed medications, and the offender's response to treatment.

16. *Mental status examination.* In this final portion of the interview, the offender's current psychological functioning should be examined. In addition to performing a formal mental status examination, the evaluator should address any current problems or symptoms, things the offender would like to change about himself, current interests and goals, and the offender's perception of any factors that might interfere with the achievement of his goals.

Psychological Testing

The decision whether to use psychological tests or how much psychological testing to include in the evaluation of the sex offender will depend on (a) the training and experience of the evaluator and (b) the purpose of the evaluation. Obviously, one must be competent to administer, score, and interpret psychological tests in general, as well as being competent to use some of the measures specifically utilized with this population. In addition, the purpose and goals of the evaluation will dictate the type of testing used. Generally speaking, if the primary goal of the assessment is risk assessment, the use of actuarial risk assessment tools such as the PCL-R, Static-99, and SORAG are all that is needed. However, if the primary goal of the evaluation is to determine the offender's treatment needs, more extensive psychological testing may be required. Generally speaking, psychological testing is of very limited utility in determining the presence of a paraphilia (APA, 1998).

Among the cognitive tests recommended for use in the assessment of sex offenders are brief intelligence measures, such as the Wechsler Abbreviated Scale of Intelligence (WASI) or the Kaufman Brief Intelligence Test (K-BIT). Rarely is it necessary to administer a more lengthy intelligence measure unless the offender is also being evaluated for learning disabilities, mental retardation, or other cognitive deficits. In addition, a brief neuropsychological screening battery such as Cognistat and the Trail Making Test, or the Brief Neuropsychological Cognitive Examination might be utilized in conjunction with or in lieu of portions of the mental status examination. More extensive neuropsychological testing is not routinely indicated at the present time despite some research evidence that suggests cerebral dysfunction in paraphiliacs (Langevin, 1990; Marshall, 1996). This could change as additional data become available.

The use of an objective personality measure is useful in determining the presence of other psychopathology and identifying a sexual offender's personality characteristics and disorders. The MMPI-2 and the MCMI-III are probably the most typically utilized self-report personality measures with sexual offenders. Despite the inability of their validity scales to distinguish dissimulators from those who are being honest, these scales can offer insight or confirmation regarding the offender's test-taking attitude. They may also be helpful in the assessment of related questions such as potential for substance abuse or to identify posttraumatic symptoms. However, in his review of the literature regarding sex offender assessment, Marshall (1996) cautioned that interviews with sex offenders offer far more information than is ever revealed in self-report measures. The Psychopathy Checklist-Revised (PCL-R) is the most valid measure of psychopathy available if this is of concern. If indicated, brief symptom-specific scales such as the Beck Depression Inventory-II (BDI-II) or the State-Trait Anger Scale (STAS) can be used. The evaluator needs to remain aware that the item content on these scales is very obvious and amenable to dissimulation. The Substance Abuse Subtle Screening Inventory (SASSI) offers a valid alternative to more obvious measures of substance abuse.

The use of projective measures in the evaluation of sex offenders can be beneficial in understanding dynamic risk factors such as interpersonal skills and expectations, reality testing, impulse control, self-esteem, and ability to manage affect, if these characteristics cannot be inferred from interview and history alone. The Rorschach will address most of these issues, while projective story-telling tests such as the Thematic Apperception Test (or for young juvenile sex offenders, the Roberts Children's Apperception Test) are good at identifying relationship and self-image issues. Occasionally, these tests offer the opportunity for the offender to unwittingly disclose his sexual deviancy or dynamics related to his sexual offenses. Projective drawings may also allow the offender to reveal sexual preoccupations through their focus on or elaboration of certain body parts or articles of clothing.

There are a variety of offense-specific measures available to the psychological evaluator. They range from brief self-report measures of cognitions such as the Abel and Becker Cognitions Scale, the Attitudes Towards Women Scale, the Burt Rape Myth Acceptance Scale, or the Hanson Sexual Attitudes Questionnaire (Hanson et al., 1994) to more comprehensive self-report measures such as the Multiphasic Sex Inventory (Nichols & Molinder, 1984). Although limited in utility because of the obvious item content of these scales, they are often helpful in confirming impressions gained through interview or in revealing inconsistencies in self-report. In addition, evaluators may wish to utilize measures of sexual history or sexual functioning, such as the Derogatis Sexual Functioning Inventory. Finally, sentence completion items combine some of the features of both objective and projective personality measures, providing structure yet allowing the offender to reveal the content of his thoughts in his own words. L. C. Miccio-Fonseca (1998) has published a useful sentence completion measure, the *Personal Sentence Completion Inventory.*

In addition, the evaluator may wish to use one of the two methods available for assessing sexual preference: the penile plethysmograph or the Abel Assessment for Sexual Interest (Abel, Huffman, Warberg, & Holland, 1998). Penile plethysmography is an unstandardized procedure that provides a continuous measure of the size of the penis and can presumably assess the wearer's degree of sexual arousal while viewing or listening to sexual material. However, Howes (1995) concluded that while phallometric results are significant in research studies, they are generally not accurate enough to use in individual diagnostic evaluations. The Abel, while more promising in the fact that it is standardized and relies on visual reaction times to viewing sexual material, nonetheless has not been researched sufficiently to ensure its accuracy in identifying the presence of deviant sexual interests (Smith & Fischer, 1999). Lanyon (2001) emphasizes that until these techniques can be further validated, the structured clinical interview remains the most reliable and straightforward way of determining the presence of paraphilias.

Interviews of Significant Others

The final aspect of evaluation is that of speaking with other people who know the sexual offender well. This may include his parents, spouse, or current sexual partner. These people are in a position to confirm or contradict information provided by the offender himself, and may also provide additional information that is helpful in determining the presence of a paraphilia. While these interviews can occur prior to meeting with the offender, it is my experience that these interviews are most useful after I have already had a chance to conduct an individual interview. This way I can follow up on information he has provided to verify its accuracy, or at least his perceptions.

In addition to serving a checks and balances function, interviewing the sex offender's family allows some insight into the kind of support that exists in the community for the offender. This information is useful both in determining risk to reoffend as well as in making recommendations regarding placement and community supervision needs. It is a very different situation when making recommendations for a sexual offender who is essentially a loner with few social supports as opposed to the man who has a loving and supportive family to help him.

Interviewing family members is also important in order to gauge the kinds of support the offender may receive regarding his attendance and participation in treatment. If the family recognizes the offender's need for help, is willing to help him keep his appointments, and willing to participate in his treatment when appropriate, this represents a more positive potential outcome than if the family shares in the offender's denial concerning his offense or his deviant sexual interests. If the sexual offender being evaluated is a juvenile, evaluation of the parents' attitudes regarding their son and his offense, their own strengths and weaknesses as individuals, and their ability to work together as a couple are often crucial in terms of risk assessment and placement issues.

Occasionally the question is raised of whether the evaluator should interview a victim as part of the assessment of a sex offender. This is contraindicated, as it could be very traumatic to the victim to be asked questions by the person evaluating his or her perpetrator. It could easily appear to the victim that the evaluator is "taking sides," or questioning the veracity of the victim's statements. If an evaluator needs information from the victim, it is best to obtain that information from police reports, child protective services interviews, or to have someone else interview that person.

RISK ASSESSMENT

Risk, Risk Assessment, and Risk Management

Among the most common questions asked when a sex offender is referred for evaluation are those of "What is the likelihood that this person will commit another sexual offense?" or "How dangerous is this person to society?" Despite the complexity and controversy surrounding our ability to predict violence or sexual reoffense, mental health professionals continue to be asked by the courts for assistance in such matters (Borum, 1996; Melton et al., 1997). While earlier professional attempts to assess risks of all types have been shown to be woefully inadequate, more recent trends in the field have been shown to be more promising and accurate (Hanson & Bussiere, 1998; Monahan, 1984).

It is useful at the outset to distinguish between the three concepts of risk, risk assessment, and risk management. Risk is closely related to the ideas of danger and probability (Bernstein, 1996). It refers to the nature of the danger, how likely that danger will occur, how frequently it will happen, the severity of the danger's consequences, and the imminence of that danger occurring (Janus & Meehl, 1997). In reviewing the literature related to the prediction of risk, however, there is often some confusion regarding which aspect of risk is being addressed. For example, when the question is "How likely is it that a known offender will reoffend?" we could be talking about sexual offenses, violent offenses, or general criminal offenses. We can also be dealing with temporal issues. For example, are we concerned with immediate risk or long-term risk? When reviewing research related to the question of risk, the critical reader must keep these questions in mind.

A second issue is that of risk assessment. Risk assessment refers to a method of predicting that a given danger will occur. Traditionally, risk assessment has relied on the clinical judgment of mental health professionals, with disappointing results. More recently, new developments in risk assessment have improved clinicians' accuracy in this area. These will be reviewed below.

A final issue is that of risk management. This involves the question of what it would take to prevent (or significantly reduce the likelihood of) a particular event occurring. If the question is "What steps can we take to ensure that this convicted child molester will not harm another child?," then a comprehensive understanding of that offender should result in recommendations that will significantly reduce the chance that this person will commit another sexual offense. Generally speaking, it is much easier to answer questions related to risk management rather than questions related to risk assessment.

Evaluating the Research Related to Risk Assessment

There is a prolific body of literature related to sexual offense recidivism (Hanson & Bussiere, 1998). The results of these studies often appear to be conflicting, largely because of significant differences in the populations studied, the research designs, and the methods used to analyze the data. Table 4 provides a summary of variables that should be evaluated in recidivism research. These issues will also be briefly reviewed so that the reader can better evaluate a given study and the information provided by that research.

What is the population being studied? The first issue has to do with the particular group of sex offenders being studied. Most researchers have relied on the population of sex offenders to which they have the most ready access, which is usually their place of employment. As a result, studies of sex offenders have utilized general criminal populations, those committed to state hospitals, or those incarcerated in maximum-security psychiatric hospitals. Only a few studies have used non-incarcerated offenders, or those who have volunteered to participate in a study. These populations differ significantly in the types of offenses they commit, the level of criminality or psychopathy present, the degree and type of comorbid psychiatric disturbance present, and their level of honesty in disclosing their offense history. At the present time, it is clear that sex offenders differ from other types of criminals in significant ways. For example, rapists show more similarities to other types of criminals and are more likely to recidivate with non-sexual violence than are child molesters (Hanson & Bussiere, 1998).

TABLE 4. Variables in Evaluating Recidivism Research

- What is the overall design of the study?
- What is the population of sexual offenders being studied?
- What criteria for recidivism are being used?
- What sources of outcome data are being relied upon?
- What is the length and consistency of the follow-up period?
- What method of data analysis is being used?

In addition, most studies lump all types of sex offenders together in a single sample without regard for offense type, level of psychopathy, or presence of paraphilias. The proportion of each offender type will also vary widely from study to study. Some studies do make an effort to distinguish one type of offender from another in examining risk of recidivism. There is some indication, however, that it may be unimportant to do this, at least with paraphiliac sex offenders, as they have typically been shown to have more than one deviant sexual interest (Abel & Rouleau, 1990a). In addition, a recent actuarial study performed equally well for rapists as it did child molesters (Hanson & Thornton, 1999).

What criteria for recidivism are used? In designing a study of recidivism, researchers must decide how they will determine what recidivism criteria they are interested in. That is, what type of reoffense do they wish to study? Most often, the research will focus on whether an offender has committed a new sexual offense. This is especially true of the most recent studies. However, they could also examine violent offenses or more general, non-violent offenses as well. Some studies look at two or three of these variables within the same study. Generally speaking, the research literature has found that sex offenders commit general criminal offenses at a higher rate than they do violent offenses, which in turn occur at a higher rate than sexual offenses (Hanson & Bussiere, 1998; Hanson & Thornton, 1999).

A second issue related to outcome studies is that of how the researcher will define recidivism. Practically speaking, there are four choices, since self-report is generally not an option. These choices range from the most stringent, reincarceration, to lesser degrees of stringency—reconviction, rearrest, or simply being charged for a new sexual offense. It is well established that the actual number of sex offenses is grossly underestimated by official reports. Relying on conviction records can be misleading, as the offenses involving sexual activity can be lost, most often through plea-bargaining. Even arrest reports are misleading, since many sex crimes are not reported to police (Furby, Weinrott, & Blackshaw, 1989) or simply go undetected (Weinrott & Saylor, 1991). In addition, the largest self-report study ever conducted using 561 sex offenders of different types (Abel et al., 1987) found that offenders who committed an offense that involved physical contact with a victim were only detected and arrested 3% of the time. Thus, the more stringent the recidivism criterion, the lower the recidivism rate will appear (Hanson & Bussiere, 1998; Prentky, Knight, & Lee, 1997).

What sources of outcome data are used? Those conducting recidivism studies of sex offenders are often limited when selecting how they will determine whether a new sexual offense has occurred. The usual choices include FBI records, probation reports, police reports, parole revocations, and other methods of tracking crimes that vary significantly in different jurisdictions and countries. A researcher runs into many problems when attempting to follow a study participant's criminal record after being released from incarceration. Many earlier studies of sex offense recidivism relied on a single source of data when tracking study participants. Furby and colleagues (1989) demonstrated that the use of multiple record sources increases study validity, and more recent recidivism studies have relied on as many sources of information as can be made available to them (Prentky, Lee, Knight, & Cerce, 1997).

What is the length and consistency of the follow-up period? The follow-up period in any study of sex offense recidivism refers to the period of time that offender is given the opportunity to commit a new sexual offense. By definition, the follow-up period cannot begin until the offender is released from incarceration, is back on the streets, and able to reoffend by being exposed to a population of potential victims.

One year is the most common observation period noted in earlier studies of sexual offense recidivism (Miller, 1984). More recently, a follow-up period of three or four years has become more common (Hanson & Bussiere, 1998). Studies that include extremely long follow-up periods are rare for obvious reasons. Two notable exceptions include those of Hanson, Steffy, and Gauthier (1993), which had follow-up periods of 15 to 30 years, and Prentky, Lee, Knight, and Cerce (1997), which followed study participants for 25 years. The results of these studies and the meta-analytic study of Hanson and Bussiere (1998) clearly indicate that most sexual reoffenses do not occur within the first five years of release into the community, with recidivism rates increasing significantly after this time. Generally speaking, rapists have been noted to commit a sexual reoffense more quickly than child molesters (Prentky, Lee, Knight, & Cerce, 1997). Child molesters in particular are at risk to reoffend sexually throughout their lives (Gibbens, Soothill, & Way, 1978; Hanson, Steffy, & Gauthier, 1993).

What is the method of data analysis? The most common method of data analysis in studies of sex offense recidivism is to calculate the simple percentage or proportion of individuals who reoffended during the study period. However, this method has been shown to underestimate recidivism rates because not all study participants are usually released into the community at the same time. Those who are in the community for a relatively shorter period of time could still reoffend if they had as much opportunity as the first offender released in the study.

Prentky, Knight, and Lee (1997), Hanson, Scott, and Steffy (1995), and Hanson and Bussiere (1998) and other leading researchers in this field now recommend the use of survival analysis to correct this problem. Using this method, all subjects can be included regardless of the length of time followed and whether or not they reoffended. Survival analyses rely on the calculation of a failure rate, which is defined as the proportion of individuals who reoffended. Failure rate is an estimate that takes into account the amount of time each offender has been on the street and thus able to reoffend.

What is the study design? The last research issue to address is that of the design of the particular study being examined. The vast majority of recidivism studies employ a retrospective design, where the behavior of a group of sex offenders is examined by looking back. For example, a study could be arbitrarily begun in 1984, and all the sex offenders released from a particular facility over the next 15 years would then be followed to see who reoffended, and data analyses conducted to see what these offenders had in common. Generally speaking, the results from these types of studies are less reliable than those of prospective studies where a group of offenders is followed from the present time through a specified period into the future (Furby et al., 1989).

Methods of Risk Assessment

In this next section, four methods of predicting sexual recidivism will be reviewed, along with a discussion of the strengths and limitations of each. Table 5 provides a brief summary of these methods.

Clinical judgment. By far the most common method used to predict whether an individual sex offender will reoffend is that of reliance on professional clinical judgment. But how reliable and accurate is this method? Judging from studies of violent recidivism, not very good. For one thing, there is little interrater reliability when clinical judgment alone is relied upon (Dawes, 1994). In addition, studies have demon-

TABLE 5. Methods of Risk Assessment

- Clinical judgment

- Empirically informed clinical judgment

- Actuarial assessment

- Anamnestic (individualized) approach

---

strated that the amount of clinical training and the experience of a given psychologist are unrelated to accuracy in the prediction of violence (Goldberg, 1970). Dawes (1994) also found that while the amount of information provided to the clinicians was highly related to the degree of confidence the clinician placed in their judgment, it was entirely unrelated to the accuracy of the prediction. One study (Quinsey & Ambtman, 1979) compared predictions of future violence made by forensic psychiatrists and high school teachers. The psychiatrists did no better than the teachers, and there was little agreement between the supposed experts.

In general, clinical judgment alone produces correlations with predictions of future violent behavior in the range of .10, with many false positive predictions (Melton et al., 1997). There are many reasons to believe that a similar lack of success would be found in relation to the prediction of future sexual offense. First, as noted above, the research literature on sexual offense recidivism is vast and complex. It is difficult to keep up with, and difficult to reconcile the varying research populations and study methods. In addition, clinicians (like everyone else) are vulnerable to bias and judgment errors. Dangerousness or risk is often viewed as a trait that somehow resides within an individual, rather than the more accurate perception that there is an interaction between an individual, a potential victim, and the situation in which they find themselves that more accurately defines risk. Studies have shown that mental health professionals have a tendency to make recommendations regarding dangerousness based upon the severity of the charges or the illusionary perception that a relationship exists between two variables when it has been shown empirically (or not yet been demonstrated at all) that no such relationship exists. For example, most clinicians would think that victim empathy would be an important variable to consider when making a risk assessment on an individual sex offender, when in fact, it has been shown to be irrelevant (Hanson & Bussiere, 1998). In addition, clinicians are not immune to cultural and socioeconomic biases. Finally, it is simply the safer road to take in reaching the conclusion that a sex offender is at high risk to reoffend, as this approach avoids negative publicity or possible legal action if the offender is released and commits a new sexual offense.

Given the state of our current knowledge and the more reliable and valid methods of risk assessment available to us, it would be unethical to rely solely on one's clinical judgment in assessing risk of recidivism in sex offenders.

Empirically informed clinical judgment. A significant improvement over reliance on clinical judgment alone is that of using a systematic method of reviewing traits or factors known to be associated with sexual recidivism through the research literature. This assessment method might include some sort of formal or informal checklist. It ensures that the clinician relies on empirically derived variables rather than their own impressions of what is important to consider, and also ensures that the clinician will consider all the relevant variables, not forgetting the ones that slip their memory that day. The difficulty with informal checklists compiled by individual clinicians lies within their lack of standardization. Even in more formal checklists, there is an unknown amount of redundancy between items. In addition, the items themselves remain subject to bias weighting on the part of the person using them.

I know of 10 such instruments currently available that are used to assess risk of sexual reoffense, but only two of them are in widespread use. The first such instrument, the Hare Psychopathy Checklist-Revised (PCL-R), was not originally intended to be used for this purpose. However, since it is well established that the presence of psychopathy is significantly associated with sexual recidivism (Gretton, McBride, & Hare, 1995; Hare, 1998), it is often utilized in risk assessment with sex offenders. This is especially true when an offender has a high PCL-R score in combination with evidence of deviant sexual arousal, both in adults (Rice & Harris, 1997), as well as in adolescents (O'Shaughnessy, Hare, Gretton, & McBride, 1994). The test consists of 20 items demonstrated to be associated with the construct of psychopathy as originally developed by Cleckly (1941) and elaborated by Hare (1991). Qualified raters assign scores of 2 (the item definitely applies to that individual), 1 (the item applies to a limited extent), or 0 (the item does not apply), resulting in a score that ranges from 0 to 40. Hanson (2000) indicates that as a risk assessment tool, gradual increases in checklist scores are associated with gradual increases in recidivism risk. He refers to the PCL-R as a modest predictor of sex offense recidivism.

The other empirically based method in relatively wide usage is the Sexual Violence Risk-20 (SVR-20), which is specifically designed to be used in sexual violent risk assessments with adult sexual offenders (Boer, Hart, Kropp, & Webster, 1997). Developed from a review of the relevant research literature, this instrument also consists of 20 items related to psychosocial adjustment, past sexual offenses, and future plans. It is coded in a manner similar to the PCL-R, only instead of using numbers, the rater assigns a score of "Yes" if the risk factor is definitely present in the individual, a "Maybe" if the risk factor may be present or is present only to a limited degree, and a "No" if the risk factor is absent or does not apply. After going through this exercise, the clinician is asked to make a summary rating indicating that the offender is at low, moderate, or high risk to commit a sexual reoffense. The test manual does not provide the results of any reliability or validity, but the results of several studies suggest that it has adequate concurrent and predictive validity (Doren, 1999). Nonetheless, the items included in the manual are consistent with the current literature, and similar approaches to violence risk assessment (Webster, Douglas, Eaves, & Hart, 1997) and spousal abuse (Kropp, Hart, Webster, & Eaves, 1995) have been found to have adequate interrater reliability and predictive validity (Kropp & Hart, 2000).

Actuarial risk assessment of sexual recidivism. It is well established that actuarial methods of risk assessment are superior to those of unstructured clinical judgment (Monahan, 1995). Actuarial tools use multiple regression formulas to derive predictions of sexual reoffense within a given period time. These instruments integrate empirically derived factors so that redundancy between items is eliminated. Such tools are very similar to those used by the life insurance industry or physicians when answering questions about life expectancy when someone is diagnosed with a particular disease.

While actuarial tools significantly improve the consistency and accuracy of risk assessment, they are limited in that they are based on only a small number of factors. In addition, these instruments are overly weighted on static or unchanging factors in the offender's life, making them of limited utility after an offender has completed a treatment program. For the instruments to perform as they should, they must be used with populations as similar as possible to the original standardization samples.

Just as there are many structured clinical judgment tools available or in development, I am aware of 22 actuarial measures of sexual reoffense. Many of them are still in various stages of development, and only 10 of them have been validated as of this writing. While an extensive review of these actuarial tools is beyond the scope of this article, I would like to discuss two of them with which I am familiar and that are in relatively widespread use.

The first of these instruments is the Sex Offender Risk Appraisal Guide (SORAG), developed along with the well-respected Violence Risk Assessment Guide by Quinsey, Harris, Rice, and Cormier (1998). It is based on a retrospective sample of 178 rapists and child molesters from a maximum-security forensic hospital in Ontario. It yields a score that can be translated into one of nine risk levels, and also provides an estimate of sexual reoffense risk over a period of 7 and 10 years. The SORAG includes the use of the PCL-R in its scoring, and is heavily weighted on the variable of psychopathy. In its initial validation studies, it was found to have moderate predictive accuracy (r = .21, ROC = .62).

The Static-99 is a relatively new instrument by Hanson and Thornton (1999) that combines the items from Hanson's Rapid Risk Assessment for Sex Offense Recidivism (RRASOR) with those from Thornton's Structured Anchored Clinical Judgment (SACJ). The resulting 10-item scale is easily scored and provides levels of risk assessment and estimates of both sexual and violent recidivism at 5, 10, and 15-year intervals. It is based on a sample of 1,086 incarcerated adult male sex offenders primarily consisting of rapists and child molesters, and was replicated on another sample of sex offenders. Since recidivism is based primarily upon convictions, it is likely to somewhat underestimate the true rate of reoffense. In its favor, however, one of the offender samples had a follow-up period of 23 years, while two others exceeded 10 years. When compared to its predecessors, the Static-99 outperformed both the RRASOR and the SACJ with a modest correlation of .33 and an ROC area of .71. This latter statistic suggests that there is a 71% chance that a randomly selected recidivist would have a more deviant score than a randomly selected non-recidivist. Rapists and child molesters performed almost identically. It is as good as or superior to all other actuarial measures of sexual recidivism available at the present time (Doren, 1999).

There have been numerous cross-validation studies on both the SORAG and the Static-99 in recent years that confirm their ability to predict sexual recidivism with at least moderate accuracy (Barbaree, Seto, Langton, & Peacock, 2001; Hanson & Thornton, 2000). In a recent study that directly compared the accuracy of the two instruments, they were found to be essentially similar in their predictive ability, but were not found to make unique contributions to the prediction of sexual recidivism (Nunes, Firestone, Bradford, Greenberg, & Broom, 2002).

The authors of several of the actuarial instruments currently in use recognize the need to include more dynamic risk factors into their assessments, augmenting the static factors contained in the actuarial instruments themselves. Hanson and Harris (2001) have developed a dynamic risk assessment scheme that will complement the Static-99. Their instrument, called the Sex Offender Need Assessment Rating (SONAR), has recently been published but has not yet been cross-validated.

Anamnestic (individualized) approach. This final type of risk assessment attempts to identify those factors that are particular to a specific individual's pattern of sexual offending. Through the review of archival data, clinical interview, and information from third-party reports that detail specific prior incidents of sexual assault, the evaluator is able to reconstruct vignettes that yield insights about repetitive themes that are present in all known offenses. In this manner, the clinician can begin to develop hypotheses about the offender's intrapsychic dynamics, cognitive distortions, and deviant sexual interests. In addition, situational variables and relevant victim characteristics can also be included in the overall risk assessment and development of a treatment and risk management plan.

An Overall Approach to Risk Assessment

Noting the relative superiority of actuarial tools over clinical judgment, Quinsey et al. (1998) have suggested that actuarial instruments be relied upon exclusively when performing risk assessments. However, most other researchers do not share this conservative view, and one recent study has even challenged the superiority of the actuarial approach to that of structured clinical judgment (Kropp & Hart, 2000).

At the present time, there are two methods widely utilized by clinicians making risk assessments. In the first method, the clinician first assesses risk of sexual reoffense by utilizing a validated actuarial measure or a structured clinical judgment tool appropriate for a given offender, and then adjusts their estimation of risk conservatively based upon either a dynamic risk assessment scale or a systematic consideration of other risk factors that have been empirically identified (Sreenivasan, Kirkish, Garrick, Weinberger, & Phenix, 2000). In the second method, the clinician utilizes two or more actuarial instruments, systematically reviews the relevant research literature relevant to recidivism, and then reaches a conclusion by integrating all of this information. While the use of an actuarial instrument is necessary, it is not sufficient, as one must consider other risk factors identified through research that are not included in the actuarial tool. In addition, it will always be necessary to look beyond those traits and factors of offenders that can easily be operationalized and subjected to research. The individual history, symptoms, and dynamics of each offender, as well as the characteristics of their preferred victims and a variety of situational variables, must be considered as well. A list of static and dynamic risk factors can be found in Table 6.

While actuarial risk assessments do provide statistical estimations of reoffense, it is often a good idea to phrase risk level in the relatively simple and easy-to-grasp terms of low, moderate, or high. For one thing,

TABLE 6. Static and Dynamic Risk Factors

Static Risk Factors

	*Correlation with Sexual Reoffense**
Victim, stranger	(.22)
Deviant sexual preference	(.20)
Prior sexual offense	(.19)
Failure to complete treatment	(.18)
Offender, age 25 or older at time of assessment	(.13)
Presence of personality disorder	(.13)
Anger problems	(.13)
Non-sexual criminal history	(.12)
Presence of a severe mental disorder	(.12)
Never married	(.11)
Negative childhood environment	(.11)
History of diverse sex crimes	(.10)
Victim, male	(.10)

Dynamic Risk Factors

- Unemployment, poor employment history, or lack of job skills
- Substance abuse
- Poor social adjustment
- Attitudes tolerant of rape or child molestation
- Poor coping skills
- Exacerbation in symptoms of a severe mental disorder
- Low self-esteem or lack of self-confidence
- Access to a potential victim
- Negative attitudes towards treatment
- Uncooperative with supervision

* based upon Hanson and Bussiere (1998)

this conveys a sense of relative risk instead of putting the estimation of risk in such absolute terms. For another, courts and other professionals who are unfamiliar with the statistical properties associated with actuarial risk prediction can better understand what clinicians are trying to convey.

As part of assessing risk to sexually reoffend, there are other important questions to address as well. These might include the likely type of reoffense; for example, exposing as opposed to child molestation. The type of (or in some instances, the specific) victim that the offender is most likely to target is also important to address, and has not been the object of much formal study thus far (Furby et al., 1989; Quinsey, Rice, & Harris, 1995). The immanence and/or severity of a sexual reoffense might also be addressed if possible, along with any warning signs that the treating clinician or supervising parole officer might want to watch out for. This latter question might also address the issue of under what circumstances a particular individual might be most likely to commit another sexual offense. Risk management issues should also be addressed.

CONCLUSION

The evaluation of sexual offenders will always require some latitude so that the evaluation can be tailored to fit the needs of the individual and his situation. There will never be a "one size fits all" evaluation any more than there can be a treatment plan that does not take into account the intrapsychic and situational variables related to a particular offender. What is important is that the assessment is comprehensive and addresses all the concerns and issues noted in this article, as overlooking almost any of the areas noted can result in the omission of essential information that could result in errors in diagnosis and recommendations regarding treatment and placement. The evaluation must integrate findings from a structured clinical interview along with as much third-party information as is available, along with the results of any psychometric testing that is deemed relevant. Such a comprehensive evaluation is more likely to ensure an accurate diagnosis along with simultaneously ensuring the safety of the community and meeting the treatment needs of the sexual offender.

REFERENCES

Abel, G. G. (1997, April). *The paraphilias.* Lecture given at the Sexual Offenders Conference in San Diego, CA.
Abel, G. G., Becker, J. V., Cunningham-Rathner, N., Rouleau, J., & Murphy, W. (1987). Self-reported sex crimes of non-incarcerated paraphiliacs. *Journal of Interpersonal Violence, 2,* 3-25.
Abel, G. G., Huffman, J., Warberg, B., & Holland, C. (1998). Visual reaction time and plethysmography as measures of sexual interest in child molesters. *Sexual Abuse: A Journal of Research and Treatment, 10,* 81-95.

Abel, G. G., Lawry, S. S., Karlstrom, E., Osborn, C. A., & Gillespie, C. F. (1994). Screening tests for pedophilia. *Criminal Justice and Behavior, 21*, 115-131.

Abel, G. G., & Rouleau, J. L. (1990a). Male sex offenders. In M. E. Thase, B. A. Edelstein, & M. Hersen (Eds.), *Handbook of outpatient therapy of adults* (pp. 271-290). New York: Plenum Press.

Abel, G. G., & Rouleau, J. L. (1990b). The nature and extent of sexual assault. In W. Marshall, D. Laws, & H. Barbaree (Ed.), *Handbook of sexual assault: Issues, theories and treatment of the offender* (pp. 9-21). New York: Plenum Press.

American Psychiatric Association. (1968). *Diagnostic and statistical manual of mental disorders* (2nd ed.). Washington, DC: Author.

American Psychiatric Association. (1994). *Diagnostic and statistical manual of mental disorders* (4th ed.). Washington, DC: Author.

American Psychiatric Association. (1998). *Task force report on sexually dangerous offenders*. Washington, DC: Author.

American Psychological Association. (1992). Ethical principles of psychologists and code of conduct. *American Psychologist, 47*, 1597-1611.

Barbaree, H., & Marshall, W. (1988). Deviant sexual arousal, offense history and demographic variables as predictors of reoffense among child molesters. *Behavioral Sciences and the Law, 6*, 267-280.

Barbaree, H., Seto, M., Langton, P., & Peacock, R. (2001). Evaluating the predictive accuracy of six risk assessment instruments for adult sex offenders. *Criminal Justice and Behavior, 28*, 490-521.

Berlin, F. S. (1999, November). *Diagnosis and treatment of sexually violent predators*. Presentation at Atascadero State Hospital for the California Department of Mental Health, Atascadero, CA.

Berlin, F. S., Lehne, G. K., Malin, H. M., Hunt, W. P., Thomas, K., & Fuhraneck, J. (1997). *The eroticized violent crime: A psychiatric perspective with six clinical examples*. Unpublished manuscript.

Bernstein, P. L. (1996). *Against the gods: The remarkable story of risk*. New York: Wiley and Sons.

Boer, D. P., Hart, S. D., Kropp, P. R., & Webster, C. D. (1997). *Manual for the sexual violence risk-20*. Vancouver, British Columbia: The British Columbia Institute Against Family Violence.

Borum, R. (1996). Improving the clinical practice of violent risk assessment. *American Psychologist, 9*, 945-956.

Carter, D. L., Prentky, R. A., Knight, R. A., & Vanderveer, P. L. (1987). Use of pornography in the criminal and developmental histories of sex offenders. *Journal of Interpersonal Violence, 2*, 196-211.

Cleckley, H. (1941). *The mask of sanity*. St. Louis, MO: Mosby.

Committee on Ethical Guidelines for Forensic Psychologists. (1991). Specialty guidelines for forensic psychologists. *Law and Human Behavior, 15*, 655-665.

Crepault, C., & Coulture, M. (1980). Men's erotic fantasies. *Archives of Sexual Behavior, 9*, 565-580.

Dawes, R. M. (1994). *House of cards: Psychology and psychotherapy built on myth*. New York: Free Press.

Doren, D. M. (1999). *The issue of accuracy of the risk assessment instruments within the context of sex offender civil commitment evaluations.* Unpublished document.

Freund, K., & Watson, R. J. (1991). Assessment of the sensitivity and specificity of a phallometric test: An update of phallometric diagnosis of pedophilia. *Psychological Assessment, 3*, 147-155.

Furby, L., Weinrott, M., & Blackshaw, L. (1989). Sex offender recidivism: A review. *Psychological Bulletin, 105*, 3-30.

Gibbens, T., Soothill, K., & Way, C. (1978). Sibling and parent-child incest offenses. *British Journal of Criminology, 18*, 40-52.

Goldberg, L. R. (1970). Man versus model of man: A rationale, plus some evidence for a method of improving on clinical inference. *Psychological Bulletin, 73*, 422-432.

Gretton, H., McBride, M., & Hare, R. (1995, February). Psychopathy in adolescent sex offenders: A follow-up study. Paper presented at the Annual Conference of the Association for the Treatment of Sexual Abusers, New Orleans, LA.

Hall, G. C. N. (1995). Sexual offender recidivism revisited: A meta-analysis of recent treatment studies. *Journal of Consulting and Clinical Psychology, 63*, 802-809.

Hanson, R. K., & Bussiere, M. (1998). Predicting relapse: A meta-analysis of sexual offender recidivism studies. *Journal of Consulting and Clinical Psychology, 66*, 348-362.

Hanson, R. K., Gizzarelli, R., & Scott, H. (1994). The attitudes of incest offenders: Sexual entitlement and acceptance of sex with children. *Criminal Justice and Behavior, 21, 2*, 187-202.

Hanson, R. K., & Harris, A. J. R. (2001). A structured approach to evaluating change among sexual offenders. *Sexual Abuse: A Journal of Research and Treatment, 13*(2), 105-122.

Hanson, R. K., Morton, K. E., & Harris, A. J. R. (2002). *Sexual offender recidivism risk: What we know and what we need to know.* Unpublished manuscript.

Hanson, R. K., Scott, H., & Steffy, R. A. (1995). A comparison of child molesters and non-sexual criminals: Risk predictors and long-term recidivism. *Journal of Research in Crime and Delinquency, 32*, 325-337.

Hanson, R. K., Steffy, R., & Gauthier, R. (1993). Long-term recidivism of child molesters. *Journal of Consulting and Clinical Psychology, 61*, 646-652.

Hanson, R. K., & Thornton, D. (1999). *Static 99: Improving actuarial risk assessment for sex offenders.* Ottawa, Canada: Department of the Solicitor General of Canada.

Hanson, R. K., & Thornton, D. (2000). Improving risk assessment for sex offenders: A comparison of three actuarial scales. *Law and Human Behavior, 24*, 119-136.

Hare, R. D. (1991). *The Hare psychopathy checklist-revised.* New York: Multi-Health Systems, Inc.

Hare, R. D. (1998). The Hare PCL-R: Some issues concerning its use and misuse. *Legal and Criminological Psychology, 3*, 99-119.

Haugaard, J. J., & Reppucci, N. D. (1988). *The sexual abuse of children.* San Francisco: Jossey-Bass Publishers.

Howes, R. J. (1995). A survey of plethysmographic assessment in North America. *Sexual Abuse: A Journal of Research and Treatment, 7*, 9-24.

Hunt, M. (1974). *Sexual behavior in the 1970s.* Chicago: Playboy Press.

Janus, E. S., & Meehl, P. E. (1997). Assessing the legal standard for the prediction of dangerousness in sex offender commitment proceedings. *Psychology, Public Policy and Law, 3*, 33-64.

Kafka, M. P. (1993). Update on paraphilias and paraphilia-related disorders. *Currents in Affective Illness, 12*, 5-13.

Kendall, P. C., & Hammen, C. (1995). *Abnormal psychology*. Boston: Houghton Mifflin Company.

Kennedy, H., & Grubin, D. (1992). Patterns of denial in sex offenders. *Psychological Medicine, 22*, 191-196.

Kinsey, A., Pomeroy, W., & Martin, C. (1948). *Sexual behavior in the human male*. Philadelphia: Saunders.

Kinsey, A., Pomeroy, W., Martin, C., & Gebhard, P. (1953). *Sexual behavior in the human female*. Philadelphia: Saunders.

Knight, R. A., Warren, J. I., Reboussin, R., & Soley, B. J. (1998). Predicting rapist type from crime-scene variables. *Criminal Justice and Behavior, 25*(1), 46-80.

Kropp, P. R., & Hart, S. D. (2000). The spousal assault risk assessment guide (SARA): Reliability and validity in adult male offenders. *Law & Human Behavior, 24*(1), 101-118.

Kropp, P. R., Hart, S. D., Webster, C. D., & Eaves, D. (1995). *Manual for the spousal assault risk assessment guide* (2nd ed.). Vancouver, British Columbia: The British Columbia Institute Against Family Violence.

Langevin, R. (1988). Defensiveness in sex offenders. In R. Rogers (Ed.), *Clinical assessment of malingering and deception* (pp. 269-290). New York: Guilford Press.

Langevin, R. (1990). Sexual anomalies and the brain. In W. L. Marshall, D. R. Laws, & H. E. Barbaree (Eds.), *Handbook of sexual assault: Issues, theories and treatment of the offender* (pp. 103-112). New York: Plenum Press.

Lanyon, R. (2001). Psychological assessment procedures in sex offending. *Professional Psychology, Research and Practice, Vol. 32, 3*, 253-260.

Marshall, W. L. (1996). Assessment, treatment and theorizing about sex offenders: Developments during the past twenty years and future directions. *Criminal Justice and Behavior, 23*(1), 162-199.

Mead, M. (1949). *Male and female: A study of the sexes in a changing world*. New York: William Morrow and Company.

Melton, G. B., Petrila, J., Poythress, N. G., & Slobogin, C. (1997). *Psychological evaluations for the courts: A handbook for mental health professionals and lawyers* (2nd ed.). New York: Guilford Press.

Miccio-Fonseca, L. C. (1998). *Personal sentence completion inventory*. Brandon, VT: Safer Society Press.

Miller, D. (1984). *A survey of recidivism research in the United States and Canada*. Boston: Massachusetts Department of Correction.

Monahan, J. (1984). The prediction of violent behavior: Toward a second generation of theory and policy. *American Journal of Psychiatry, 141*, 10-15.

Monahan, J. (1995). *The clinical prediction of violent behavior*. Northvale, NJ: Jason Aronson.

Mott, F. L., & Haum, R. J. (1988). Linkages between sexual activity and alcohol and drug use among American adolescents. *Family Planning Perspectives, 20*, 128-136.

Murphy, W. D., & Peters, I. M. (1992). Profiling child sexual abusers: Psychological considerations. *Criminal Justice and Behavior, 19*, 24-37.

Nichols, H. R., & Molinder, I. (1984). *Multiphasic sex inventory manual.* Tacoma, WA: Nichols and Molinder.

Nunes, K. L., Firestone, P., Bradford, J. M., Greenberg, D. M., & Broom, I. (2002). A comparison of modified versions of the static-99 and the sex offender risk appraisal guide. *Sexual Abuse: A Journal of Research and Treatment, 14*, 253-269.

O'Shaughnessy, R., Hare, R. D., Gretton, H., & McBride, M. (1994). Psychopathy and adolescent sex offending. Unpublished data. Published in R. D. Hare (1998), The Hare PCL-R: Some issues concerning its use and misuse. *Legal and Criminological Psychology, 3*, 99-119.

People v. Stoll, 89 DAR 15164 (1989).

Prentky, R. A., Knight, R., & Lee, A. (1997). Risk factors associated with recidivism among extrafamilial child molesters. *Journal of Consulting and Clinical Psychology, 65*, 141-149.

Prentky, R. A., Lee, A., Knight, R., & Cerce, R. (1997). Recidivism rates among child molesters and rapists: A methodological analysis. *Law and Human Behavior, 21*, 635-659.

Quinsey, V. L. (1984). Sexual aggression: Studies of sex offenders against women. In D. Weisstub (Ed.), *Law and mental health: International perspectives*, Vol. 1 (pp. 84-122). New York: Pergamon Press.

Quinsey, V. L. (1986). Men who have sex with children. In D. Weisstub (Ed.), *Law and mental health: International perspectives*, Vol. 2 (pp. 140-172). New York: Pergamon Press

Quinsey, V. L., & Ambtman, R. (1979). Variables affecting psychiatrist's and teacher's assessments of the dangerousness of mentally ill offenders. *Journal of Consulting and Clinical Psychology, 47*, 353-362.

Quinsey, V. L., Harris, G. T., Rice, M. E., & Cormier, C. A. (1998). *Violent offenders: Appraising and managing risk.* Washington, DC: American Psychological Association.

Quinsey, V. L., Rice, M. E., & Harris, G. T. (1995). Actuarial prediction of sexual recidivism. *Journal of Interpersonal Violence, 10*, 85-105.

Rice, M. E., & Harris, G. T. (1997). Cross-validation and extension of the Violent Risk Assessment Guide for child molesters and rapists. *Law and Human Behavior, 21*, 231-241.

Rind, B., Tromovitch, P., & Bauserman, R. (1998). A meta-analytic examination of assumed properties of child sexual abuse using college samples. *APA Bulletin, 124*, 22-53.

Sewall, K. W., & Salekin, R. T. (1997). Understanding and detecting dissimulation in sex offenders. In R. Rogers (Ed.), *Clinical assessment of malingering and deception* (2nd ed.) (pp. 328-350). New York: Guilford Press.

Smith, G., & Fischer, L. (1999). Assessment of juvenile sexual offenders: Reliability and validity of the Able Assessment for Interest in Paraphilias. *Sexual Abuse: A Journal of Research and Treatment, 11*, 217-232.

Sreenivasan, S., Kirkish, P., Garrick, T., Weinberger, L., & Phenix, A. (2000). Actuarial risk assessment models: A review of critical issues related to violence and sex-offender recidivism assessments. *Journal of the American Academy of Psychiatry and Law, 28*, 438-448.

Templeman, T. L., & Stinnett, R. D. (1991). Patterns of sexual arousal and history in a "normal" sample of young men. *Archives of Sexual Behavior, 10*, 137-150.

Webster, C. D., Douglas, K. S., Eaves, D., & Hart, S. D. (1997). *HCR-20: Assessing risk for violence, version 2.* British Columbia: Mental Health, Law and Policy Institute at Simon Fraser University.

Weinrott, M. R., & Saylor, M. (1991). Self-report of crimes committed by sex offenders. *Journal of Interpersonal Violence, 6*, 286-300.

Zelnik, M., & Kanter, J. F. (1980). Sexual activity, contraceptive use and pregnancy among metropolitan-area teenagers: 1971-1979. *Family Planning Perspectives, 12*, 230-237.

The Current Role of Post-Conviction Sex Offender Polygraph Testing in Sex Offender Treatment

Ron Kokish

SUMMARY. Polygraph testing is becoming increasingly important in sex offender treatment. Polygraph advocates cite dramatic increases in historical disclosures that presumably allow more precise targeting of treatment interventions, earlier detection of risky behaviors that often lead to new offenses, and improved treatment and supervision compliance. Based on this, they believe the procedure supports desirable behavior that continues to various degrees after treatment and supervision end. Opponents cite ethical problems related to inaccurate results, unproven accuracy rates, and the risk that examinees may be coerced into making false admissions. To counter these criticisms, proponents have developed standards, best practices, and examiner training and certification programs intended to reduce error rates and address ethical issues. Opponents argue that these measures have not been tested and that empirically established error rates and best practices may not be possible for a variety of reasons. This article reviews the current situation, leaving readers to decide the wisdom and ethics of using polygraph testing in their own practices. *[Article copies available for a fee from The Haworth Document Delivery Service: 1-800-HAWORTH. E-mail address: <docdelivery@haworthpress.com> Website: <http://www.HaworthPress.com> © 2003 by The Haworth Press, Inc. All rights reserved.]*

Address correspondence to: Ron Kokish, PO Box 476, Trinidad, CA 95570 (E-mail: ron@delko.net).

[Haworth co-indexing entry note]: "The Current Role of Post-Conviction Sex Offender Polygraph Testing in Sex Offender Treatment." Kokish, Ron. Co-published simultaneously in *Journal of Child Sexual Abuse* (The Haworth Maltreatment & Trauma Press, an imprint of The Haworth Press, Inc.) Vol. 12, No. 3/4, 2003, pp. 175-194; and: *Identifying and Treating Sex Offenders: Current Approaches, Research, and Techniques* (ed: Robert Geffner et al.) The Haworth Maltreatment & Trauma Press, an imprint of The Haworth Press, Inc., 2003, pp. 175-194. Single or multiple copies of this article are available for a fee from The Haworth Document Delivery Service [1-800-HAWORTH, 9:00 a.m. - 5:00 p.m. (EST). E-mail address: docdelivery@haworthpress.com].

Digital Object Identifier: 10.1300/J070v12n03_07

KEYWORDS. Polygraph, sex offenders, post-conviction sex offender testing, sex offender treatment

HOW POLYGRAPHY WORKS

Polygraph testing consists of taking physiological measurements, interpreting the results, and offering a professional opinion as to whether the examinee was attempting deception when she/he answered certain ("relevant") questions. In practice, heart rate, blood pressure, breathing patterns, and galvanic skin response are the most typical measures used. This is because they are easily accessible and affordable, and accurate instrumentation is available. Changes in these physiological measures are believed to be associated with involuntary arousal in response to fear. This arousal is often called the "fight/flight response." Theoretical underpinnings for the procedure include a hypothesis that almost all people experience fear of being discovered when they lie. Polygraph examiners attempt to isolate and measure this fear in relation to the issue in question. Since the measurements are physiological and their interpretation is based on psychological theory, polygraphy is considered a "psycho-physiological" procedure (Hassett, 1978).

POLYGRAPH TESTING AND TREATMENT GOALS

We treat sex offenders to achieve three major goals. These are, in order of importance:

1. To reduce the number of sexual reoffenses committed by treated offenders;
2. To reduce the number of general criminal offenses, but especially violent offenses committed by treated offenders; and
3. To change treated offenders in ways that lead to increased social fulfillment for them and those whose lives they touch.

Several recent meta-analyses indicate that we are doing a credible job reaching the first two goals. Based on these studies, we can reasonably claim to be achieving an overall 40% treatment effect for 5-10 years following discharge (Alexander, 1999; Grossman, Martis, & Fichtner, 1999;

Hall, 1995; Hanson et al., 2002), though this effect certainly varies between offender categories (e.g., incest offenders, rapists) and from program to program. Our third goal is more difficult to measure. Only subjective reports from therapists, supervision officers, patients, and their families inform us about the degree to which we are attaining it, but this does not detract from its importance.

During treatment, we look at certain objectives that we believe are related to achieving our goals. Among these are:

1. Patient honesty with therapists, group members, family, and other important people;
2. Patient compliance with treatment procedures; and
3. Patient compliance with supervision conditions.

Proponents of Post Conviction Sex Offender (polygraph) Testing (PCSOT) assert that PCSOT significantly enhances their ability to attain these objectives, and that its use is thus in the community's and the offenders' best interests.

Polygraph examinations have been used to monitor probationers and particularly child abusers since the mid 1960s (Abrams, 1989b). Sex offender treatment programs (SOTPs) began using polygraph examinations to obtain more complete sexual histories and to monitor program compliance as long ago as 1975 (Wolfe, personal communication, May 10, 1999). Over the years, polygraph examinations have become an increasingly important tool for sexual offender treatment. A 1996 survey found that over 30% of 960 responding programs utilized PCSOT to varying degrees (Burton & Smith-Darden, 2000). A more recent survey found that at least some SOTPs in 33 of the 50 United States, Germany, and Canada use periodic polygraph examinations (Abrams & Simmons, 2000). The survey reported that 9.8% of probation and parole supervisors surveyed in 1994 said their agencies often or always used polygraph with adult sex offenders on their caseloads. This number rose to 16.3% in a similar 1998 survey. By 2000, approximately one-fourth of respondents reported often or always using polygraph with their agencies' adult sex offender probationers and parolees. At least one state (Colorado) now requires state recognized treatment programs to utilize polygraph examinations, and polygraphy use is encouraged by the Association for the Treatment of Sexual Abusers (ATSA) (ATSA, 2001).

ELICITING INCREASED INFORMATION

Polygraph utility flows from its ability to elicit information from offenders who might be less forthcoming with traditional interviewing techniques (ATSA, 1997). Sex offender treatment providers report significant, often dramatic increases in information disclosed by offenders who anticipate taking a polygraph examinations. For example, one study (English, Jones, Pasini-Hill, Patrick, & Cooley-Towell, 2000) comparing 180 offenders before and after testing found the following:

1. An 80% increase in the number of offenders admitting male victims;
2. A 190% increase in the number of offenders admitting to both male and female victims;
3. A 230% increase in admission of both juvenile and adult victims;
4. A 60% increase in admission of high-risk behaviors;[1] and
5. A 196% increase in admission of more than one kind of high risk behavior.

Another study (Hindman & Peters, in press) compared 98 intra-familial sex offenders treated without PCSOT between 1978 and 1983 to 129 comparable offenders who were treated with polygraphy by the same program between 1983 and 1988. When they entered treatment, the non-polygraph group reported an average of 1.2 victims. This increased to 1.5 victims by the time they completed their sexual histories. The polygraph group reported an average of 1.3 victims at program entry with an increase to 9 victims by the time they completed their sexual histories. In addition to admitting fewer victims, 67% of the non-polygraph group reported being sexually abused as minors, and 21% reported sexually abusing others as minors. Those figures were nearly reversed for the polygraph group, with only 29% reporting they were sexually abused as minors, and 71% admitting they sexually abused others as minors.

In a later replication study using data gathered between 1988 and 1994, the same researchers (Hindman & Peters, 2000) reported the non-polygraph group ($n = 76$) admitting an average of 2.5 victims, with 65% of the offenders claiming they were abused as minors, and 22% admitting they had sexually abused others. The polygraph group ($n = 152$) admitted a mean average of 13.6 victims, only 32% claimed they were sexually abused as minors, and 68% admitted abusing others. Additionally, 17%

of the non-polygraphed (primarily male) offenders admitted sexually abusing a male victim. Among the otherwise comparable polygraphed offenders, 30% admitted sexually abusing males.

Treatment providers who use polygraphy argue that complete historical information allows them to hold offenders more accountable and helps them to target treatment interventions more precisely, all of which ultimately helps lower reoffense rates for treated offenders. Many offenders apparently agree. Kokish, Blasingame, and Plaud (2002) conducted an anonymous survey of 95 sex offenders being treated in three separate programs that use PCSOT regularly and adhere to current standards. Respondents stated by nearly 7-to-1 that periodic polygraph testing was more helpful than harmful. Many commented that being coerced into truthfulness with therapists and fellow group members was a new and positive experience that often carried over into everyday life, making them more honest with loved ones as well. Some said that if their programs stopped testing they would likely return to their former, more devious ways. However, they hoped that testing for the duration of treatment would eventually make honesty easier, perhaps even habitual. Even respondents who reported experiencing erroneous "deception indicated" (DI) ratings on one or more examinations considered polygraphy more helpful than harmful by a ratio of 4.3-to-1.

It appears, then, that polygraph examinations integral to sex offender treatment help achieve the objective of increased honesty within and outside the treatment setting. One study addressed the possibility that learning openness and honesty helps offenders and their loved ones lead more fulfilling lives (Kokish et al., 2002). It found strong, albeit subjective support.

But does increased disclosure during treatment result in better post-treatment outcomes? Many treatment providers assert that full disclosure of deviant sexual history is essential for effective treatment. How, they ask, can we focus on modifying behaviors we are not fully aware of? But, while this assertion has obviously attractive face validity, no controlled studies have been published comparing post-treatment recidivism between programs that use PCSOT and those that do not. Additionally, recidivism rates in Canada and Great Britain, where PCSOT is rarely used, do not appear substantially different from recidivism rates in the United States, where PCSOT is in wider use (Hanson & Bussière, 1996).

ACHIEVING INCREASED TREATMENT
AND SUPERVISION COMPLIANCE

Polygraph examinations have been used to monitor probationers and particularly child abusers since at least 1966 (Consigli, 2001). Abrams (1986) reported on 21 experimental subjects monitored by polygraph between 1983 and 1985, comparing them to 243 comparable control subjects. Sixty-nine percent of the experimental subjects successfully completed their probationary periods, compared to only 26% of controls. This result is all the more remarkable when one considers that polygraph monitoring made experimental subjects more vulnerable than control subjects to detection. The likelihood of false positives in this experiment is mitigated by the fact all Deception Indicated (DI) charts were verified by subsequent admissions. There were no known instances of unreliable "No Deception Indicated" (NDI) charts, but it is of course impossible to ascertain how many experimental subjects successfully lied to examiners. Abrams' (1986) experimental group included seven sex offenders. Five of them (71%) successfully completed probation, compared to only three of the seven sex offender control subjects (43%). Although the small number of experimental subjects limits the value of this investigation, it does provide significant evidence for the effectiveness of polygraph monitoring as a deterrent to reoffending during supervision.

Abrams and Abrams (1993) also cite other studies reflecting impressive probation success rates when offenders (sexual and other) are monitored via polygraphy. For example, 173 polygraphed offenders supervised and treated by sex offender specialists in Jackson County, Oregon, were (a) 95% free of new sex crime convictions, (b) 96% free of new felony convictions, (c) 89% free of any new criminal convictions, and (d) 65% free of parole/probation violations. Unfortunately, although local officials agreed that failure rates would have been considerably higher without polygraphy, the data are weakened by the absence of a control group.

According to Abrams (1993), the Oregon Polygraph Licensing Advisory Committee held two days of public hearings in July of 1990. The majority of those who spoke about sex offender testing were therapists, probation officers, and judges. They almost unanimously agreed about the value of PCSOT and were anxious to avoid proposed restrictions. Altogether, available evidence suggests that polygraph monitoring is an effective way to maximize supervision and treatment compliance while minimizing reoffense risk with sex offenders.

ACCURACY ESTIMATES

That polygraph examinations can generate increased disclosures is not surprising to social scientists. Roese and Jamieson (1993) summarized 20 years of research indicating that a mere belief that questioners have an independent "pipeline" to the truth is an effective way to obtain information that might not be offered up in the absence of that belief. However, belief that polygraph examiners can ascertain truth is obviously not synonymous with an ability to do so. The actual degree of that ability has been hotly debated for nearly a century. As recently as 2001, Iacono (2001) maintained that Comparison Questions Tests (CQT)[2] have no scientific validity. However, Raskin and Honts (2001) argue that CQT sensitivity and specificity likely exceed 90% when charts are scored by examiners who administer the examinations. They also assert that sensitivity is unchanged while specificity remains respectable at 75% when independent examiners score the same charts.

Examining literature relevant to polygraph use by National Security Agencies, the National Research Council of the National Academies (2002) recently concluded, ". . . in populations of examinees such as those represented in the polygraph literature, untrained in counter-measures, specific incidents polygraph tests can discriminate lying from truth telling at rates well above chance, though well below perfection" (p. 4).

For PCSOT specifically, the scientific debate is just beginning. Since PCSOT utilizes virtually no test format other than CQT (Abrams & Abrams, 1993; Blasingame, 1998; Consigli, 2001), the following discussion is limited to the CQT format.

Meaningful consideration of polygraph accuracy should address at least the following issues.

Laboratory versus Field Data

Laboratory studies have the advantage of being able to control conditions so that ground truth is known with absolute certainty. However, since polygraph testing attempts to measure physiological reactions to a psychological phenomenon (fear of being caught in a lie), these studies are often criticized on the basis that laboratory conditions cannot simulate the psychological milieu of real-life testing.

Field studies have the advantage of looking at tests administered under real-life psychological conditions. However, since they look at tests given in cases where ground truth was unknown at time of testing, it is difficult to establish valid criteria for ground truth against which to compare examination results.

All Examiners Are Not Alike

Raskin, Barland, and Podlesny (in Blasingame, 1998), for example, reported a study wherein one examiner was accurate 53% of the time while fellow examiners with the same training were accurate 100% of the time. Many studies agree that examiners who score charts "blindly" (i.e., without interviewing the examinee and administering the actual examination) are usually less accurate than the examiner who administered the test (Raskin & Honts, 2001). This seems to underscore the fact that all examiners are not the same and that "art" may still play a significant role in polygraph accuracy.

All Examinees Are Not Alike

There is general agreement that actively psychotic people are inappropriate polygraph subjects and that test accuracy drops as examinee IQ goes into and below the borderline range (Blasingame, 1998). Guilt complex responding,[3] although an apparently rare phenomenon, cannot always be discounted. During a 10-year period, the present author encountered two suspected guilt complex responders and verified both cases with guilt complex tests (Abrams, 1989a).

All Tests Are Not Alike

Federal law no longer permits private sector pre-employment testing because of its alleged inaccuracy and the serious consequences (i.e., not getting the job) that usually follow from DI charts. Yet, even the most severe polygraph critics like David Lykken acknowledge high accuracy for Guilty Knowledge Tests[4] (Lykken, 1981).

There are four kinds of sex offender tests (California Association of Polygraph Examiners [CAPE], 2001):

1. Specific issue examinations inquire into whether a particular act was committed at a particular time.
2. History examinations inquire into whether the examinee has fully disclosed his/her sexual and/or criminal history to the examiner and/or treatment program.

3. Maintenance examinations inquire into supervision, treatment, or safety plan violations.
4. Monitoring examinations inquire into the commission of unidentified sexual offenses while under supervision or since entering treatment.

Monitoring and maintenance issues have historically been addressed in a single examination (Blasingame, 1998; Consigli, 2001). However, some experts now think that separating those issues will yield more accurate results (K. English, personal communication, November 29, 2001), and some professional organizations are incorporating this belief into their PCSOT standards (CAPE, 2001).

There is general agreement that narrow questions inquiring about specific acts at specific times produce the most accurate test charts. These narrow tests are suitable investigative tools. However, sex offender treatment programs (SOTPs) use polygraphy to obtain information for treatment leverage. Hence, there is a tendency to ask broad questions (e.g., "Since your 18th birthday, have you sexually touched anyone under the age of 18 other than . . . ?"). While generating more information, broad questions can reduce chart accuracy.

Base Rates of Truthfulness and Attempted Deception

Professionals and examinees have distinct though related concerns about test accuracy. Professionals want to know the probability of a particular chart representing that examinee's truthfulness (or lack of it) regarding the relevant questions (i.e., chart accuracy). Examinees already know how well their chart rating matches their truthfulness. What they want to know is the probability of their truthful or deceptive answers being accurately assessed by the examiner on each examination they are required to undergo (i.e., test "sensitivity" and "specificity"). These two sets of probabilities differ from one another. The former varies with base rates of truth telling and deception in the population being examined; the latter does not.

The Federal Government, which often relies on polygraphy for security and intelligence purposes, asked the Office of Technology Assessment (OTA) to conduct a major inquiry into polygraph accuracy and practices (Saxe, Dougherty, & Cross, 1983). OTA investigators found 10 CQT field studies with sufficient scientific merit to warrant inclusion in their analysis. Correct detection of guilt (sensitivity) ranged from 70.6% to 98.6% and averaged 86.3% when inconclusive results were counted as errors. Correct detection of innocence (specificity) ranged from 12.5% to 94.1% and averaged 76% when inconclusive results were counted as errors. The OTA study elected to count inconclusive results as errors on grounds that a guilty or innocent person had not been correctly identified.

However, many experts do not consider inconclusive charts erroneous, arguing that an error is a mistaken belief, while an inconclusive result is a correct belief about the limitation of one's knowledge. Raskin (1988) discarded inconclusive results from OTA's data. He calculated 90% accuracy for detection of guilt and 80% for correct identification of innocent subjects. There have been technological advances since the OTA report. Some more recent reports claim that correct identification of both guilty and innocent examinees exceeds 95% (Forensic Research, 1997; Raskin & Honts, 2001). Nonetheless, the OTA report is still cited as a conservative and reasonable estimate of CQT accuracy.

Laboratory studies included in the OTA report were less accurate. Counting inconclusive results as errors, sensitivity ranged from 35.4% to 100% (mean average 63.7%) and specificity from 32% to 91% (mean average 57.9%). However, when Raskin and Honts (2001) looked at nine laboratory studies conducted between 1978 and 1997, omitting inconclusive charts they arrived at average overall accuracy of 90%. None of these nine studies detected innocent subjects with less than 75% accuracy, although one study only detected guilt at the 53% level. Had Raskin and Honts omitted this "outlier," accuracy would have been even higher.

Altogether, it is fair to say there remains considerable disagreement in the scientific community about the accuracy of CQT polygraph examinations, OTA accuracy estimates (90%/80%) remain approximately midway between the most pessimistic and most optimistic scientific opinions. If SOTPs operate from a working hypothesis that OTA rates are realistic, they appear to have a very good clinical tool; indeed, many respected medical tests are not so accurate. Unfortunately, the matter is not as simple as it first appears, because base rates of truthfulness and deception still have to be accounted for. Consider the following scenario.

An SOTP persuades its participants to answer examiners truthfully on four of every five examinations and tests 100 participants. According to Raskin's OTA projections, 80% (64) of the 80 truthful examinees will be correctly identified and 10% (4) deceptive examinees will be misidentified as truthful, yielding 68 NDI charts. From the program's point of view, over 94% of its truthful charts (64/68) will be accurate and 9 of every 10 lies will be detected. Unfortunately, 16 truthful examinees will be misidentified as deceptive, producing, in combination with 4 correct assessments of deception, 20 DI charts.

Thus, when the base rate of deception is relatively low (10%), many if not most examinees accused of deception will actually have been truthful. Paradoxically, then, the more successful a program is at persuading its participants to be truthful, the higher its false positive rate becomes. To make matters worse, all studies included in the OTA report were based on specific issue examinations about real or mock crimes. Most PCSOT examinations focus on sexual histories or attempt to monitor a range of behaviors over time (e.g., "Since your last examination, have you . . . ?"). Such examinations can be more akin to "screening tests," a format that is considered less accurate than the specific issue examinations typically administered in the criminal justice system (Krapohl, 2001; Saxe et al., 1983).

We have only one scientific study that examined PCSOT accuracy specifically (Kokish et al., 2002). The study asked participants in three SOTPs to complete an anonymous questionnaire that included questions about accuracy. The 95 study participants had taken 333 tests. They reported being truthful on 287 with examiners correctly identifying 265 and misclassifying 22 as DI. They reported attempting deception on 39 examinations, with examiners correctly detecting 28 and misclassifying 11 as NDI. This yields the following accuracy rates:

1. Correct identification of truthful examinees: 92.3% (265/287)
2. Correct identification of deceptive examinees: 71.8% (28/39)
3. NDI chart accuracy: 96.3% (287/298)
4. DI chart accuracy: 66.6% (11/33)

Interestingly, this study differs from most Criminal Justice and Intelligence studies in that reported specificity exceeded sensitivity. This may be a function of repeatedly testing the same group of examinees. The study is of course open to criticism in that offender self-report is, on its face, a poor way to establish ground truth. Nonetheless, the information was carefully collected to insure anonymity, and the accuracy claims are not very far from OTA accuracy rates. Only 12 of these 95 offenders had been in treatment less than a year, and mean time in treatment was nearly 30 months (SD = 18.12 months). We would expect low rates of attempted deception from examinees immersed in a treatment culture that repeatedly reinforces the value of compliance and honesty while quickly sanctioning non-compliance and attempted deception. This expectation is supported by the fact that 85% of charts produced by examinees in these programs were rated NDI by examiners. This is very close to the 90% truthfulness claim from the anonymous respondents themselves. Finally, study credibility is further enhanced in that over 81% of respondents reporting experience with incorrect DI ratings nonetheless said periodic polygraph testing had a positive effect on their therapy and should be continued.

Altogether, available scientific data seem to suggest that SOTPs can have high but not absolute confidence in NDI charts. However, DI charts are more problematic and should be given less weight when case management decisions need to be made.

Critics caution that the coercive nature of polygraph testing may generate false confessions (Cross & Saxe, 1992, 2001). Kokish and colleagues (2002) appear to have conducted the only study that examined this question empirically. Five of 22 individuals (23%) who anonymously reported experiencing incorrect DI ratings said they reacted by admitting things they had not done. Four of these five individuals reported passing their next examination. It seems then that concern over coercing fictitious confessions bears further investigation.

POLYGRAPH IN CONTEXT

Although the term "therapy" is often used, mental health work with sex offenders is distinctly different from traditional psychotherapy. Traditionally, the patient-psychotherapist relationship is voluntary and patient oriented, in that patients take initiative to seek help regarding subjective distress. Sex Offender Treatment (SOT) is more community oriented. Community agents refer offenders because the community perceives the offenders' criminal behavior as a source of distress for others. Traditional patients are free to discontinue treatment at any time. They have discretion to decline certain procedures, and therapists are primarily accountable to their patients. Community agents, however, require sex offenders to remain in therapy regardless of their wishes and may require them to complete procedures they dislike, because the whole purpose of sex offender therapy is to modify "patient" behavior outside the therapy room. This is occurs whether or not the patients are in agreement with the desired modifications.

Sex offender therapists are accountable to their patients for competence and ethical behavior, but are accountable to the community for treatment results. Thus, SOT is, in a word, coercive. Given all this, one could even argue that the term "therapy" is not appropriate for sex offender work. The term "treatment," however, is certainly appropriate when defined simply as acting on something for the purpose of change (e.g., one can "treat" steel to harden or cloth to change its ability to resist stains, etc.).

There is wide consensus in the field that SOT success is improved when change efforts are made, not by a single treatment agent but by a team that has strong community support. This approach has come to be known as the "containment model" (California Coalition on Sexual Offending [CCOSO], 2001). English and Jones (1998) conceptualized Containment Teams as a metaphorical triangle consisting of supervision agents, therapists, and polygraph examiners. Team members engage in a variety of coordinated activities intended to achieve treatment goals and have distinct though overlapping roles. They share information as needed to support one another in fulfilling these roles. They consult regularly to assess progress, identify problems, plan treatment strategies, and make major case decisions.

Polygraphy is rooted in investigative work, but containment based SOTPs use it as a clinical tool for obtaining diagnostic information and to monitor and shape offender behavior outside the treatment setting. Whereas opponents criticize polygraphy for its coercive nature (Cross & Saxe, 1992, 2001), proponents working within a containment framework embrace it for that very reason (English, Jones, Pasini-Hill et al., 2000; English, Jones, Patrick, Pasini-Hill, & Gonzalez, 2000). However, given its coercive nature and still uncertain accuracy, a majority of proponents recognize certain ethical concerns, especially protection from self-incrimination and appropriate responses to DI charts.

Blasingame (1998) addressed these concerns with a list of 16 recommendations for ethical and effective use. The American Polygraph Association (APA) sets national standards for sex offender testing (APA, 1995), some state organizations have followed (CAPE, 2001), and ATSA includes a section on polygraph in its practice standards and guidelines (ATSA, 1997, 2001). The various documents are essentially consistent with one another and generally address the following issues:

1. Maximizing accuracy and reliability by adhering to explicit standards for (a) examiner training and experience; (b) instrumentation and instrument calibration; (c) pre- and post-test interview procedures and formats; (d) chart scoring and interpretation; (e) examinee fitness; and (f) test format, environment, and frequency.
2. Appropriate and inappropriate application for making case decisions.
3. Protecting the treatment setting and examinee by (a) proper advisements and informed consents; (b) accurate record keeping

and secure record storage; (c) limiting privilege and confidentiality in regard to new crimes and program violations; and (d) careful management of disclosures related to criminal acts committed before entering treatment.

The last item (3d) warrants further discussion. SOTPs use polygraph examinations for persuading examinees to disclose information about their behavior. Since allowing offenders to break rules and perhaps even reoffend with impunity would make little sense, there is general agreement that self-disclosure of illicit behavior during supervision and treatment will not remain confidential or privileged (e.g., non-approved contact with a minor). Programs advise participants accordingly, but ask them to disclose illicit behavior anyway. Participants are told that failed examinations will lead to increased surveillance and restrictions as well as thorough investigations, making discovery of illicit behavior quite likely. However, consequences may be mitigated if offenders self-disclose rather than waiting to be independently discovered. This argument can be persuasive within a carefully managed treatment culture. The present author has seen offenders self-report many program violations and even some felonious acts. Additionally, the author has seen several offenders report violations committed by other participants because they were afraid keeping the knowledge to themselves would weigh on their minds, causing them to fail their next examination.

Reporting of pre-treatment crimes is another matter. As we saw earlier in this chapter, what sex offenders are prosecuted for rarely represents the true depth of their deviance or full extent of their criminal behavior. Polygraphy's usefulness as a clinical tool derives from its ability to elicit historical information, presumably allowing psycho-behavioral patterns to be more fully uncovered, better understood, and more effectively managed and changed. However, officially reporting incriminating historical information usually leads to additional prosecution, often ending the very treatment it was designed to enhance. This paradox assumes critical importance because all states have laws requiring therapists to report child abuse to law enforcement.

One way of resolving the dilemma is for local prosecutors to enter into various kinds of immunity agreements with the sex offenders being treated in their jurisdictions (English, Jones, Pasini-Hill et al., 2000). Typically, these immunity agreements stay in effect only so long as offenders comply with supervision and treatment conditions. If conditional release is revoked or, in the prison setting, if the offender is unsuccessfully discharged from treatment, the information can be used as a basis for investigation leading to prosecution.

When no immunity agreement is in place, programs can collect historical information, sans details that identify specific victims. Some programs prefer this strategy, because they believe it is the most effective way of providing the confidentiality necessary for effective treatment. Others prefer the immunity route because it allows for treatment outreach to unreported victims and because they believe encouraging offenders to conceal anything at all supports victim objectification (English, Jones, Pasini-Hill et al., 2000). Some examiners are also concerned that directing offenders to withhold incriminating information could affect test accuracy (K. English, personal communication, November 29, 2001), although this is an empirical issue that should be amenable to scientific inquiry.

When it comes to PCSOT, issues of accuracy and ethics are inseparably intertwined. Many PCSOT proponents believe that adhering to standards will increase accuracy, thereby mitigating ethical dilemmas around managing examinees who produce DI charts. Staunch critics, however, believe that polygraphy is inherently flawed (Oksol & O'Donahue, 2001). They point out that in spite of efforts spanning more than a century, accuracy is still not firmly established. These critics fear that setting standards for such a flawed procedure may yield only a more powerful illusion of scientific credibility and argue that under such circumstances it may be better to avoid polygraphy altogether (Cross & Saxe, 1992, 2001).

WHERE ARE WE NOW, WHERE ARE WE GOING?

Available evidence suggests that PCSOT application is growing in the United States, with between 30-40% of existing SOTPs presently using it. User satisfaction appears high. ATSA sponsors a very active professional e-mail discussion list for credentialed SOT professionals. The list has over 700 subscribers, has been in existence since 1998, and often averages between 10 and 20 posts per day. The present author sent an inquiry to that list asking whether any members who had, at some point, integrated polygraphy into their treatment work became dissatisfied with the procedure and abandoned it. No one responded affirmatively. The one relevant study to date suggests that offenders are nearly as satisfied as professionals (Kokish et al., 2002). However, many issues and questions remain.

Polygraph utility for eliciting information has been studied and is well documented, though Kokish and colleagues (2002) suggest that eliciting false confessions may be a problem in some programs. Accuracy has also been widely studied, but both laboratory and field studies can be criticized, and firmly established accuracy rates remain elusive even for the criminal justice setting. Given psychological theory underlying polygraph practice, it seems likely that accuracy is somewhat context dependent and has simply not been scientifically studied in the PCSOT context. For that context, we have only one study submitted for peer review and nothing published to date. PCSOT-specific research is needed to maximize precision and help resolve ethical dilemmas around managing reportedly deceptive offenders in circumstances where base rates may combine with accuracy limitations to produce high false positive rates.

For the time being then, SOTPs are faced with a series of dilemmas that will have to be endured. Those that choose to incorporate polygraphy will gain much pertinent information about their offender-patients. Arguably, this information can make treatment more effective, helping lower post-treatment reoffense rates and perhaps even contributing to improved quality of life for the offenders and their families. Available information also suggests that polygraph monitoring increases program compliance and serves as a deterrent to reoffending during treatment. But there is no empirical evidence thus far that PSCOT reduces post-treatment recidivism, and programs that employ PCSOT risk generating false admissions and wrongfully sanctioning substantial numbers of program participants whose charts are incorrectly rated as being consistent with attempted deception.

Programs that decline polygraphy will avoid these ethical risks, but will almost certainly have to function with less information about their offender patients. Consequently, they will likely assume a higher risk of undetected program violations and reoffenses during treatment, and perhaps higher rates of post-treatment reoffending. In such circumstances, it falls to each SOTP to determine which advantages and liabilities to choose.

Kohlberg (in Weinrich-Haste, 1983) theorized that moral maturity is characterized by a person's ability to make ethical decisions relevant to context and to recognize and resolve moral dilemmas. It may be then, that those SOT providers who are most uncomfortable with their decision to use or not use polygraphy are modeling high levels of moral maturity for program participants. And it may be that their uncertainty is helping move the field to an ultimately satisfactory, though still elusive, resolution of the dilemmas PCSOT poses for sex offender therapists, supervision officers, examiners, and SOTP participants. Until these dilemmas are resolved, this author offers the following recommendations for ethical PCSOT use to those who choose to include PCSOT in their treatment repertoire:

1. Polygraph efficacy is maximized when examinees experience appropriate positive and negative consequences as a result of the charts they produce. It is advisable to share responsibility for such consequences across several disciplines. Therefore, treatment providers should work as members of Containment Teams (English, 1998).

2. Treatment providers should work with examiners who adhere to training and practice guidelines established by the American Polygraph Association and other professional polygraph organizations.

3. All crimes and rule violations committed during treatment, including but not limited to new crimes, should be immediately reported to appropriate officials. Patients should be informed in writing before beginning treatment that such reports will be made.

4. It is unreasonable to expect offenders to fully disclose as disclosure is likely to lead to additional prosecutions. Therefore, patients should be protected from prosecution for self-disclosed crimes committed prior to beginning treatment. Written use immunity agreements with prosecutors, not collecting victim identities, and legal consultation to patients regarding Fifth Amendment rights can contribute to appropriate protections for patients without unduly jeopardizing community safety.

5. Polygraphy should not be the only form of monitoring used by a treatment team. Other methods such as electronic surveillance, collateral contacts, chemical testing, and unannounced field visits should be employed on a regular basis.

6. NDI charts appear to be highly reliable. Together with other measures of patient progress, NDI charts can play an important role in supporting case management decisions.

7. DI charts do not appear to be as reliable at this time. Their primary value is to highlight a need for cautious case management and to trigger independent investigations of alleged facts and perceived risks. DI charts alone should never be the primary basis for case management decisions that could have significant adverse effects on a patient and/or her/his family.

8. Neither NDI nor DI charts should be used as the sole basis for decisions requiring court action (e.g., probation violations, early termination of probationary status, family reunification).

9. Some patients produce less reliable charts than others. Particular caution is warranted when testing patients who (a) are 13 years of age or younger; (b) manifest impaired reality testing; (c) take medications known to effect the physiological responses on which polygraphy relies; (d) appear unable to produce DI charts even when independent information makes it highly unlikely they are being deceptive; and/or (e) have an IQ less than 80.

10. Polygraph, corrections, and psychotherapy professionals should actively cooperate in joint research and other ventures to enhance PSCOT accuracy, utility, and ethical practice.

NOTES

1. For example, bestiality, giving victim alcohol or drugs, drug abuse on offender's part, urination with sexual act, etc.

2. There are various types of comparison question tests but all ask "relevant" and some form of "comparison" questions. Relevant questions are straightforward, focusing on what the examiner actually wants to find out. Comparison questions are about the same general subject as relevant questions (e.g., sex) but not about specific events relevant to the examination (e.g., whether a particular child's genitals were fondled or how many children the examinee victimized during the previous five years). Truthfulness or deception is inferred from numerical comparison of measured physiological responses to the two types of questions.

3. A "guilt complex responder" (misnamed, because the phenomenon relates less to guilt than anxiety) is an individual who cannot pass a test because of the extreme anxiety generated by the mere question as to whether she/he committed a particular act. A "guilt complex test" utilizes an issue that holds some threat to the examinee while the examiner knows ground truth in advance of the examination. If the truthful subject produces DI charts, he/she is presumed to be a guilt complex responder.

4. A test limited to situations in which only authorities and the guilty individual are likely to have knowledge of certain facts (e.g., the type of gun used in a crime, the number of times a victim was shot, etc.).

REFERENCES

Abrams, S. (1986). Polygraph surveillance of probationers. *Polygraph, 13*(3), 174-182.
Abrams, S. (1989a). *The complete polygraph handbook*. Lexington, KY: Lexington Books.
Abrams, S. (1989b). Probation polygraph surveillance of child abusers. *The Prosecutor, 22*(3), 29-36.

Abrams, S., & Abrams, J. B. (1993). *Polygraph testing of the pedophile* (1st ed.). Portland, OR: Ryan Gwynner Press.

Abrams, S., & Simmons, G. (2000). Post-conviction polygraph testing: Then and now. *Polygraph, 29*(1), 63-67.

Alexander, M. A. (1999). Sexual offender treatment efficacy revisited. *Sexual Abuse: A Journal of Research & Treatment, 11*(2), 101-116.

American Polygraph Association. (1995). *Standards for post conviction sex offender testing: Practice guidelines.* Chattanooga, TN: Author.

Association for the Treatment of Sexual Abusers. (1997). *Ethical standards and principles for the management of sexual abusers.* Beaverton, OR: Author.

Association for the Treatment of Sexual Abusers. (2001). *Practice standards and guidelines for members of the association for the treatment of sexual abusers.* Beaverton, OR: Author.

Blasingame, G. (1998). Suggested clinical uses of polygraphy in community-based sexual offender treatment programs. *Sexual Abuse: A Journal of Research and Treatment, 10*(1), 37-45.

Burton, D. L., & Smith-Darden, J. P. (2000). *1996 nationwide survey of treatment programs and models.* Brandon, VT: Safer Society Foundation.

California Association of Polygraph Examiners. (2001). *CAPE guidelines for clinical polygraph examination of sex offenders: Post conviction.* Redlands, CA: Author.

California Coalition on Sexual Offending. (2001). *Effective management of sex offenders residing in open communities.* Sacramento, CA: Author.

Consigli, J. (2001). Post-conviction sex offender testing and the American polygraph association. In M. Kleiner (Ed.), *Handbook of polygraph testing* (pp. 237-250). New York: Academic Press.

Cross, T. P., & Saxe, L. (1992). A critique of the validity of polygraph testing in child sexual abuse cases. *Journal of Child Sexual Abuse, 1*(4), 19-33.

Cross, T. P., & Saxe, L. (2001). Polygraph testing and sexual abuse: The lure of the magic lasso. *Child Maltreatment, 6*(3), 195-206.

English, K. (1998). The containment approach: An aggressive strategy for the community management of adult sex offenders. *Psychology, Public Policy and Law, 4*(1/2), 218-235.

English, K., Jones, L., Pasini-Hill, D., Patrick, D., & Cooley-Towell, S. (2000). *The value of polygraph testing in sex offender management* (Research Report Submitted to the National Institute of Justice No. D97LBVX0034). Denver, CO: Department of Public Safety, Division of Criminal Justice, Office of Research and Statistics.

English, K., Jones, L., Patrick, D., Pasini-Hill, D., & Gonzalez, S. (2000). We need you to become experts in post-conviction polygraph. *Polygraph, 29*(1), 44-62.

English, K. S. P., & Jones, L. (1998). The containment approach: An aggressive strategy for community management of adult sex offenders. *Psychology, Public Policy, and Law, 4*(1/2), 218-235.

Forensic Research. (1997). *The validity and reliability of polygraph testing* (industry Saturday). Severna Park, MD: American Polygraph Association.

Grossman, L. S., Martis, B., & Fichtner, C. G. (1999). Are sex offenders treatable? A research overview. *Psychiatric Services, 50*(3), 349-361.

Hall, G. C. N. (1995). Sexual offender recidivism revisited: A meta-analysis of recent treatment studies. *Journal of Consulting & Clinical Psychology, 63*(5), 802-809.

Hanson, K. R., & Bussière, M. T. (1996). *Predictors of sexual offender recidivism: A meta-analysis* (No. Cat. No. JS4-1/1996-4E). Ottawa: Public Works and Government Services Canada, Department of the Solicitor General of Canada.

Hanson, K. R., Thornton, D., Gordon, A., Harris, A. J. R., Marques, J. et al. (2002). First report of the collaborative outcome data project on the effectiveness of psychological treatment for sex offenders. *Sexual Abuse, A Journal of Research and Treatment, 14*(2), 169-194.

Hassett, J. (1978). *A primer of psychophysiology.* San Francisco: W. H. Freeman and Company.

Hindman, J., & Peters, J. M. (in press). How polygraphing adult sex offenders can lead us to better understanding the juvenile sex offender. *Federal Probation.*

Iacono, W. G. (2001). Forensic "lie detection": Procedures without scientific basis. *Journal of Forensic Psychology Practice, 1*(1), 75-86.

Kokish, R., Blasingame, G., & Plaud, J. (2002). An exploration of the accuracy, benefits and detriments of post-conviction sex-offender polygraph testing using offender self-report. Manuscript in progress.

Krapohl, D. J. (2001). The polygraph in personnel screening. In M. Kleiner (Ed.), *Handbook of polygraph testing* (pp. 217-236). New York: Academic Press.

Lykken, D. (1981). *A tremor in the blood.* New York: McGraw-Hill.

Oksol, E. M., & O'Donahue, W. T. (2001). *A critical analysis of the polygraph.* Unpublished manuscript.

National Research Council of The National Academies; Division of Behavioral and Social Sciences and Education. (2002). *The polygraph and lie detection.* Washington, DC: Author.

Raskin, D. C. (1988). Does science support polygraph testing? In A. Gale (Ed.), *The polygraph test: Lies, truth and science* (pp. 96-110). Thousand Oaks, CA: Sage Publications.

Raskin, D. C., & Honts, C. R. (2001). The comparison question test. In M. Kleiner (Ed.), *Handbook of polygraph testing* (pp. 1-47). New York: Academic Press.

Roese, N. J., & Jamieson, D. W. (1993). Twenty years of bogus pipeline research: A critical review and meta-analysis. *Psychological Bulletin, 114*(2), 363-375.

Saxe, L., Dougherty, D., & Cross, T. (1983). *Scientific validity of polygraph testing: A research review and evaluation: A technical memorandum* (No. OTA-TM-H-15). Washington, DC: U.S. Congress Office of Technology Assessment.

Weinrich-Haste, H. (1983). Moral development. In R. Harre & R. Lamb (Eds.), *The encyclopedic dictionary of psychology* (pp. 398-400). Cambridge, MA: The MIT Press.

Treatment of Adult Sexual Offenders: A Therapeutic Cognitive-Behavioural Model of Intervention

Pamela M. Yates

SUMMARY. Recent research indicates that, of the various forms of treatment available to sexual offenders, cognitive-behavioural methods are likely to have the greatest impact in reducing rates of sexual re-offending. Cognitive-behavioural treatment typically targets attitudes that support sexual offending, anger management, victim empathy, deviant sexual arousal, and relapse prevention. More recently, treatment has targeted cognitive processes more generally, management of other emotional states in addition to anger, intimacy deficits, and risk self-management (Marshall, Anderson, & Fernandez, 1999; Yates, Goguen, Nicholaichuk, Williams, & Long, 2000). This article describes the components of cognitive-behavioural treatment with sexual

Address correspondence to: Pamela M. Yates, Manager, Sex Offender Programs, Correctional Service of Canada, 340 Laurier Avenue West, Ottawa, ON Canada K1A 0P9 (E-mail: yatespm@csc-scc.gc.ca).

[Haworth co-indexing entry note]: "Treatment of Adult Sexual Offenders: A Therapeutic Cognitive-Behavioural Model of Intervention." Yates, Pamela M. Co-published simultaneously in *Journal of Child Sexual Abuse* (The Haworth Maltreatment & Trauma Press, an imprint of The Haworth Press, Inc.) Vol. 12, No. 3/4, 2003, pp. 195-232; and: *Identifying and Treating Sex Offenders: Current Approaches, Research, and Techniques* (ed: Robert Geffner et al.) The Haworth Maltreatment & Trauma Press, an imprint of The Haworth Press, Inc., 2003, pp. 195-232. Single or multiple copies of this article are available for a fee from The Haworth Document Delivery Service [1-800-HAWORTH, 9:00 a.m. - 5:00 p.m. (EST). E-mail address: docdelivery@haworthpress.com].

offenders, including recent developments, assessment, treatment methods, and the importance of therapist characteristics on the therapeutic process and on treatment outcome. *[Article copies available for a fee from The Haworth Document Delivery Service: 1-800-HAWORTH. E-mail address: <docdelivery@haworthpress.com> Website: <http://www.HaworthPress.com>*

KEYWORDS. Sexual offenders, treatment, assessment, cognitive-behavioural treatment

Sexual aggression, with its significant impact on victims, their families, and the community, is a serious problem and a growing public concern. During the past decade, increased attention has been paid to the problem of sexual violence by the criminal justice system, resulting in substantial increases in the sexual offender population in correctional systems (e.g., Becker, 1994; Becker & Murphy, 1998; Fisher & Beech, 1999; Gordon & Porporino, 1990; McGrath, Hoke, & Vojtisek, 1998; Motiuk & Belcourt, 1996; Prentky, 1995). Given the growing number of sexual offenders within the criminal justice system, there has been a concurrent need for interventions that are effective in reducing the likelihood of sexual re-offending (Becker, Harris, & Sales, 1993; Marshall, 2001; Pithers, 1993).

Treatment has included, either singularly or in some combination, general psychotherapy, organic and physical treatments, such as neurosurgery and physical and chemical castration, pharmacological interventions to reduce sexual arousal, behavioural reconditioning, multi-faceted cognitive-behavioural interventions, and some form of relapse prevention programming (Abel et al., 1984; Abel & Blanchard, 1974; Barbaree & Seto, 1997; Becker & Murphy, 1998; Bradford, 1985, 1990; Cooper, 1986; Fedoroff, Wisner-Carlson, Dean, & Berlin, 1992; Freeman-Longo & Knopp, 1992; Grossman, Martis, & Fichtner, 1999; Hansen & Lykke-Olesen, 1997; Heim & Hursch, 1979; Langevin, 1983; Laws, 1989; Laws & Marshall, 1990; Lockhart, Saunders, & Cleveland, 1989; Maletzky, 1980, 1991; Marques, Day, Nelson, & Miner, 1989; Marques, Day, Nelson, & West, 1994; Marshall, Jones, Ward, Johnson, & Barbaree, 1991; McGrath et al., 1998; Meyer, Cole, & Emory, 1992; Pithers & Cumming, 1989). These interventions have demonstrated varying degrees of success in terms of treatment outcome, including re-offense rates with recent, sex offender specific, skills-based, cognitive-behavioural programs appropriately matched to offender risk and need demonstrating the greatest efficacy in reducing recidivism (Barbaree & Seto, 1997; Hanson, 1999; Hanson et al., 2002; Looman, Abracen, & Nicholaichuk, 1999; Marques et al., 1989; Marques et al., 1994; Marshall, Eccles, & Barbaree, 1991; McGrath et al., 1998; Nicholaichuk, Gordon, Gu, & Wong, 2000).

More recently, treatment of sexual offenders has been revised to include models of self-regulation (Ward & Hudson, 2000a, 2000b; Ward, Hudson, & Keenan, 1998) and self-management (Yates, Goguen, Nicholaichuk, Williams, & Long, 2000), and attention has been paid to the therapeutic processes and methods by which treatment is implemented (Fernandez, Marshall, Serran, Anderson, & Marshall, 2001; Marshall, Anderson, & Fernandez, 1999; Yates et al., 2000). Finally, a variety of approaches have been utilized with special populations of sexual offenders, such as holistic approaches with First Nations and female sexual offenders (e.g., Correctional Service of Canada, 2001a, 2001b), and family and systems interventions with juvenile sexual offenders (e.g., Becker et al., 1993; Becker & Hunter, 1997).

The present article provides an overview of a comprehensive cognitive-behavioural approach to the treatment of adult male sexual offenders. Prior to describing this model, a brief review of the importance of attending to risk, need, and responsivity factors is discussed. Finally, two relatively recent developments are described, namely, the self-regulation model and the influence of process issues and therapist characteristics on the effectiveness of treatment.

RISK, NEED, AND RESPONSIVITY FACTORS IN SEXUAL OFFENDER TREATMENT

As indicated above, research suggests that cognitive-behavioural treatment of sexual offenders may be effective in reducing recidivism rates, as compared to control groups of untreated or otherwise treated sexual offenders (Alexander, 1999; Hall, 1995; Hanson et al., 2002; Nicholaichuk et al., 2000). However, research has also found differential treatment effects for different types of offenders and for offenders with different levels of risk (e.g., Alexander, 1999; Hanson & Bussière, 1998; Nicholaichuk, 1996; Nicholaichuk et al., 2000). Given this evident heterogeneity among sexual offenders, appropriate and effective treatment is that which is differentially applied based upon offenders' individual risk and need levels, and which is implemented taking into account individual dynamic risk factors and responsivity issues. These principles and their implementation in practice are described below.

It is well documented in the general criminal behaviour literature that effective interventions are those that are matched to offender risk, need, and responsivity characteristics (Andrews & Bonta, 1998). Risk, which varies across individual offenders and groups of offenders, refers to the likelihood or probability that an individual will commit an offense. *Risk factors* are those factors that are known, both generally and for individual offenders, to be associated with variation in the probability of committing an offense or a re-offense. The presence or absence of these factors will increase or decrease the probability of occurrence of an offense. When changed through some form of intervention such as treatment, these risk factors are associated with concurrent changes in the likelihood of re-offending, either increasing or decreasing this probability (Andrews & Bonta, 1998).

A distinction is made between static and dynamic risk factors. *Static risk factors* are those that cannot be influenced or changed through intervention, such as previous offense history and age. *Dynamic risk factors*, or criminogenic needs, are those factors which are also associated with risk to offend, but which can be changed through intervention and which, when changed, are associated with changes in the likelihood of offending sexually (Andrews & Bonta, 1998). The need principle of effective correctional intervention states that the most effective interventions are those that target these criminogenic needs (Andrews & Bonta, 1998; Gendreau & Goggin, 1996, 1997; Gendreau, Little, & Goggin, 1996).

Among sexual offenders, several static and dynamic risk factors have been reliably found to be associated with variations in rates of sexual offending. Static risk factors for sexual offending include (a) a prior history of sexual and non-sexual offending, (b) early onset of sexual offending behaviour, (c) young age (under 25 years), (d) never having been married, (e) diversity in sexual offenses, (f) a history of non-contact sexual offenses, (g) non-sexual violence in addition to sexual violence at the time of the offense, (h) previous violent offenses, (i) having unrelated, male, stranger, or child victims, and (j) previous treatment failure or non-completion (Hanson, 2000; Hanson & Bussière, 1998; Hanson & Thornton, 1999).

Dynamic risk factors for sexual offending include (a) attitudes supportive of sexual offending, (b) cognitive distortions, (c) deviant sexual preference or arousal, (d) sexually deviant lifestyle, (e) intimacy deficits, (f) deficits in sexual and general self-regulation, (g) negative mood, (h) lack of community support, (i) impulsivity, (j) release to high risk circumstances in the community, (k) compliance with community supervision, (l) compliance with treatment, (m) tendency toward interpersonal aggression, (n) criminal personality, (o) intimacy and relationship problems, (p) viewing oneself as low risk, (q) antisocial lifestyle, (r) access to victims, and (s) possibly, substance abuse (Gordon, Nicholaichuk, Olver, & Wong, 2000; Hanson, 2000; Hanson & Thornton, 1999; Haynes, Yates, Nicholaichuk, Gu, & Bolton, 2000).

Although there is overlap, it is important to note that the predictors of sexual recidivism will be differentially evident for individual offenders and will also differ from the predictors of non-sexual violent and non-violent offending. Specifically, more general factors, such as juvenile delinquency, unemployment, and antisocial personality, are associated with general, rather than sexual, recidivism, while sexual offending specific factors, such as deviant sexual preference, are associated with sexual re-offending. Some factors, such as psychopathy, are associated with both sexual and non-sexual violent recidivism (Hare, 1999; Seto & Barbaree, 1999). In addition, sexual offenders are more likely to re-offend non-violently and violently (non-sexually) than they are to re-offend sexually (Hanson & Bussière, 1998; Motiuk & Brown, 1996; Nicholaichuk et al., 2000). As such, in addition to variations in risk for sexual offending among individuals and groups of offenders, risk for specific criminal acts can also vary (Hanson & Bussière, 1998).

Given that many risk factors for sexual offending are known through research, risk can be said to be predictable and can therefore be influenced through intervention, including treatment (Andrews & Bonta, 1998). The principle of attending to risk suggests that the most intensive levels of intervention should be reserved for higher risk offenders, while lower levels of intervention or no intervention should be applied to lower risk offenders. Treatment of offenders, including sexual offenders, has been found to be most effective for higher risk offenders (Andrews & Bonta, 1998; Gendreau & Goggin, 1996, 1997; Gendreau et al., 1996; Gordon & Nicholaichuk, 1996), while treatment of lower risk offenders has a lesser likelihood of demonstrating a treatment effect (Nicholaichuk, 1996), and is not the best use of limited financial and personnel resources (Prentky, 1995; Prentky & Burgess, 1990).

Finally, in addition to matching risk and targeting criminogenic needs, effective interventions are those that are applied according to the responsivity principle, which states that interventions should be delivered in a manner that is consistent with offenders' learning styles and abilities (Andrews & Bonta, 1998; Gendreau & Goggin, 1996, 1997; Gendreau et al., 1996). In the treatment of offenders, individual responsivity factors, such as language, culture, personality style and disorders, mental disorders, intelligence, anxiety levels, and cognitive abilities, can affect the manner in which the offender interacts with the treatment process and, in turn, can influence the effectiveness of the intervention for that offender. According to the responsivity principle, treatment must be varied and adapted according to these learning styles–that is, tailored to meet the needs and abilities of offenders in order to maximize the potential effectiveness of the intervention and to reduce the likelihood of re-offending.

In treatment of sexual offenders, attending to risk, need, and responsivity factors implies that interventions are applied at a rate and frequency that is appropriate to individual offenders. In practice, this involves offering a variety of treatment programs, at varying levels of intensity, matched to the risk and need levels of sexual offenders participating in the program (Andrews & Bonta, 1998; Hanson, Yates, & Marshall, 2000). Within a given treatment program, regardless of intensity level, it is important to attend to responsivity factors by using a variety of implementation styles, continually working to find methods which are most effective with individual offenders (Fernandez et al., 2001; Yates et al., 2000). Thus, treatment providers must be flexible and must adapt their style and mode of service delivery so as to maximize engagement with treatment on the part of the offender. This principle is reviewed in more detail in a later section.

ASSESSMENT OF SEXUAL OFFENDERS

Given the above, effective treatment of sexual offenders begins with assessment of risk, need, and responsivity to determine the most appropriate intervention for individual offenders. Prior to commencing treatment, assessment of static and dynamic risk factors, including the use of actuarial measures, must be conducted in order to determine the offender's long-term level of risk to re-offend and, thus, the level of intervention that has the maximum likelihood of effecting change for a given offender (i.e., the risk principle). Once the most appropriate level of intervention is established, assessment of dynamic risk factors, or criminogenic needs, is conducted to establish treatment targets for that individual, which forms the basis of intervention with the client (i.e., the need principle). Finally, responsivity issues are evaluated and plans for addressing these during treatment are developed (Yates et al., 2000).

Assessment should be conducted both prior to and following treatment, with changes in dynamic risk factors, progress with respect to intermediate treatment targets, and risk for recidivism, each re-evaluated on the basis of treatment performance. In the community, the individual's circumstances, such as community support, willingness to comply with supervision, access to victims, and so forth, are also evaluated to assess risk of re-offending and to establish post-treatment follow-up and supervision needs. This also includes elucidation of the conditions under which the offender can be expected to manage his risk to re-offend, as well as the conditions under which risk would be expected to increase for a particular offender (Yates et al., 2000). Finally, as there is variation in sexual, non-sexual violent, and non-violent re-offending among sexual offenders, as described above, risk in each of these areas should be evaluated separately (Hanson & Bussière, 1998).

A variety of actuarial measures have been developed to measure static and dynamic risk for sexual recidivism, such as the Rapid Risk Assessment of Sexual Recidivism (RRASOR; Hanson, 1997), Static 99 (Hanson & Thornton, 1999), Structured Anchored Clinical Judgment-Minimum (SACJ-Min; Grubin, 1998), Violence Risk Appraisal Guide (VRAG; Quinsey, Harris, Rice, & Cormier, 1998), Minnesota Sex Offender Screening Tool (MnSOST; Huot, 1997), Sexual Violence Risk Scale (SVR-20; Boer, Wilson, Gauthier, & Hart, 1997), Sex Offender Need Assessment Rating (SONAR; Hanson & Harris, 2000b), and Violence Risk Scale: Sex Offender Version (VRS:SO; Gordon et al., 2000). While a complete discussion of each of these tools is beyond the scope of the present article, these are some of the tools which may be used to assess risk, determine appropriate program placement, evaluate changes in risk following intervention, and to re-assess risk. For example, the SONAR includes both chronic and acute dynamic risk factors for sexual offending and may be used throughout treatment to assess changes in immediate risk as well as to aid in supervision of the offender.

Polygraph is also increasingly used in the treatment and management of sexual offenders, despite inconsistent support for the reliability and validity of this tool (e.g., Blasingame, 1998). It has been suggested that this tool may be promising for the supervision of sexual offenders (Wilcox, 2000) since it increases the amount and nature of information available to the probation or parole officer providing supervision to the offender. In so doing, polygraph may aid in risk assessment and perhaps in treatment as well (Blasingame, 1998; Wilcox, 2000). However, research has not yet assessed the impact of the use of polygraph on treatment outcome, particularly recidivism. As such, it is not known whether treatment programs utilizing this procedure demonstrate significantly different outcome as compared to those not using this procedure. More research is needed to determine the utility of polygraph in the treatment of sexual offenders.

In addition to assessment of sexual offense risk, treatment planning and post-treatment risk assessment and evaluation should include assessment of risk for non-sexual violent and non-violent (general) re-offending since, as indicated previously, sexual offenders are more likely to reoffend non-sexually than sexually, and because sexual offender subtypes vary in their rates of re-offending. It should also be noted that, while the baseline rate of re-offending among sexual offenders is relatively low, this tends to increase over time (Hanson, Steffy, & Gauthier, 1993). As such, it is important to re-assess risk over the long-term in order to maximize public safety. It is also important to assess risk using multiple methods, given the programs associated with establishing rates of recidivism among this group of offenders (Yates, 2002).

COGNITIVE-BEHAVIOURAL TREATMENT OF SEXUAL OFFENDERS

This section provides a review of the components of cognitive-behavioural treatment programs designed for adult sexual offenders. It should be noted that this is an overview, and does not describe specific treatment methodologies. In addition, adjunctive interventions, such as pharmacological interventions, and treatment for special needs sexual offenders, such as juvenile, mentally disordered, cognitively impaired, or female sexual offenders are beyond the scope of this article and are also not reviewed, although components of cognitive-behavioural treatment may be applied to these groups. For additional information, the reader is referred to Marshall and colleagues (1999) and Yates and colleagues (2000). Finally, a distinction is made between *treatment* of sexual offenders and *supervision* of these offenders. While both are integral to the effective management of sexual offenders, the discussion that follows describes elements of treatment and does not address the external supervision, for example, by parole or probation officers, of these offenders.

Cognitive-behavioural treatment is based on social learning theory (Bandura, 1986) and, as indicated previously, is the most widely accepted and effective type of intervention with sexual offenders (Barbaree & Seto, 1997; Becker & Murphy, 1998; Freeman-Longo & Knopp, 1992; Laws, 1989; Looman et al., 1999; Marshall et al., 1991; Marshall et al.,

1999; Nicholaichuk et al., 2000; Yates, 2002). Cognitive-behavioural interventions are based on the premise that cognitive processes and behaviour are linked, and that cognition influences behaviour. Within this model, sexual offending is viewed as a pattern of behaviour that has developed and been maintained through learning and reinforcement and that results from entrenched maladaptive responses and coping mechanisms. Cognitive-behavioural interventions, therefore, aim to replace maladaptive or deviant responses with adaptive, prosocial beliefs and behaviour by targeting specific areas in which offenders are deficient. Cognitive-behavioural interventions also involve skills acquisition and rehearsal, reducing cognitive distortions, developing effective problem-solving strategies, improving social and victim perspective-taking, improving sexual and social relationships, managing affective states, reducing deviant sexual arousal, and developing adaptive thinking processes, affect, and behaviour (Marshall et al., 1999; Yates et al., 2000). In addition, there is a strong focus on skills acquisition and rehearsal of both existing adaptive skills and new skills learned during treatment. Extensive rehearsal is required, as new skills require considerable practice and repetition in order to become well entrenched in the individual's behavioural repertoire (Hanson, 1999).

The following discussion provides an introduction to the components of cognitive-behavioural treatment programs with sexual offenders, based upon reviews of the literature and existing treatment programs (e.g., Marshall et al., 1999; Yates et al., 2000). What follows is a discussion of components typically included in cognitive-behavioural treatment of adult male sexual offenders in both institutional (e.g., prison) and community settings.

Cognitive distortions and cognitive processes. More than two decades of research have well established the notion that attitudes and beliefs, and their resulting cognitive processes, have a direct influence on behaviour, including sexual offending behaviour (Hanson & Scott, 1995; Johnston & Ward, 1996; Ward, Hudson, Johnston, & Marshall, 1997). Cognitive distortions reflect attitudes and beliefs that support sexual aggression and that facilitate the occurrence of sexual offending by reducing cognitive dissonance, providing justification for offending, and allowing the offender to absolve himself of responsibility for his actions and to grant himself permission to engage in the offending behavior. Examples of cognitive distortions include blaming the victim, denying or minimizing the harm caused by behaviour, and rationalizing sexual aggression. Targeting cognitive distortions is based upon the assumption that underlying learned attitude and belief systems, and the resultant cognitions, play a significant role in the instigation and continuation of sexually assaultive behaviour among both offenders against adults and children (Abel et al., 1984; Hanson, Gizzarelli, & Scott, 1994; Hanson & Scott, 1996; Johnston & Ward, 1996; Laws, 1989; Marshall & Pithers, 1994; Murphy, 1990; Plaud & Newberry, 1996; Stermac & Segal, 1989).

It is important to note that global cognitive processes are hypothesized as being similar for both sexual offenders and non-offenders (Ward, Hudson, Johnston, & Marshall, 1997). Specifically, the combination of distorted beliefs, attitudes, and affective components (e.g., deviant sexual arousal, heightened emotional arousal) associated with sexual offending are regulated by normal cognitive operations that result in the offending behaviour. In other words, the distorting process is one that is common to most people. However, the difference between offenders and non-offenders lies in the content and specific distortions surrounding a given behaviour, in this instance, sexual aggression.

Although there is some discrepancy in the literature, research supports the notion that sexual offenders generally demonstrate some aspects of cognitive distortions and/or distorted underlying belief systems which support sexual aggression (Hanson et al., 1994; Marolla & Scully, 1986; Pollack & Hashmall, 1991; Stermac & Segal, 1989; Veach, 1999; Ward et al., 1997). Thus, one important component of cognitive-behavioural treatment for sexual offenders involves addressing cognitive distortions and their underlying attitudinal and belief structures, as well as changing global thinking processes generally (Becker & Murphy, 1998; Marshall et al., 1999; Yates et al., 2000). Cognitive-behavioural treatment of cognitive distortions involves challenging and altering these beliefs and replacing them with ones that do not support sexual aggression, as well as changing global dysfunctional thinking patterns, such as impulsivity.

Victim empathy. Empathy is postulated to regulate behaviour by functioning as a mechanism that inhibits aggression and by its association with prosocial and altruistic behaviour (Hildebran & Pithers, 1989; Miller & Eisenberg, 1988; Moore, 1990; Pithers, 1993; Prentky, 1995). With regard to sexual offending behaviour, it is hypothesized that a lack of empathy facilitates sexual offending by permitting cognitive distortions that allow sexual offending to occur despite clear indications of distress on the part of the victim (Marshall, O'Sullivan, & Fernandez, 1996). Thus, lack of empathy, at least indirectly, may be associated with sexual offending (Barbaree & Marshall, 1991; Mulloy, Smiley, & Mawson, 1997; Rice, Chaplin, Harris, & Coutts, 1994).

Although empathy has traditionally been regarded as an important target of treatment for sexual offenders and is included in many treatment programs (Knopp, Freeman-Longo, & Stevenson, 1992; Pithers, 1993; Schwartz, 1992; Wormith & Hanson, 1992), there is controversy regarding the appropriateness of this treatment target. This controversy arises in part from equivocal research support regarding its efficacy in reducing the likelihood of sexual aggression, and in part from a lack of a consistent definition of the construct of empathy. Specifically, although some studies suggest that empathy can be positively influenced by treatment, as evidenced by changes on measures of empathy pre- to post-treatment (e.g., Pithers, 1994; Williams & Khanna, 1990), other research indicates that sexual offenders do not consistently demonstrate empathy deficits, as compared to other non-sexual offenders or non-offender populations (Hudson et al., 1993; Langevin, Wright, & Handy, 1988; Pithers, 1994; Rice et al., 1994). Similarly, research is inconsistent with respect to the relationship between empathy deficits, empathy enhancement, and recidivism.

Empathy has been variously regarded as either a trait or disposition or, alternatively, as a process of perspective-taking which is dependent upon situational elements. Many theorists regard empathy as an innate trait that is assumed to be displayed across most, if not all, situations and toward most, if not all, persons (Marshall et al., 1996). Empathy as a trait, therefore, is viewed as non-specific to an individual or situation and as an innate characteristic that is either exhibited in all situations and toward all persons, or not at all. It is difficult, however, to design a treatment component capable of changing such a trait-like disposition. When empathy is viewed as a state that is changeable across individuals and circumstances rather than as a trait, however, there appears to be some value in targeting empathy in treatment. As a state, empathy may be defined as the cognitive ability to understand and identify with another's perspective and the emotional capacity to experience the same feelings as another (Marshall et al., 1996; Pithers, 1994). Empathy may also be conceptualized as an interaction between cognitive, affective, and behavioural factors and as a behaviour that is learned in a socio-cultural context. When viewed in this way, it is easy to see how empathy may be influenced by factors such as cognitive distortions, negative emotions, deviant sexual arousal, and other factors known to be associated with sexual offending. Thus, although the research is equivocal, when empathy is defined as a response or a state which varies across situations and which influences other known factors for sexual offending, empathy may be an appropriate target of treatment for sexual offenders.

It has also been suggested that targeting victim-specific empathy, rather than general empathy, may be more relevant to sexual offenders (Marshall et al., 1999). Although this is a relatively recent perspective, research suggests that this approach to empathy with sexual offenders may have some merit. For example, research has found that child molesters appear to demonstrate significantly greater empathy deficits toward victims of their own sexual offenses, as compared to levels of empathy toward the victims of others' sexual offenses or empathy in a non-sexual context (Fernandez, Marshall, Champagne, Brown, & Miller, 1997; Fernandez, Marshall, Lightbody, & O'Sullivan, 1999; Marshall, Champagne, Sturgeon, & Bryce, 1997; Marshall et al., 1996). Similar findings have been found among rapists (Marshall et al., 1999). Given that sexual offenders may not demonstrate global empathy deficits, but rather deficits specifically in relation to victims of their own offenses, it has been suggested that rather than a lack of empathy *per se*, these deficits may be evidence of cognitive distortions which aid the offender in avoiding the personal distress, cognitive dissonance, and threats to self-esteem associated with the sexual offending behaviour (Marshall et al., 1999). Conversely, for other offenders, such as sadistic sexual offenders, the ability to identify victim distress and harm can facilitate sexual aggression by meeting the specific needs of the offending behaviour (i.e., to inflict harm and humiliate) and by supporting cognitive distortions. Thus, what appears to be a lack of empathy on the part of sexual offenders may, in fact, represent cognitive processes and distortions (Marshall et al., 1999). In support of this theory, cognitive distortions and lack of empathy have been found in research to be strongly correlated with each other (Marshall et al., 1999), and treatment that aims at increasing empathy also reduces cognitive distortions (e.g., Bumby, 1994; Pithers, 1994).

In summary, although there is a sound theoretical rationale for the inclusion of a component targeting empathy among sexual offenders in cognitive-behavioural treatment, treatment processes to achieve this are typically unclear and ill defined (Marshall et al., 1999). Although the research support is equivocal at present, it is suggested that empathy is best conceptualized as a constellation of factors, including perspective-taking, the emotional capacity to experience another's feelings, and an interaction between cognition, affect, behaviour, and the environment. In this context, empathy is considered as variable and changeable depending upon context, is linked to cognitive distortions, and is potentially victim-specific. Thus, specific targets for treatment can be delineated, and the offender can develop and rehearse skills in these areas.

Intimacy and relationships. Early treatment programs were based upon the assumption that sexual offenders displayed deficits in general social skills, such as communication or assertiveness (Becker & Murphy, 1998; Marshall, 1996). More recent research suggests, however, that social functioning deficits among sexual offenders are more specific, and include deficits in the areas of intimacy and attachment, self-confidence in relationships, self-esteem, loneliness, and coping with stress (Cortoni, Heil, & Marshall, 1996; Cortoni & Marshall, 1995; Garlick, Marshall, & Thornton, 1996; Keenan & Ward, 2000; Marshall, 1996; Marshall et al., 1996; Marshall et al., 1999; Marshall, Serran, & Cortoni, 2000; Seidman, Marshall, Hudson, & Robertson, 1994; Smallbone & Dadds, 2000; Ward, Hudson, Marshall, & Siegert, 1995; Ward, Keenan, & Hudson, 2000). In addition, these intimacy deficits among sexual offenders appear to generalize to a pervasive lack of intimacy in all relationships (Bumby & Hansen, 1997).

It is hypothesized that as a result of early developmental and learning experiences, sexual offenders develop inadequate attachment styles, resulting in an inability to relate to others, ineffective ways of relating to others, apprehension in relationships, and lack of satisfaction in relationships (Fernandez et al., 2001; Marshall et al., 1999; Ward et al., 2000). Attachment patterns that reflect fear or rejection of relationships result in loneliness and a lack of intimacy, which has been shown by research to be predictive of sexual aggression (Fernandez et al., 2001; Marshall et al., 1999). Research has also found that sexual offenders are more lacking in intimacy and suffer from greater loneliness than either other types of offenders or non-offenders (Marshall et al., 1999). In fact, sexual offenders against children describe their desire to offend as motivated by a need for affection, intimacy, and closeness (Finkelhor, 1986; Hudson, Wales, & Ward, 1998; Ward, Hudson, & France, 1993).

Research also indicates that self-esteem is significantly lower in sexual offenders than in matched controls (Marshall, 1996; Marshall & Mazzucco, 1995) and that improved self-esteem following treatment is significantly correlated with changes in other treatment targets, such as empathy, intimacy, loneliness, and deviant sexual preference (Marshall, Champagne, Brown et al., 1997; Marshall, Champagne, Sturgeon et al., 1997). In addition, sexual offenders are characterized by a lack of self-confidence, brought about by a variety of events, including the commission of the offense itself, as well as the erosion of dignity and self-respect resulting from the personal, social, and legal processes they have experienced (Marshall, 1996). These events and lack of self-confidence can facilitate cognitive distortions and justifications for offending behaviour (Marshall, 1996). In this manner, low self-esteem may be a contributing factor to the maintenance of sexual offending behaviour (Fernandez et al., 2001; Marshall et al., 1999; Marshall & Barbaree, 1990). In addition, low self-esteem or lack of self-efficacy (Bandura, 1977), that is, a belief that one is not capable of change, can inhibit the change process. In order to change their cognitive and behavioural patterns, sexual offenders must have the requisite confidence to give up beliefs, which while dysfunctional and favorable to sexual offending, are nonetheless, secure to the individual (Marshall, 1996).

As indicated above, sexual offenders tend to have a variety of relationship and intimacy deficits, and frequently lack the skills necessary to develop and maintain relationships and intimacy. In addition, sexual offenders may also have difficulty identifying and managing emotions and coping with stress, and may use sex as a strategy to cope with stress and negative affect (Cortoni et al., 1996; Cortoni & Marshall, 1995). For example, a rapist who is angry but is unable to express this anger may use coercive sexuality as a mechanism by which to express and cope with this anger. Some offenders may also use sex to relieve feelings of boredom or anxiety, for example, the individual who masturbates several times a day and does little else to address these emotional states. For this individual, sex offers temporary relief from negative feelings. However, for those individuals with deviant sexual arousal, negative feelings often intensify to the point at which masturbation is no longer effective in reducing symptoms, and other forms of sexual activity that may be more arousing (and more distracting) are sought, a process which may serve to increase risk to offend sexually. Although the notion that sexual offenders may use sex as a coping strategy is presently at the theoretical stage, this is worth exploration with sexual offenders, with treatment focusing on the development of more adaptive coping methods and strategies.

Emotion management. Because sexual violence was initially presumed to result predominantly from anger, many programs for sexual offenders have included an anger management component as part of treatment. While it is true that some sexual offenders are, at least in part, motivated by anger in the commission of their offenses, it has become evident that a variety of other emotional states and processes are associated with sexual offending behaviour at various stages during an offense (Hall & Hirschman, 1991; Johnston & Ward, 1996; Marshall, Hudson, Jones, & Fernandez, 1995; Ward, Louden, Hudson, & Marshall, 1995). These may include either negative or positive affective states or both (Johnston & Ward, 1996).

Different types of offenders are characterized by different affective states at different times throughout the offending process. For example, some offenders exhibit consistently high levels of positive affect throughout their sexual offenses (Johnston & Ward, 1996). For these offenders, sexual offending behaviour is likely to occur more frequently because it is desirable and pleasurable and is, therefore, positively reinforced. Other offenders are driven to deviant sexual behaviour in an attempt to escape negative emotional states (Ward, Louden et al., 1995) or due to a lack of affective control. For example, pedophiles who report low self-esteem, lack of confidence or fear in relationships with adults, or loneliness, may feel more comfortable with children and, through relationships with children, can avoid the negative emotions associated with relationships with adults. Sexual offending behaviour is positively reinforcing, therefore, as it alleviates these negative affective states, at least temporarily. Conversely, some sexual offenders anticipate sexually aggressive behaviour and achieve gratification from the behaviour, thereby also rendering the behaviour reinforcing.

The manner in which sexual offenders experience and manage emotions òther than anger, however, has received comparatively little attention in research and clinical practice. This has occurred despite the widely held opinion that sex offenders are generally lacking in the skills necessary to effectively identify and manage emotions (Miner, Day, & Nafpaktitis, 1989) and the knowledge that an individual's ability to cope with negative affect plays a major role in an individual's general psychological well-being when confronted with negative or stressful life events (Endler & Parker, 1990). In addition, negative emotional states other than anger, such as anxiety, guilt, and loneliness, are often reported by offenders to be precursors to sexual offending and to be associated with deviant sexual arousal and fantasy (Hanson & Bussière, 1998; McKibben, Proulx, & Lusignan, 1994). Given these findings, addressing a variety of emotional states in treatment is warranted if sexual offenders with emotional control deficits are to develop skills to manage the various emotional states that may be associated with sexual offending behaviour.

Deviant sexual preference. Deviant sexual arousal and preference are hypothesized to develop as a result of early developmental factors, observational learning, modeling, reinforcement, early pairing of deviant stimuli with sexual arousal, and cognitive processes such as attitudes, which influence the development of sexual behaviour (Abel & Rouleau,

1986; Hanson, 1999; Laws & Marshall, 1990). Once it occurs, deviant sexual behaviour, including sexual offending behaviour, may later be used in fantasy and masturbation. Therefore, it may continue to be associated with positive reinforcement, thereby increasing the probability of continued deviant arousal to inappropriate stimuli and subsequent sexual offending behaviour (Abel & Rouleau, 1986).

It is important to note that the behavioural pairing of deviant stimuli with sexual arousal does not represent the full picture with respect to the development and expression of deviant sexual preference and arousal. Rather, research indicates that deviant sexual arousal *per se* does not explain sexual offending behaviour, but that deviant sexual arousal occurs in conjunction with cognitive and affective factors which result in the expression of sexually aggressive behaviour (Blader & Marshall, 1989; McKibben et al., 1994; Proulx, 1993). More specifically, sexually aggressive behaviour occurs as a function of a host of contextual, affective, and cognitive factors, such as the expression of anger (Groth, 1979), humiliation and degradation of the victim (Marshall & Darke, 1982), negative mood (McKibben et al., 1994; Proulx, McKibben, & Lusignan, 1996), self-esteem (Marshall et al., 1999), power and control (Yates, 1996), sexual preference (Johnston, Ward, & Hudson, 1997) and alcohol intoxication (Barbaree, Marshall, Yates, & Lightfoot, 1983).

Early treatment interventions for sexual offenders focused predominantly on treating deviant sexual preferences using behavioral methods. This was assumed to be the sole or primary motivation for sexual aggression (Marshall et al., 1999). However, these interventions are now reserved for those sexual offenders displaying deviant sexual preference and arousal, and are implemented within comprehensive cognitive-behavioural treatment including other components such as those described within this article, as well as adjunctive medical interventions where required (e.g., Bradford, 1990; Marshall, Eccles et al., 1991). Thus, research supports a broader, more integrated approach to treatment than targeting deviant sexual preference or arousal in isolation (Barbaree & Marshall, 1991; Langevin, Lang, & Curnoe, 1998; Marshall, Eccles et al., 1991; Proulx et al., 1996).

Deviant sexual preference or arousal is typically assessed prior to treatment using phallometric assessment. If present, sexual arousal reconditioning techniques are implemented to reorient arousal to appropriate stimuli. It is important to note that phallometric procedures suffer from substantial methodological and psychometric limitations, including unreliability and lack of validity, and should be interpreted with caution. A review of these limitations is beyond the scope of the present article. For a thorough review, the reader is referred to Fernandez and Marshall (2000). Assessment of sexual interest (Abel, 1995; Abel, Huffman, Warberg, & Holland, 1998) has been proposed as an alternative to phallometric assessment in the measurement of deviant sexuality. Rather than measuring changes in penile tumescence in response to stimuli, visual response time is measured as an indicator of sexual interest in lieu of sexual arousal. While this area may be promising, research suggests that this measure may not be superior to phallometric assessment and that additional evaluation is required (e.g., Fischer & Smith, 1999; Letourneau, 2002).

Research is equivocal with respect to the reliability and validity of phallometric and sexual interest procedures, as well as whether or not deviant sexual arousal can, in fact, be reduced through treatment. The impact of arousal reconditioning practices on recidivism in the long-term is also questionable, and these practices are replete with ethical and professional concerns. Nonetheless, there is some evidence that methods such as covert sensitization and aversion therapy may be associated with positive post-treatment outcome, including reduced recidivism (Haynes, Yates, & Nicholaichuk, 1998; Haynes et al., 2000; Maletzky, 1980, 1991; Quinsey, Chaplin, & Carrigan, 1980; Quinsey & Marshall, 1983). In addition, given that deviant sexual preference is a strong predictor of recidivism (Hanson & Bussière, 1998), treatment should attempt to address this risk factor when it is present.

Self-management. The theory of self-regulation of behaviour among sexual offenders was developed as an alternative to traditional relapse prevention approaches in order to overcome deficiencies in this model (Hudson & Ward, 1996a, 1996b; Ward & Hudson, 1998, 2000a, 2000b; Ward et al., 1998; Ward, Louden et al., 1995). Relapse prevention was initially developed as a follow-up intervention for continuing abstinence from addictive behaviours achieved during treatment (Marlatt, 1982; Marlatt & Gordon, 1985; Miller, 1980) and was subsequently applied to sexual offenders (Anechiarico, 1998; George & Marlatt, 1989; Hanson, 1996; Hudson & Ward, 1996a, 1996b; Knopp et al., 1992; Laws, 1995; Marshall et al., 1999; Wormith & Hanson, 1992). It is important to note that, although relapse prevention was developed as a follow-up to treatment and was not designed to comprise a treatment approach, it has been routinely applied in both treatment and follow-up programming contexts with sexual offenders.

The application of the relapse prevention model to sexual offenders has been problematic and has been criticized for a variety of reasons. Specifically, over time, it has become evident that sexual offending behaviour is less similar to addictive behaviour than had been previously believed (Marshall et al., 1999; Marshall & Marshall, 1998). There is no clear evidence to suggest that the dynamics of sexual offending behaviour follow the same processes of abstinence, lapse, and relapse as addictive behaviours (Marshall et al., 1999). In addition, theoretical inconsistencies in the structure of the model (Ward & Hudson, 1996, 1998, 2000a; Ward, Hudson, & Marshall, 1994; Ward, Louden et al., 1995) and lack of flexibility and lack of applicability of concepts to some sexual offenders (Ward, Louden et al., 1995), have led to the misapplication of constructs and intervention procedures in treatment programs for sexual offenders (Marshall & Anderson, 1996). Although various modifications to the model have been made by several authors (e.g., Laws, 1989, 1995; Marques, 1982; Pithers, Marques, Gibat, & Marlatt, 1983; Ward, Hudson et al., 1995), the traditional relapse prevention approach within sexual offender treatment programs remains problematic. Finally, empirical support for the effectiveness of this model in the treatment of sexual offending is limited (Marshall & Anderson, 1996; Marshall et al., 1999; Ward & Hudson, 1998, 2000a, 2000b; Ward, Hudson, & Siegert, 1995).

Hudson, Ward, and their colleagues have developed an alternative approach to the traditional relapse prevention model, which was specifically designed for sexual offenders (Hudson & Ward, 1996b; Ward & Hudson, 1998, 2000a; Ward et al., 1998; Ward, Louden et al., 1995). This model, a self-regulation model, is reviewed briefly below. For a more comprehensive review of this model and its operationalization with sexual offender treatment, see Ward and Hudson (2000a) and Yates and colleagues (2000), respectively.

The self-regulation model is a nine-stage model which includes perceptions, cognitive distortions, proximal planning of the offense, and post-offense evaluation of behaviour. Whereas traditional relapse prevention approaches focus predominantly on negative emotional states associated with the undesirable behaviour (alcohol or drug addiction), Ward and Hudson's model of self-regulation allows for both positive and negative emotional states and evaluations in the offense process. Thus, this model addresses pathways to sexual offending which have traditionally been ignored in research, theory, and intervention with sex offenders, and approaches sexual offending behaviour from a broader perspective (Ward & Hudson, 2000a).

According to the model, sexual offending results from the manner in which behaviour is self-regulated by the individual. Specifically, the individual's behaviour may be disinhibited as a function of a failure to control behaviour or emotional states. Alternatively, individuals may misregulate their behaviour through the use of ineffective strategies for achieving goals, resulting in a loss of control. Finally, self-regulation may not be dysfunctional but, rather, based upon problematic or inappropriate goals. The first two processes reflect what has been traditionally applied in treatment with sexual offenders, with treatment focusing upon managing negative emotions and learning effective strategies to cope with negative life events or skill deficits. The third process, however, speaks to approach behaviour on the part of sexual offenders whose aim is to engage in offending behaviour, typically to achieve a specific goal, such as sexual gratification. This latter process has typically not been addressed with sexual offenders in treatment, and appears to be more common among some sexual offenders, particularly sexual offenders against children (Ward & Hudson, 2000a).

A central tenet in the self-regulation model involves the delineation of various pathways that individuals may follow during a given sexual offending sequence and that vary both across and within individuals (Ward & Hudson, 2000a). Specifically, individuals may have *approach* or *avoidance* goals with respect to sexual offending behaviour. Approach goals are focused upon achieving a desired state, whereas avoidance goals are focused upon avoiding an undesired state (Ward & Hudson, 2000a). For example, offenders with approach goals approach sexual offending behaviour with a specific goal, such as gratification or the alleviation of negative emotional states. In these cases, the individual is not attempting to refrain from offending. By contrast, offenders with avoidance goals attempt to prevent themselves from offending sexually; however, they lack the skills necessary to do so or do not utilize these skills in a particular situation (i.e., loss of control).

In attempting to achieve either approach or avoidance goals, individuals may be comparatively active or passive in their efforts. Specifically, offenders may variously attempt to approach or avoid offending, and may do so in a manner that is relatively passive, automatic, or explicit, depending upon whether the individual's goal is to offend or to avoid offending. For example, while the goal of individuals following an avoidant pathway is to avoid offending, these individuals may either make no active efforts to avoid engaging in an offense or pre-offense behaviour (passive) or, alternatively, these individuals may engage in behaviours designed to avoid offending (active) but which are ineffective. By contrast, the goal of individuals following an approach pathway may be achieved either impulsively (automatic) or in a manner which is predatory and which involves careful planning of the offense (explicit).

Taken together, the four pathways to sexual offending behaviour described by Hudson and Ward and their colleagues (avoidant-passive, avoidant-active, approach-automatic, and approach-explicit) explain the various dynamics and motivations of sexual offending. In addition, individuals may change pathways as the offense progression unfolds, for example, by switching from an avoidance strategy to approaching offending (Ward & Hudson, 2000a).

This self-regulation model has several advantages over the traditional relapse prevention approach with sexual offenders. First, the model is more applicable to this population, as it has been developed specifically from research with sexual offenders. In addition, the model more accurately allows for examination of the various motivations and dynamics of sexual offending, and is considerably more flexible. The model also allows for both positive and negative affective states to be associated with sexual offending behaviour, and for a more active decision-making role on the part of the individual. The model acknowledges that the dynamics and motivations to offend may change over time, with history, or during a given offense progression. With respect to treatment, this model allows for greater integration of the number and variety of risk factors an individual offender may present. In addition, the model allows for increased opportunities for intervention and for the development of strategies to prevent re-offending. Finally, rather than focussing solely upon deficits, as has been traditional in the treatment of sexual offenders, this model also allows treatment to focus upon existing strengths and self-regulation skills that an individual offender may possess and, thus, provides greater opportunity to rehearse and reinforce these pre-existing skills.

The self-regulation model developed by Ward and Hudson and colleagues has been operationalized for implementation as the core component of treatment within a cognitive-behavioural treatment program for sexual offenders within the Correctional Service of Canada (Yates et al., 2000). Treatment focuses upon both assisting offenders to understand their progression to sexual offending and the various pathways followed in this progression. Offenders analyze their previous sexual offenses in a structured manner to determine the various dynamics and motivations for offending. This is a systematic analysis that includes perceptions, interpretations of events, cognitive distortions and cognitive processes, affective states associated with offending, and deviant sexual arousal and fantasy. This analysis also includes individuals' pathways to offending behaviour, decision-making during the progression to offending, and points during the progression when the offenders were inhibited from acting out.

Each of these processes is specifically linked for individual offenders to the other components described above, in a personalized and individualized analysis of the progression to offending. Once the offender has developed a comprehensive understanding of his patterns of behaviour, cognition, and affect, and the relationship of these to sexual offending behaviour and dynamics, he then develops offense-specific strategies for preventing a return to sexual offending behaviour. A strong emphasis is placed both on the development of new strategies and the reinforcement of existing strategies, as it is not assumed that offenders are deficient in all areas. Rather, offenders' existing skills and those factors that have inhibited aggression in the past are delineated and reinforced. A strong emphasis is also placed upon rehearsing new and existing prosocial skills, as considerable time and practice is required to entrench new behaviours and to reach the point at which these skills for self-managing behaviour are as well-entrenched as misregulation skills have been (Hanson, 1999). Finally, offenders prepare individualized self-management plans to prevent re-offending, based upon their analysis of the behavioural progression to offending.

In this plan, which includes strategies to intervene at all potential points during the progression, offenders develop strategies to avoid situations that may present a risk for re-offending, to effectively cope with problematic or high-risk situations as they arise, and to change goals with respect to sexual offending (Yates et al., 2000). The focus of self-management planning involves the delineation of prosocial goals and strategies to achieve these goals, rather than solely on avoiding problematic or high-risk situations, as such approach goals are more easily attainable than avoidance goals (Mann, 1998). Finally, there is a strong reliance on reinforcement of prosocial and non-offending verbalizations and behaviour made by the offender. When treatment is provided in the community, these plans are shared with those individuals providing supervision to the offender as part of a comprehensive management strategy of the offender.

Post-treatment follow-up programming. Treatment for sexual offenders should not continue indefinitely, but should be followed by some form of maintenance follow-up programming. As described above, the goal of treatment is to effect change on specific treatment targets for individual offenders, and to reduce the risk for future re-offending. In so doing, treatment will vary in intensity, duration, frequency, and treatment targets, according to the risk and need levels of offenders. Once the goals of treatment have been met (i.e., the offender has made sufficient progress and demonstrates the ability to manage his risk to offend), treatment should be terminated, and follow-up maintenance programming instituted. For those offenders who demonstrate sound abilities to manage their risk and for whom supervision will be a sufficient intervention, follow-up programming will not be required. When implemented, maintenance can entail follow-up after release to the community from a prison-based program, or follow-up programming which continues after completion of community-based treatment. This follow-up typically includes a combination of maintenance programming by sex offender therapists and supervision by probation or parole staff. Research indicates that the risk that some sexual offenders pose to re-offend increases over time, as evidenced by studies with longer follow-up periods (Hanson et al., 1993), so extended follow-up, particularly supervision, may be required with some offenders.

Although there is little research on the impact of follow-up maintenance programming, there is a high degree of consensus among researchers and therapists with regard to the benefits of maintenance, and many treatment programs for sexual offenders routinely include a follow-up or maintenance element (Cumming & McGrath, 2000; Green, 1995; Hanson & Harris, 2000a; Laws, Hudson, & Ward, 2000; Marshall et al., 1999; Spencer, 1999; Wilson, Stewart, Stirpe, Barrett, & Cripps, 2000; Yates et al., 2000). Of the few studies that have been conducted, findings are generally promising in that combining supervision with community intervention has been found to be effective in preventing a return to sexual offending, improving the manageability of the offender during supervision, and in reducing the rates of post-intervention recidivism (McGrath et al., 1998).

Within prison settings, maintenance is provided to ensure that treatment gains do not erode before release. To facilitate the generalization of skills beyond the institution, reinforcement must also take place in the community, as the effects of treatment may decrease over time without ongoing supervision and intervention in the community (Cumming & McGrath, 2000). Thus, it is suggested that a combination of supervision and maintenance programming is the most effective approach for the management of sex offenders in the community (Cumming & McGrath, 2000).

PROCESS ISSUES IN TREATMENT OF SEXUAL OFFENDERS

Each of the components of treatment described above form a comprehensive cognitive-behavioural intervention for sexual offenders based upon research suggesting appropriate targets of treatment for this heterogeneous group. Providing effective intervention to sexual offenders to reduce re-offending and the likelihood of future victimization requires not only treatment components validated by research, but also attention to the processes and dynamics of treatment. Until recently, the importance of process issues, the working relationship between the client and therapist, and a therapeutic approach to working with sexual offenders have been ignored, despite substantial evidence that this approach accounts for considerable variance in treatment outcome among non-correctional populations (Fernandez et al., 2001; Marshall et al., 1999). Specifically, in the areas of addictions, depression, mental health, and therapy, research clearly indicates that therapist characteristics and approach are integral to effective treatment (Fernandez et al., 2001; Marshall et al., 1999). In addition, rapport among group members and with the therapist, the establishment of a positive therapeutic working alliance, and group cohesiveness, have each been long known to be important to the effectiveness of treatment (e.g., Budman, Soldz, Demby, Davis, & Merry, 1989; Yalom, 1985).

Creating a positive and therapeutic treatment atmosphere and attending to process issues in treatment requires a commitment on the part of the therapist to the belief that treatment is effective and that sexual offenders can change, as well as abandoning the traditionally held punitive approach to these offenders. This latter approach derives from the belief that these offenders cannot change and that they are fundamentally dishonest (Fernandez et al., 2001; Frank, 1971, 1973; Marshall et al., 1999; Quinsey, Khanna, & Malcolm, 1996). This punitive treatment approach frequently results in an aggressive, confrontational style of relating to the offender, forcing the offender to accept the label of sexual offender, and creating power struggles between the therapist and the offender (Fernandez et al., 2001; Marshall et al., 1999). Such interactions result in increased resistance to treatment, argumentativeness (both on the part of the offender and the therapist), denial, decreased self-esteem and self-confidence on the part of the offender, and lack of cooperation and compliance with treatment (Fernandez et al., 2001; Marshall et al., 1999). A punitive, confrontational style of relating also erodes or completely prevents the development of a positive therapeutic working alliance between the therapist and the offender. Each of these results can negatively affect treatment progress (Fernandez et al., 2001; Marshall et al., 1999), leading to insufficient reductions in risk to re-offend or in non-completion of treatment, both of which can obviously function to increase the risk of future victimization.

Since research clearly indicates that offenders who do not complete treatment re-offend at significantly higher rates than offenders who complete treatment (Hanson & Bussière, 1998; Hanson et al., 2002), the importance of a treatment process which functions to keep offenders in treatment is immediately evident. As such, a confrontational style can result in limited benefits from treatment and, in fact, has been found to have a significant negative impact in both non-offender and offender populations (Annis & Chan, 1983; Beech & Fordham, 1997; Fernandez et al., 2001; Kear-Colwell & Pollack, 1997; Lieberman, Yalom, & Miles, 1973; Marshall et al., 1999; Miller, 1995; Miller & Sovereign, 1989). Importantly, this aggressive, confrontational style of treatment also renders the therapist's work with sexual offenders, which can be challenging at the best of times, all the more difficult.

Attending to process issues in the treatment of sexual offenders also entails attending to the characteristics and training of therapists. Recently, a variety of therapist characteristics and behaviours have been shown to maximize treatment gains (Fernandez et al., 2001; Marshall et al., 1999; Marshall, Mulloy, & Serran, 1998). These include empathy, respect, warmth, friendliness, sincerity, genuineness, directness, confidence, and interest in the client. An effective therapist is also one who is a prosocial model, who communicates clearly, who is appropriately self-disclosing, rewarding, encouraging, and non-collusive, who deals appropriately with frustration and other difficulties, and who spends an appropriate amount of time on issues, asks open-ended questions, and is appropriately challenging without being aggressively confrontational (Fernandez et al., 2001). Effective therapists actively listen to their clients, support their clients without being collusive, are open and interested in their clients, hold and express the belief that the client is capable of change, create opportunities for success, motivate the offender to change, and create a treatment atmosphere which is secure for the offender (Fernandez et al., 2001; Marshall et al., 1998; Marshall et al., 1999). It is evident that establishing security, safety, and openness in treatment is extremely important with sexual offenders, given the nature of their offenses and the degree of self-disclosure required during treatment. Other hypothesized important therapist features include trustworthiness, acceptance, supportiveness, flexibility, emotional responsiveness, ability to enhance clients' self-esteem, and the creating of favorable expectancies during treatment (Fernandez et al., 2001; Marshall et al., 1998; Marshall et al., 1999).

These characteristics and features allow the therapist to challenge offenders on important risk factors, such as cognitive distortions, without being collusive and without creating a negative, unproductive, and punitive treatment atmosphere. In addition, the value of such characteristics is readily evident. For example, if we expect clients to adopt prosocial attitudes and behaviour and to demonstrate empathy, it is evident that we as therapists must model and display such characteristics. In addition, the processes and features described in this section are essential to the development and maintenance of self-esteem, which is hypothesized to be important to both the treatment process and the reduction of risk to re-offend (Fernandez et al., 2001; Marshall et al., 1999). A complete discussion of the influence of self-esteem and its relationship to the process and features of treatment for sexual offenders is beyond the scope of this article. However, Marshall and colleagues (1999) provide a thorough review of this area, as well as process issues in treatment generally.

In addition to the general processes described above, it is important that therapists reinforce positive and prosocial expressions made by the client during treatment (Fernandez et al., 2001). Traditionally, as a result of the punitive approach to sexual offenders, therapists have focussed predominantly or solely upon offenders' deficits and upon negative expressions and behaviours, ignoring existing strengths, skills, and prosocial verbalizations and behaviour. This has occurred despite the knowledge that, according to basic principles of learning, reinforcement of desired behaviour is more effective in developing and maintaining the behaviour than is punishment of undesirable behaviour (Akers, 1985). Thus, if we are to effect positive change, it is essential that therapists reinforce desired behaviours and successive approximations of these behaviours, in accordance with principles of effective reinforcement (Fernandez et al., 2001). That is, to be effective, reinforcement of a desired behaviour must immediately follow the behaviour, must be contingent upon the behaviour, must be proportional to the behaviour, and must be relevant to the individual receiving the reinforcement (Fernandez et al., 2001).

It has been argued that sexual offenders do not demonstrate verbalizations and behaviours which are prosocial and which could, therefore, be reinforced. Obviously, this is not always the case. However, for those offenders who demonstrate predominantly negative behaviour, it is the responsibility of the therapist to create opportunities for the offender to demonstrate positive behaviour that the therapist then reinforces immediately, while concurrently ignoring the negative behaviour (Fernandez et al., 2001). This process simultaneously functions to extinguish the undesirable behaviour and increase the probability that the desirable behaviour will recur.

Part of this process in treatment also involves examination of those situations in which the individual *did not* offend, which have historically been ignored in treatment. That is, sexual offenders do not offend all the time, but rather have had periods, often lengthy, during which they did not engage in sexual offending behaviours. As such, one goal of treatment is to uncover the skills the individual used during these periods of non-offending behaviour, and to build upon and reinforce these skills in order to increase the likelihood of engaging in *non-offending* behaviour in the future (Yates et al., 2000). As can be seen, this is a significant change from the orientation and processes to which treatment programs for sexual offenders typically adhere. However, it is a change that is associated with a greater likelihood of success (Fernandez et al., 2001; Marshall et al., 1999).

In addition to increasing the possibility of a positive treatment outcome, a therapeutic approach to the treatment of sexual offenders is more compatible with the self-regulation or self-management model of treatment described above. Specifically, while traditional relapse approaches have held a negative orientation and have focussed on avoidance goals, the more positive self-management orientation allows for the development of approach goals to prosocial behaviour, which are more readily attained than avoidance goals (Mann, 1998). That is, in attempting to prevent a return to sexual offending behaviour, it is easier for offenders to approach and successfully achieve a prosocial goal than it is to sustain avoidance of problematic or high-risk situations over the long-term. With approach goals, prosocial non-offending skills are more likely to be reinforced and to become habitual elements of the behavioural repertoire than are avoidance behaviours. As indicated above, the self-management approach focuses on building, strengthening and reinforcing skills and allowing individuals to meet their needs in prosocial ways, rather than simply avoiding situations that may pose a risk.

This section provides only a very brief overview of process issues and important therapist characteristics. However, the importance of these issues cannot be overstated. The goal of treatment for sexual offenders is to reduce the likelihood of re-offending and the future victimization of others. Community safety is a foremost concern for therapists providing this important service to this sometimes difficult client group, and therapists strive to ensure that the treatment they provide is as effective as possible. Providing effective treatment not only involves appropriately addressing risk, need, and responsivity factors, and implementing treatment based upon what is known to be effective in the research literature. It also entails providing treatment in a manner which will be most productive and which will allow the offender to maximize progress and reduce risk. Recent research and theorizing suggests that the most effective approach is to abandon traditionally held punitive and confrontational approaches to treatment and to adopt an approach that is more therapeutic.

EFFECTIVE INTERVENTION: AN INTEGRATED MODEL

In conclusion, research indicates that cognitive-behavioural, skills- based treatment for sexual offenders is effective in reducing re-offending. Treatment effects are also enhanced when attention is paid to the process of treatment and therapist characteristics in addition to the content and procedures utilized. The foundation of treatment is based upon pre-treatment assessment of risk, need, and responsivity, and treatment is variously applied depending upon the outcome of this assessment. Higher levels of intervention are reserved for higher risk offenders, and targets of treatment and treatment goals are individualized and personalized for individual offenders. Follow-up maintenance programming is utilized in order to maintain and strengthen treatment gains, to resolve difficulties and problems as they arise, and to reinforce non-offending behaviour. It is integrated into the supervision of sexual offenders in the community as part of a comprehensive management strategy of the offender.

With respect to process issues in treatment, sexual offender therapists should be selected on the basis of those characteristics of effective therapists described above. Furthermore, they should be well-trained in assessment, treatment, and the use of positive therapeutic techniques to maximize treatment gain and, hence, reduce the probability of re-offending. Finally, a self-management model of treatment has been proposed which overcomes some of the problems associated with the traditional relapse prevention model and which is more amenable to a positive therapeutic approach to treatment. Treatment involves the development and reinforcement of new skills, as well as reinforcement of existing skills, to prevent a reoccurrence of sexual offending to aid in achieving the ultimate goal of reduced victimization.

REFERENCES

Abel, G. G. (1995). *Abel screening system manual.* Atlanta, GA: Abel Screening Inc.

Abel, G. G., Becker, J. V., Cunningham-Rathner, J., Rouleau, J., Kaplan, M., & Reich, J. (1984). *The treatment of child molesters.* Atlanta, GA: Behavioral Medicine Laboratory, Emory University.

Abel, G. G., & Blanchard, E. B. (1974). The role of fantasy in the treatment of sexual deviation. *Archives of General Psychiatry, 30,* 467-475.

Abel, G. G., Huffman, J., Warberg, B., & Holland, C. L. (1998). Visual reaction time and plethysmography as measures of sexual interest in child molesters. *Sexual Abuse: A Journal of Research and Treatment, 10*(2), 81-96.

Abel, G. G., & Rouleau, J. L. (1986). Sexual disorders. In G. Winokur, & P. Clayton (Eds.), *The medical basis of psychiatry* (pp. 246-267). Philadelphia: W.B. Saunders.

Akers, R. L. (1985). *Deviant behavior: A social learning approach* (3rd ed.). Belmont, CA: Wadsworth.

Alexander, M. A. (1999). Sexual offender treatment efficacy revisited. *Sexual Abuse: A Journal of Research and Treatment, 11,* 101-116.

Andrews, D. A., & Bonta, J. (1998). *The psychology of criminal conduct.* Cincinnati, OH: Anderson.

Anechiarico, B. (1998). A closer look at sex offender character pathology and relapse prevention: An integrative approach. *International Journal of Offender Therapy and Comparative Criminology, 42*(1), 16-26.

Annis, H. M., & Chan, D. (1983). The differential treatment model: Empirical evidence from a personality typology of adult offenders. *Criminal Justice and Behaviour, 10,* 159-173.

Bandura, A. (1977). Self-efficacy: Toward a unifying theory of behaviour change. *Psychological Review, 84,* 191-215.

Bandura, A. (1986). *Social foundations of thought and action: A social cognitive theory.* Englewood Cliffs, NJ: Prentice-Hall.

Barbaree, H. E., & Marshall, W. L. (1991). The role of male sexual arousal in rape: Six models. *Journal of Consulting and Clinical Psychology, 59,* 621-630.

Barbaree, H. E., Marshall, W. L., Yates, E., & Lightfoot, L. O. (1983). Alcohol intoxication and deviant sexual arousal in male social drinkers. *Behaviour Research and Therapy, 21,* 365-373.

Barbaree, H. E., & Seto, M. C. (1997). Pedophilia: Assessment and treatment. In D. R. Laws, & W. T. O'Donoghue (Eds.), *Sexual deviance: Theory, assessment, and treatment* (pp. 175-193). NewYork: Guilford.

Becker, J. V. (1994). Offenders: Characteristics and treatment. *The Future of Children, 4,* 176-197.

Becker, J. V., Harris, C. D., & Sales, B. D. (1993). Juveniles who commit sexual offenses: A critical review of research. In G. C. N. Hall, & R. Hirschman (Eds.), *Sexual aggression: Issues in etiology, assessment, and treatment* (pp. 215-228). Washington, DC: Taylor and Francis Group.

Becker, J. V., & Hunter, J. A. (1997). Understanding and treating child and adolescent sexual offenders. *Advances in Clinical Child Psychology, 19*, 177-197.

Becker, J. V., & Murphy, W.D. (1998). What we know and do not know about assessing and treating sex offenders. *Psychology, Public Policy, and Law, 4*, 116-137.

Beech, A., & Fordham, A. S. (1997). Therapeutic climate of sexual offender treatment programs. *Sexual Abuse: A Journal of Research and Treatment, 9*, 219-237.

Blader, J. C., & Marshall, W. L. (1989). Is assessment of sexual arousal in rapists worthwhile? A critique of current methods and the developments of a response compatibility approach. *Clinical Psychology Review, 9*, 569-587.

Blasingame, G. D. (1998). Suggested clinical uses of polygraphy in community-based sexual offender treatment programs. *Sexual Abuse: A Journal of Research and Treatment, 10*, 37-45.

Boer, D. P., Wilson, R. J., Gauthier, C. M., & Hart, S. D. (1997). Assessing risk of sexual violence: Guidelines for clinical practice. In C. D. Webster, & M. A. Jackson (Eds.), *Impulsivity: Theory, assessment, and treatment* (pp. 326-342). New York: Guilford Press.

Bradford, J. M. W. (1985). Organic treatments for the male sexual offender. *Behavioural Sciences and the Law, 3*, 355-375.

Bradford, J. M. W. (1990). The antiandrogen and hormonal treatment of sex offenders. In W. L. Marshall, & H. E. Barbaree (Eds.), *Handbook of sexual assault: Issues, theories, and treatment of the offender* (pp. 297-310). New York: Plenum.

Budman, S. H., Soldz, S., Demby, A., Davis, M., & Merry, J. (1989). What is cohesiveness? An empirical examination. *Small Group Research, 24*, 199-216.

Bumby, K. (1994, November). *Cognitive distortions of child molesters and rapists.* Paper presented at the 13th Annual Research and Treatment Conference of the Association for the Treatment of Sexual Abusers, San Francisco, CA.

Bumby, K., & Hansen, D.J. (1997). Intimacy deficits, fear of intimacy, and loneliness among sex offenders. *Criminal Justice and Behaviour, 24*, 315-331.

Cooper, A. J. (1986). Progesterones in the treatment of male sex offenders: A review. *Canadian Journal of Psychiatry, 31*, 73-79.

Correctional Service of Canada. (2001a). *Women who sexually offend: A protocol for assessment and treatment.* Ottawa, ON: Correctional Service of Canada.

Correctional Service of Canada. (2001b). *Tupiq: Corrections for inuit offenders.* Kingston, ON: Correctional Service of Canada.

Cortoni, F., Heil, P., & Marshall, W. L. (1996, November). *Sex as a coping mechanism and its relationship to loneliness and intimacy deficits in sexual offending.* Paper presented at the 15th Annual Research and Treatment Conference of the Association for the Treatment of Sexual Offenders, Chicago, IL.

Cortoni, F., & Marshall, W. L. (1995, October). *Childhood attachments, juvenile sexual history and adult coping skills in sex offenders.* Paper presented at the 14th Annual Research and Treatment Conference of the Association for the Treatment of Sexual Abusers, New Orleans, LA.

Cumming, G. F., & McGrath, R. J. (2000). External supervision. In D. R. Laws, S. M. Hudson, & T. Ward (Eds.), *Remaking relapse prevention with sex offenders: A sourcebook* (pp. 236-253). Thousand Oaks, CA: Sage.

Endler, N. S., & Parker, D. A. (1990). Multidimensional assessment of coping: A critical evaluation. *Journal of Personality and Social Psychology, 58*(5), 844-854.

Fedoroff, J. P., Wisner-Carlson, R., Dean, S., & Berlin, F. S. (1992). Medroxy-progesterone acetate in the treatment of paraphilic sexual disorders: Rate of relapse in paraphilic men treated in long-term group psychotherapy with or without medroxy-progesterone acetate. *Journal of Offender Rehabilitation, 18*, 109-123.

Fernandez, Y. M., & Marshall, W. L. (2000). Phallometric testing with sexual offenders: Limits to its value. *Clinical Psychology Review, 20*, 807-822.

Fernandez, Y. M., Marshall, W. L., Lightbody, S., & O'Sullivan, C. (1999). The child molester empathy measure. *Sexual Abuse: A Journal of Research and Treatment, 11*, 17-31.

Fernandez, Y. M., Marshall, W. L., Serran, G., Anderson, D., & Marshall, L. (2001). *Group process in sexual offender treatment.* Ottawa, ON: Correctional Service of Canada.

Finkelhor, D. (1986). *A sourcebook on child sexual abuse.* Beverly Hills, CA: Sage.

Fischer, L., & Smith, G. (1999). Statistical adequacy of the Abel assessment for interest in paraphilias. *Sexual Abuse: A Journal of Research and Treatment, 11*, 195-205.

Fisher, D., & Beech, A. R. (1999). Current practice in Britain with sexual offenders. *Journal of Interpersonal Violence, 14*, 240-256.

Frank, J. D. (1971). Therapeutic factors in psychotherapy. *American Journal of Psychotherapy, 25*, 350-361.

Frank, J. D. (1973). *Persuasion and healing* (2nd edition). Baltimore, MD: Johns Hopkins University Press.

Freeman-Longo, R. E., & Knopp, H. F. (1992). State-of-the-art sex offender treatment: Outcome and issues. *Annals of Sex Research, 5*, 141-160.

Garlick, Y., Marshall, W. L., & Thornton, D. (1996). Intimacy deficits and attribution of blame among sexual offenders. *Legal and Criminological Psychology, 1*, 251-258.

Gendreau, P., & Goggin, C. (1996). Principles of effective correctional programming. *Forum on Corrections Research, 8*, 38-41.

Gendreau, P., & Goggin, C. (1997). Correctional treatment: Accomplishments and realities. In P. Van Voorhis et al. (Eds.), *Correctional counseling and rehabilitation* (pp. 271-279). Cincinnati, OH: Anderson.

Gendreau, P., Little, T., & Goggin, C. (1996). A meta-analysis of the predictors of adult offender recidivism: What works! *Criminology, 34*, 3-17.

George, W. H., & Marlatt, G. A. (1989). Introduction. In D. R. Laws (Ed.), *Relapse prevention with sex offenders* (pp. 1-31). New York: Guilford.

Gordon, A., & Nicholaichuk, T. (1996). Applying the risk principle to sex offender treatment. *Forum on Corrections Research, 8*, 36-38.

Gordon, A., Nicholaichuk, T., Olver, M., & Wong, S. (2000). *The violence risk scale: Sex offender version.* Saskatoon, SK: Correctional Service of Canada.

Gordon, A., & Porporino, F. J. (1990). *Managing the treatment of sexual offenders: A Canadian perspective* (Research Report No. B-05). Ottawa, ON: Correctional Service of Canada.

Green, R. (1995). Comprehensive treatment planning for sex offenders. In B. K. Schwartz, & H. R. Cellini (Eds.), *The sex offender: Corrections, treatment and legal practice* (pp. 10-1 to 10-8). New Jersey: Civic Research Institute.

Grossman, L. S., Martis, B., & Fichtner, C. G. (1999). Are sex offenders treatable? A research review. *Psychiatric Services, 50,* 349-361.

Groth, A. N. (1979). The adolescent sexual offender and his prey. *International Journal of Offender Therapy and Comparative Criminology, 21,* 249-254.

Grubin, D. (1998). *Sex offending against children: Understanding the risk.* Police Research Series Paper 99. London: Home Office.

Hall, G. C. N. (1995). Sexual offender recidivism revisited: A meta-analysis of recent treatment studies. *Journal of Consulting and Clinical Psychology, 63,* 802-809.

Hall, G. C. N., & Hirschman, R. (1991). Toward a theory of sexual aggression: A quadripartite model. *Journal of Consulting and Clinical Psychology, 59,* 662-669.

Hansen, H., & Lykke-Olesen, L. (1997). Treatment of dangerous sexual offenders in Denmark. *Journal of Forensic Psychiatry, 8,* 195-199.

Hanson, R. K. (1996). Evaluating the contribution of relapse prevention theory to the treatment of sexual offenders. *Sexual Abuse: A Journal of Research and Treatment, 8,* 201-208.

Hanson, R. K. (1997). *The development of a brief actuarial risk scale for sexual offense recidivism* (User Report 97-04). Ottawa: Department of the Solicitor General of Canada.

Hanson, R. K. (1999). Working with sex offenders: A personal view. *Journal of Sexual Aggression, 4,* 81-93.

Hanson, R. K. (2000). *Risk assessment: Association for the treatment of sexual abusers (ATSA) information package.* Beaverton, OR: Association for the Treatment of Sexual Abusers.

Hanson, R. K., & Bussière, M. (1998). Predicting relapse: A meta-analysis of sexual offender recidivism studies. *Journal of Consulting and Clinical Psychology, 66,* 348-362.

Hanson, R. K., Gizzarelli, R., & Scott, H. (1994). The attitudes of incest offenders: Sexual entitlement and acceptance of sex with children. *Criminal Justice and Behavior, 21,* 187-202.

Hanson, R. K., Gordon, A., Harris, A. J. R., Marques, J. K., Murphy, W., Quinsey, V. L., & Seto, M. C. (2002). First report of the collaborative outcome data project on the effectiveness of psychological treatment for sexual offenders. *Sexual Abuse: A Journal of Research and Treatment, 14,* 169-194.

Hanson, R. K., & Harris, A. J. R. (2000a). Where should we intervene? Dynamic predictors of sexual offence recidivism. *Criminal Justice and Behaviour, 27,* 6-35.

Hanson, R. K., & Harris, A. J. R. (2000b). *The sex offender need assessment rating (SONAR): A method for measuring change in risk levels.* Ottawa: Department of the Solicitor General of Canada.

Hanson, R. K., & Scott, H. (1995). Assessing perspective taking among sexual offenders, non-sexual criminals and non-offenders. *Sexual Abuse: A Journal of Research and Treatment, 7,* 259-277.

Hanson, R. K., & Scott, H. (1996). Social networks of sexual offenders. *Psychology, Crime and Law, 2,* 249-258.

Hanson, R. K., Steffy, R. A., & Gauthier, R. (1993). Long-term recidivism of child molesters. *Journal of Consulting and Clinical Psychology*, *61*, 646-652.

Hanson, R. K., & Thornton, D. (1999). *Static-99: Improving actuarial risk assessment
for sex offenders*. Ottawa, ON: Department of the Solicitor General of Canada.

Hanson, R. K., Yates, P. M., & Marshall, W. L. (2000, September). *Implementing what
works with sex offenders*. Paper presented at the 36th Annual Conference of the International Community Corrections Association, Ottawa, ON.

Hare, R. D. (1999). Psychopathy as a risk factor for violence. *Psychiatric Quarterly*,
70, 181-197.

Haynes, A. K., Yates, P. M., & Nicholaichuk, T. P. (1998, October). *Relationship between response to phallometric stimuli and recidivism following sex offender treatment*. Paper presented at the 17th Annual Convention of the Association for the
Treatment of Sexual Abusers, Vancouver, BC.

Haynes, A. K., Yates, P. M., Nicholaichuk, T. P., Gu, D., & Bolton, R. (2000, June).
*Sexual deviancy, risk, and recidivism: The relationship between deviant sexual
arousal, the rapid risk assessment for sexual offense recidivism (RRASOR) and sexual recidivism*. Paper presented at the 61st Annual Conference of the Canadian Psychological Association, Ottawa, ON.

Heim, N., & Hursch, C. J. (1979). Castration for sex offenders: Treatment or punishment? A review and critique of recent European literature. *Archives of Sexual Behaviour*, *8*, 281-304.

Hildebran, D., & Pithers, W. D. (1989). Enhancing offender empathy for sexual abuse
victims. In D. R. Laws (Ed.), *Relapse prevention with sex offenders* (pp. 236-243).
New York: Gilford.

Hudson, S. M., Marshall, W. L., Wales, D. S., McDonald, E., Bakker, L. W., &
McLean, A. (1993). Emotional recognition skills of sex offenders. *Annals of Sex
Research*, *6*, 199-211.

Hudson, S. M., Wales, D. S., & Ward, T. (1998). Kia Marama: A treatment program for
child molesters in New Zealand. In W. L. Marshall, & Y. M. Fernandez (Eds.),
Sourcebook of treatment programs for sexual offenders (pp. 17-28). New York:
Plenum.

Hudson, S. M., & Ward, T. (1996a). Introduction to the special issue on relapse prevention. *Sexual Abuse: A Journal of Research and Treatment*, *8*, 173-175.

Hudson, S. M., & Ward, T. (1996b). Relapse prevention: Future directions. *Sexual
Abuse: A Journal of Research and Treatment*, *8*, 249-256.

Huot, S. J. (1997). *Minnesota sex offender screening tool (MnSOST): Research summary*. St. Paul, MN: Minnesota Department of Corrections.

Johnston, L., & Ward, T. (1996). Social cognition and sexual offending: A theoretical
framework. *Sexual Abuse: A Journal of Research and Treatment*, *8*, 55-80.

Johnston, L., Ward, T., & Hudson, S. (1997). Deviant sexual thoughts: Mental control
and the treatment of sexual offenders. *The Journal of Sex Research*, *34*, 121-130.

Kear-Colwell, J., & Pollock, P. (1997). Motivation or confrontation: Which approach
to the child sex offender? *Criminal Justice and Behaviour*, *24*, 20-33.

Keenan, T., & Ward, T. (2000). A theory of mind perspective on cognitive, affective,
and intimacy deficits in child sexual offenders. *Sexual Abuse: A Journal of Research and Treatment*, *12*, 49-58.

Knopp, F. H., Freeman-Longo, R. E., & Stevenson, W. (1992). *Nationwide survey of juvenile and adult sex offender treatment programs.* Orwell, VT: Safer Society Press.

Langevin, R. (1983). *Sexual strands.* Hillsdale, NJ: Erlbaum.

Langevin, R., Lang, R., & Curnoe, S. (1998). The prevalence of sex offenders with deviant fantasies. *Journal of Interpersonal Violence, 13*, 315-327.

Langevin, R., Wright, M. A., & Handy, L. (1988). Empathy, assertiveness, aggressiveness, and defensiveness among sex offenders. *Annals of Sex Research, 1*, 533-547.

Laws, D. R. (1989). *Relapse prevention with sex offenders.* New York: Guilford.

Laws, D. R. (1995). Central elements in relapse prevention procedure with sex offenders. *Psychology, Crime and Law, 2*, 41-53.

Laws, D. R., Hudson, S. M., & Ward, T. (2000). *Remaking relapse prevention with sex offenders: A sourcebook.* Thousand Oaks, CA: Sage Publications, Inc.

Laws, D. R., & Marshall, W. L. (1990). A conditioning theory of the etiology and maintenance of deviant sexual preference and behaviour. In W. L. Marshall, & H. E. Barbaree (Eds.), *Handbook of sexual assault: Issues, theories, and treatment of offenders* (pp. 103-113). New York: Plenum.

Letourneau, E. J. (2002). A comparison of objective measures of sexual arousal and interest: Visual reaction time and penile plethysmography. *Sexual Abuse: A Journal of Research and Treatment, 14*, 207-223.

Lieberman, M. A., Yalom, I. D., & Miles, M. B. (1973). *Encounter groups: First facts.* New York: Basic Books.

Lockhart, L. L., Saunders, B. E., & Cleveland, P. (1989). Adult male sexual offenders: An overview of treatment techniques. In J. S. Wodarski (Eds.), *Treatment of sex offenders in social work and mental health settings* (pp. 1-32). Binghamton, NY: The Haworth Press, Inc.

Looman, J., Abracen, J., & Nicholaichuk, T. P. (1999). Recidivism among treated sexual offenders and matched controls: Data from the regional treatment centre (Ontario). *Journal of Interpersonal Violence, 15*, 279-320.

Maletzky, B. M. (1980). Self-referred versus court-referred sexually deviant patients: Success with assisted covert sensitization. *Behaviour Therapy, 11*, 306-314.

Maletzky, B. M. (1991). *Treating the sexual offender.* Newbury Park, CA: Sage.

Mann, R. E. (1998, October). *Relapse prevention? Is that the bit where they told me all of the things that I couldn't do anymore?* Paper presented at the 17th Annual Research and Treatment Conference of the Association for the Treatment of Sexual Abusers, Vancouver, BC.

Marlatt, G. A. (1982). Relapse prevention: A self-control program for the treatment of addictive behaviours. In R. B. Stuart (Ed.), *Adherence, compliance and generalization in behavioural medicine* (pp. 329-378). New York: Brunner/Mazel.

Marlatt, G. A., & Gordon, J. R. (1985). *Relapse prevention: Maintenance strategies in the treatment of addictive behaviours.* New York: Guilford.

Marolla, J., & Scully, D. (1986). Attitudes towards women, violence, and rape: A comparison of convicted rapists and other felons. *Deviant Behaviour, 7*, 337-355.

Marques, J. K. (1982, March). *Relapse prevention: A self-control model for the treatment of sex offenders.* Paper presented at the 7th Annual Forensic Mental Health Conference, Asilomar, CA.

Marques, J. K., Day, D. M., Nelson, C., & Miner, M. H. (1989). The sex offender treatment and evaluation project: California's relapse prevention program. In D. R. Laws (Eds.), *Relapse prevention with sex offenders* (pp. 247-267). New York: Guilford.

Marques, J. K., Day, D. M., Nelson, C., & West, M. (1994). Effects of cognitive-behavioural treatment on sex offender recidivism: Preliminary results of a longitudinal study. *Criminal Justice and Behaviour, 21*, 28-54.

Marshall, W. L. (1996). Assessment, treatment and theorizing about sex offenders: Developments during the past twenty years and future directions. *Criminal Justice and Behaviour, 23*, 162-199.

Marshall, W. L. (2001, November). *Research, theory and practice: Thoughts on twenty years of accomplishment and what lies ahead.* Paper presented at the 20th Annual Conference of the Association for the Treatment of Sexual Abusers, San Antonio, TX.

Marshall, W. L., & Anderson, D. (1996). An evaluation of the benefits of relapse prevention programs with sexual offenders. *Sexual Abuse: A Journal of Research and Treatment, 8*, 209-229.

Marshall, W. L., Anderson, D., & Fernandez Y. M. (1999). *Cognitive behavioural treatment of sexual offenders.* Toronto, ON: John Wiley & Sons.

Marshall, W. L., & Barbaree, H. E. (1990). Outcome of comprehensive cognitive behavioural treatment programs. In W. L. Marshall, D. R. Laws, & H. E. Barbaree (Eds.), *Handbook of sexual assault: Issues, theories, and treatment of the offender* (pp. 363-385). New York: Plenum.

Marshall, W. L., Champagne, F., Brown, C., & Miller, S. (1997). Empathy, intimacy, loneliness, and self-esteem in non-familial child molesters. *Journal of Child Sexual Abuse, 6*, 87-97.

Marshall, W. L., Champagne, F., Sturgeon, C., & Bryce, P. (1997). Increasing the self-esteem of child molesters. *Sexual Abuse: A Journal of Research and Treatment, 9*, 321-333.

Marshall, W. L., & Darke, J. (1982). Inferring humiliation as motivation in sexual offenses. *Treatment of Sexual Aggressives, 5*, 1-3.

Marshall, W. L., Eccles, A., & Barbaree, H. E. (1991). The treatment of exhibitionists: A focus on sexual deviance versus cognitive and relationship features. *Behaviour Research and Therapy, 29*, 129-136.

Marshall, W. L., Hudson, S. M., Jones, R., & Fernandez, Y. M. (1995). Empathy in sex offenders. *Clinical Psychology Review, 15*, 99-113.

Marshall, W. L., Jones, R., Ward, T., Johnson, P., & Barbaree, H. E. (1991). Treatment outcome with sex offenders. *Clinical Psychology Review, 11*, 465-485.

Marshall, W. L., & Marshall, L. (1998, October). *Sexual addiction and substance abuse in sexual offenders.* Paper presented at the 17th Annual Research and Treatment Conference of the Association for the Treatment of Sexual Abusers, Vancouver, BC.

Marshall, W. L., & Mazzucco, A. (1995). Self-esteem and parental attachments in child molesters. *Sexual Abuse: A Journal of Research and Treatment, 7*, 279-285.

Marshall, W. L., Mulloy, R., & Serran, G. (1998). *The identification of treatment facilitative behaviours enacted by sexual offender therapists.* Unpublished manuscript.

Marshall, W. L., O'Sullivan, C., & Fernandez, Y. M. (1996). The enhancement of victim empathy among incarcerated child molesters. *Legal and Criminological Psychology, 1,* 95-102.

Marshall, W. L., & Pithers, W. D. (1994). A reconsideration of treatment outcome with sex offenders. *Criminal Justice and Behaviour, 21,* 10-27.

Marshall, W. L., Serran, G. A., & Cortoni, F. A. (2000). Childhood attachments, sexual abuse and their relationship to adult coping in child molesters. *Sexual Abuse: A Journal of Research and Treatment, 12,* 17-26.

McGrath, R. J., Hoke, S. E., & Vojtisek, J. E. (1998). Cognitive-behavioural treatment for sex offenders. *Criminal Justice and Behaviour, 25,* 203-225

McKibben, A., Proulx, J., & Lusignan, R. (1994). Relationships between conflict, affect, and deviant sexual behaviours in rapists and paedophiles. *Behaviour Research and Therapy, 32,* 571-575.

Meyer, W. J., Cole, C., & Emory, E. (1992). Depo provera treatment for sex offending behaviour: An evaluation of outcome. *Bulletin of the American Academy of Psychiatry and Law, 20,* 249-259.

Miller, W. R. (1980). The addictive behaviours. In W. R. Miler (Ed.), *The addictive behaviours: Treatment of alcoholism, drug abuse, smoking and obesity* (pp. 3-10). New York: Plenum.

Miller, W. R. (1995). Increasing motivation for change. In R. K. Hester, & W. R. Miller (Eds.), *Handbook of alcoholism treatment approaches: Effective alternatives* (pp. 89-104). New York: Allyn & Bacon.

Miller, P. A., & Eisenberg, N. (1988). The relationship of empathy to aggressive and externalizing/antisocial behaviour. *Psychological Bulletin, 103,* 234-344.

Miller, W. R., & Sovereign, R. G. (1989). The check-up: A model for early intervention in addictive behaviours. In T. Loberg, W. R. Miller, P. E. Nathan, & G. A. Marlatt (Eds.), *Addictive behaviours: Prevention and early intervention* (pp. 219-231). Amsterdam: Swets & Zeitlinger.

Miner, M. H., Day, D. M., & Nafpaktitis, M. K. (1989). Assessment of coping skills: Development of a situational competency test. In D. R. Laws (Ed.), *Relapse prevention with sex offenders* (pp. 127-136). New York: Guilford.

Moore, B. S. (1990). The origins and development of empathy. *Motivation and Emotion, 14,* 75-79.

Motiuk, L., & Belcourt, R. (1996). Profiling the Canadian federal sex offender population. *Forum on Corrections Research, 8,* 3-7.

Motiuk, L., & Brown, S. L. (1996, August). *Factors related to recidivism among released federal sex offenders.* Paper presented at the 26th International Congress of Psychology, Montreal, QC.

Mulloy, R., Smiley, W. C., & Mawson, D. L. (1997, June). *Empathy and the successful treatment of psychopaths.* Poster presented at the Annual Meeting of the Canadian Psychological Association, Toronto, ON.

Murphy, W. D. (1990). Assessment and modification of cognitive distortions in sex offenders. In W. L. Marshall, D. R. Laws, & H. E. Barbaree (Eds.), *Handbook of sex-*

ual assault: Issues, theories, and treatment of the offender (pp. 331-342). New York: Plenum.

Nicholaichuk, T. P. (1996). Sex offender treatment priority: An illustration of the risk/need principle. Forum on Corrections Research, 8, 30-32.

Nicholaichuk, T. P., Gordon, A., Gu, D., & Wong, S. (2000). Outcome of an institutional sexual offender treatment program: A comparison between treated and matched untreated offenders. Sexual Abuse: A Journal of Research and Treatment, 12, 139-153.

Pithers, W. D. (1993). Treatment of rapists: Reinterpretation of early outcome data and exploratory constructs to enhance therapeutic efficacy. In G. C. Nagayama Hall, & R. Hirschman et al. (Eds.), Sexual aggression: Issues in etiology, assessment, and treatment. Series in applied psychology: social issues and questions (pp. 167-196). Washington, DC: Taylor and Francis Group.

Pithers, W. D. (1994). Process evaluation of a group therapy component designed to enhance sex offenders' empathy for sexual abuse survivors. Behaviour Research and Therapy, 32, 565-570.

Pithers, W. D., & Cumming, G. F. (1989). Can relapse be prevented? Initial outcome data from the Vermont treatment program for sexual aggressors. In D. R. Laws (Eds.), Relapse prevention with sex offenders (pp. 313-325). New York: Guilford.

Pithers, W. D., Marques, J. K., Gibat, C. C., & Marlatt, G. A. (1983). Relapse prevention with sexual aggressives: A self-control model of treatment and maintenance of change. In J. G. Greer, & I. R. Stuart (Eds.), The sexual aggressor: Current perspectives on treatment (pp. 214-239). New York: Van Nostrand Reinhold.

Plaud, J. J., & Newberry, D. E. (1996). Rule-governed behaviour and pedophilia. Sexual Abuse: A Journal of Research and Treatment, 8, 143-159.

Pollack, N. L., & Hashmall, J. M. (1991). The excuses of child molesters. Behavioural Sciences and the Law, 9, 53-59.

Prentky, R. A. (1995). A rationale for the treatment of sex offenders: Pro Bono Publico. In J. McGuire (Ed.), What works: Reducing re-offending–Guidelines from research and practice (pp. 155-172). New York: Wiley.

Prentky, R. A., & Burgess, A. W. (1990). Rehabilitation of child molesters: A cost-benefit analysis. American Journal of Orthopsychiatry, 60, 108-117.

Proulx, J. (1993). Les théories comportementales. In J. Aubut (Ed.), Les agresseurs sexuels: Théories, évaluation et traitement (pp. 35-43). Montréal, QC: Les Editions de la Chenelière.

Proulx, J., McKibben, A., & Lusignan, R. (1996). Relationships between affective components and sexual behaviors in sexual aggressors. Sexual Abuse: A Journal of Research and Treatment, 8, 279-289.

Quinsey, V. L., Chaplin T. C., & Carrigan, W. F. (1980). Biofeedback and signalled punishment in the modification of inappropriate sexual age preferences. Behaviour Therapy, 11, 567-576.

Quinsey, V. L., Harris, G. T., Rice, M. E., & Cormier, C. A. (1998). Violent offenders: Appraising and managing risk. Washington, DC: American Psychological Association.

Quinsey, V. L., Khanna, A., & Malcolm, P. B. (1996, August). *A retrospective evaluation of the RTC sex offender treatment program.* Paper presented at the World Congress of Psychology, Montreal, QC.
Quinsey, V. L., & Marshall, W. L. (1983). Procedures for reducing inappropriate sexual arousal: An evaluation review. In J. G. Greer, & I. R. Stuart (Eds.), *The sexual aggressor: Current perspectives on treatment* (pp. 267-289). New York: Van Nostrand Reinhold.
Rice, M. E., Chaplin, T. E., Harris, G. T., & Coutts, J. (1994). Empathy for the victim and sexual arousal among rapists and nonrapists. *Journal of Interpersonal Violence, 9,* 435-449.
Schwartz, B. K. (1992). Effective treatment techniques for sex offenders. *Psychiatric Annals, 22,* 315-319.
Seidman, B. T., Marshall, W. L., Hudson, S. M., & Robertson, P. J. (1994). An examination of intimacy and loneliness in sex offenders. *Journal of Interpersonal Violence, 9,* 518-534.
Seto, M. C., & Barbaree, H. E. (1999). Psychopathy, treatment behavior, and sex offender recidivism. *Journal of Interpersonal Violence, 14,* 1235-1248.
Smallbone, S. W., & Dadds, M. R. (2000). Attachment and coercive sexual behaviour. *Sexual Abuse: A Journal of Research and Treatment, 12,* 3-15.
Spencer, A. (1999). *Working with sex offenders in prisons and through release to the community: A handbook.* London: J Kingsley.
Stermac, L. E., & Segal, Z. V. (1989). Adult sexual contact with children: An examination of cognitive factors. *Behaviour Therapy, 20,* 573-584.
Veach, T. A. (1999). Child sexual offenders' attitudes toward punishment, sexual contact and blame. *Journal of Child Sexual Abuse, 7,* 43-58.
Ward, T., & Hudson, S. M. (1996). Relapse prevention: A critical analysis. *Sexual Abuse: A Journal of Research and Treatment, 8,* 177-200.
Ward, T., & Hudson, S. M. (1998). A model of the relapse process in sexual offenders. *Journal of Interpersonal Violence, 13,* 700-725.
Ward, T., & Hudson, S. M. (2000a). A self-regulation model of relapse prevention. In D. R. Laws, S. M. Hudson, & T. Ward (Eds.), *Relapse prevention with sex offenders: A sourcebook* (pp. 79-101). Thousand Oaks, CA: Sage.
Ward, T., & Hudson, S. M. (2000b). Sexual offenders' implicit planning: A conceptual model. *Sexual Abuse: A Journal of Research and Treatment, 12,* 189-202.
Ward, T., Hudson, S. M., & France, K. G. (1993). Self-reported reasons for offending behaviour in the child molester. *Annals of Sex Research, 6,* 139-148.
Ward, T., Hudson, S. M., Johnston, L., & Marshall, W. L. (1997). Cognitive distortions in sex offenders: An integrative review. *Clinical Psychology Review, 17,* 479-507.
Ward, T., Hudson, S. M., & Keenan, T. (1998). A self regulation model of the sexual offense process. *Sexual Abuse: A Journal of Research and Treatment, 10,* 141-157.
Ward, T., Hudson, S. M., & Marshall, W. L. (1994). The abstinence violation effect in child molesters. *Behaviour Research and Therapy, 32,* 431-437.
Ward, T., Hudson, S. M., Marshall, W. L., & Siegert, R. (1995). Attachment style and intimacy deficits in sexual offenders: A theoretical framework. *Sexual Abuse: A Journal of Research and Treatment, 7,* 317-335.

Ward, T., Hudson, S. M., & Siegert, R. (1995). A critical comment on Pithers' relapse prevention model. *Sexual Abuse: A Journal of Research and Treatment, 7,* 167-175.

Ward, T., Keenan, T., & Hudson, S. M. (2000). Understanding cognitive, affective, and intimacy deficits in sexual offenders. A developmental perspective. *Aggression and Violent Behaviour, 5,* 41-62.

Ward, T., Louden, K., Hudson, S. M., & Marshall, W. L. (1995). A descriptive model of the offence chain for child molesters. *Journal of Interpersonal Violence, 10,* 452-472.

Wilcox, D. T. (2000). Application of the clinical polygraph to the assessment, treatment and monitoring of sex offenders. *Journal of Sexual Aggression, 5,* 134-152.

Williams, S. M., & Khanna, A. (1990, June). *Empathy training for sex offenders.* Paper presented at the Third Symposium on Violence and Aggression, Saskatoon, SK.

Wilson, R. J., Stewart, L., Stirpe, T., Barrett, M., & Cripps, J. E. (2000). Community-based sexual offender management: Combining parole supervision and treatment to reduce recidivism. *Canadian Journal of Criminology, 42,* 177-188.

Wormith, J. S., & Hanson, R. K. (1992). The treatment of sexual offenders in Canada. *Canadian Psychology, 33,* 180-198.

Yalom, I. D. (1985). *The theory and practice of group psychotherapy* (3rd ed.). New York: Basic Books.

Yates, P. M. (1996). *An investigation of factors associated with definitions and perceptions of rape, propensity to commit rape, and rape prevention.* Ottawa, ON: Carleton University, Unpublished doctoral dissertation.

Yates, P. M. (2002). What works: Effective intervention with sex offenders. In H. E. Allen (Ed.), *What works: Risk reduction interventions for special needs offenders* (pp. 115-163). MD: American Correctional Association.

Yates, P. M., Goguen, B. C., Nicholaichuk, T. P., Williams, S. M., & Long, C. A. (2000). *National sex offender programs.* Ottawa, ON: Correctional Service of Canada.

Sex Hormones, Neurotransmitters, and Psychopharmacological Treatments in Men with Paraphilic Disorders

Fabian M. Saleh
Fred S. Berlin

SUMMARY. Paraphilic disorders are psychiatric syndromes primarily characterized by deviant sexual thoughts, cravings, urges, and/or behaviors. Paraphilic men may engage in inappropriate sexual behaviors when cravings for socially unacceptable sexual acts become overpowering. These often chronic disorders may not only cause emotional distress and social embarrassment to the afflicted patient but also to the targets of their paraphilic focus. The primary objective of this article is to examine and review data on the efficacy and tolerability of the testosterone-lowering agents medroxprogesterone acetate, cyproterone acetate, and leuprolide acetate. The secondary goal is to review data on less conventional and more innovative pharmacological treatments, particularly the serotonin-specific reuptake inhibitors. *[Article copies available for a fee from The Haworth Document Delivery Service: 1-800-HAWORTH. E-mail address: <docdelivery@haworthpress.com> Website: <http://www.HaworthPress.com> © 2003 by The Haworth Press, Inc. All rights reserved.]*

Address correspondence to: Fabian M. Saleh, MD, UMass Memorial Medical Center, Inc., Department of Psychiatry, 55 Lake Avenue North, Worcester, MA 01655.

[Haworth co-indexing entry note]: "Sex Hormones, Neurotransmitters, and Psychopharmacological Treatments in Men with Paraphilic Disorders." Saleh, Fabian M., and Fred S. Berlin. Co-published simultaneously in *Journal of Child Sexual Abuse* (The Haworth Maltreatment & Trauma Press, an imprint of The Haworth Press, Inc.) Vol. 12, No. 3/4, 2003, pp. 233-253; and: *Identifying and Treating Sex Offenders: Current Approaches, Research, and Techniques* (ed: Robert Geffner et al.) The Haworth Maltreatment & Trauma Press, an imprint of The Haworth Press, Inc., 2003, pp. 233-253. Single or multiple copies of this article are available for a fee from The Haworth Document Delivery Service [1-800-HAWORTH, 9:00 a.m. - 5:00 p.m. (EST). E-mail address: docdelivery@haworthpress.com].

http://www.haworthpress.com/web/JCSA
© 2003 by The Haworth Press, Inc. All rights reserved.
Digital Object Identifier: 10.1300/J070v12n03_09

KEYWORDS. Paraphilias, neurotransmitters, testosterone, pharmacotherapy

Paraphilic disorders are sexual deviation syndromes characterized by aberrant sexual fantasies, urges, and/or behaviors. The revised fourth edition of the *Diagnostic and Statistical Manual of Mental Disorders* (DSM-IV-TR; American Psychiatric Association [APA], 2000) distinguishes nine distinct paraphilic categories (see Table 1). Though the etiology and pathophysiology of the paraphilias is still under investigation, numerous scientific studies suggest abnormalities at a biological level (Hendricks et al., 1988; Mendez, Chow, Ringman, Twitchell, & Hinkin, 2000). Readily identifiable biological abnormalities, such as inherited genetic disorders, hormonal abnormalities, and neuropsychiatric disorders have been associated and linked to paraphilic and paraphilic-like phenomena (Berlin, 1983; Fedoroff, Peyser, Franz, & Folstein, 1994; Gaffney & Berlin, 1984). While there is no known cure for these often debilitating conditions, these disorders can be managed and treated effectively with one of the available biological and/or psychotherapeutic treatments.

CASE 1

"Mr. B, a 27-year-old, stated that he was preoccupied with erotic fantasies to such a degree that they interfered with work and family relationships. His wife confirmed his report that he sometimes demanded intercourse as often as 15 times a single day. There was a family history of andrenogenital syndrome, which results from an excess of androgens in a fetus with an XX genotype and causes virilization of the external genitalia. Mr. B's mother had taken thyroid medication when pregnant. The patient's serum testosterone level was 880 ng/100ml, above the

TABLE 1. Paraphilic Disorders as Classified in DSM-IV-TR

Exhibitionism	Fetishism
Frotteurism	Pedophilia
Sexual masochism	Sexual sadism
Transvestic fetishism	Voyeurism Paraphilia N.O.S.

normal (i.e., more than 2 SD) postpubertal range of 275-875 ng/100ml as reported by the laboratory performing the assay. No cause could be detected, although receptor site sensitivity to testosterone has not yet been tested. Treatment with 400 mg per week medroxyprogesterone acetate reduced the elevated testosterone level to prepubertal value of 70 ng/100ml. The patient reported relief from intrusive fantasies, as well as improved work and interpersonal relationships" (Berlin, & Schaerf, 1985, pp. 276-277).

CASE 2

"Mr. B, a 30-year-old single white male, reported a 7-year history of regular exhibitionism that increased during times of stress. His sexual fantasies centered around images of dominance, violence, and exhibitionism. When not exposing himself, Mr. B spent hours driving and masturbating while flirting with female drivers. Inpatient and outpatient psychotherapy with both psychodynamic and behavioral approaches had not been consistently helpful. Covert sensitization temporarily led to decreases in exhibitionism, but the behavior returned generally within a few months. He experienced low-frustration tolerance and irritability but denied ongoing dysphoria, sleep and appetite disturbance, and other obsessions and compulsions.

Fluoxetine 40 mg b.i.d. significantly decreased Mr. B's urges. His violent sexual fantasies diminished in intensity and intrusiveness. Overall, his sexual desire was somewhat diminished. Although he experienced retarded ejaculation, this did not interfere with pleasurable sexual experience. Follow-up after six additional months on a regimen of fluoxetine reveled that improvement had been sustained" (Perilstein, Lipper, & Friedman, 1991, pp. 169-70).

THE ROLE OF NEUROTRANSMITTERS
IN SEXUAL BEHAVIORS

This section reviews the fundamental biochemical aspects of the serotonin and catecholamine systems. Additionally, it examines and discusses the findings of those studies that are considered relevant to the discussion on sexual phenomenology.

The amino acid precursor tryptophan is converted via hydroxylation and decarboxylation to the indolamine serotonin (5-HT), which is also known as 5-hydroxytryptamine. The rate-limiting enzyme in the synthesis of 5-HT is tryptophan hydroxylase. 5-HT is principally metabolized to 5-hydroxyindolacetic acid (5-HIAA) by the enzyme monoamine oxydase (MAO). In the central nervous system (CNS), serotonin-producing neurons are found in midbrain structures. They are most abundant in the dorsal raphe nuclei and to a lesser extent in the caudal raphe nuclei. Both nuclei project up and downward to various CNS regions, including the cerebral cortex, cerebellum, limbic system, striatum, and spinal cord. After being released into the synaptic cleft, 5-HT influences through its effects on the 5-HT receptors: mood, cognition, sensory perception, temperature regulation, nociception, as well as neurovegetative drives, such as appetite, sleep, and sex (Bradford, 1996; Sjoerdsma & Palfreyman, 1990).

The catecholamine neurotransmitters norepinephrine, epinephrine, and dopamine form the noradrenergic (norepinephrine), adrenergic system (epinephrine), and dopaminergic system (dopamine), respectively. All three monoamines have the amino acid tyrosine as their precursor. Tyrosine is synthesized from phenylalanine by phenylalanine hydroxylase. The rate-limiting enzyme in the synthesis of the catecholamines is tyrosine hydroxylase, which converts tyrosine into DOPA. DOPA subsequently is converted to dopamine by the enzyme DOPA decarboxylase. The four major dopaminergic tracts that have been identified include the (a) nigrostriatal-, (b) mesolimbic-, (c) mesocortical-, and (d) tuberoinfundibular tract, respectively (see Table 2). Once released into the synaptic cleft, dopamine exerts its characteristic effects by binding to the dopaminergic receptors. Norepinephrine and epinephrine are end products of the dopamine pathway (see Figure 1). Indeed, dopamine is converted to norepinephrine and epinephrine via dopamine hydroxylase and phenylethanolamine N-methyl-transferase (PNMT), respectively.

Norepinephrine-producing neurons are mainly located in the locus ceruleus (midbrain structure). These neurons contain the enzyme dopamine hydroxylase, which converts dopamine into norepinephrine. The locus ceruleus gives rise to the noradrenergic tract which projects to the neocortex, limbic system, thalamus, and hypothalamus. At the level of the adrenal gland PNMT converts norepinephrine into epinephrine. Norepinehrine, through its effects on the CNS, also influences mood, cognition, learning, and memory. In addition, norepinephrine is involved in regulatory processes of the hypothalamic-pituitary axis and the sympathetic nervous system (SNS). Through their effects on the adrenergic receptors (α-1, α-2, β-1, β-2, and β-3) and receptor subtypes, both neurotransmitters, norepinephrine and epinephrine participate in the regulation of most organ systems.

Dysfunctions at the level of the 5-HT and dopaminergic systems have been implicated in the etiology of several psychiatric and neurological conditions. 5-HT activity is thought to be low in depressive disorders, Parkinson's or Alzheimer's disease, and high in psychotic disorders. Although the relationship between 5-HT and violence in general appears to be quite complex, numerous antemortem and postmortem studies have demonstrated a link between low cerebrospinal fluid (CSF) 5-HIAA levels and impulsive aggression, irritability, violence and suicide (Asberg, Schalling, & Traskman, 1987; Lee & Coccaro, 2001; Mann, Arango, Marzuk, Theccanat, & Rtes, 1989; Van Praag, 1983). On the other hand, a dysfunctional dopaminergic system apparently contributes to the etiology of psychotic disorders, as conjectured in the dopamine hypothesis of schizophrenia.

Data derived from animal, pharmacological, and surgical castration studies show that normative and deviant sexual behavior is modulated and influenced by intricate neurobiological systems, involving monoamines, indolamines, neuropeptides, hormones, and the opiates (Berlin et al., 1988; Bradford, 1999, 2001; Kafka, 1997; Maes et al., 2001; Tucker & File, 1983). Data from animal studies showed an inverse relationship between central serotonergic and dopaminergic concentrations and sexual behavior and sexual drive. In fact, low CNS 5-HT levels augment sexual appetite, while high 5-HT levels decrease sexual desire. Quite the opposite appears to be true for CNS dopamine. Indeed, decreased dopaminergic neurotransmission has attenuating effects on sexual drive,

TABLE 2. Schematic Representation of the Major Central Dopaminergic Tracts

---

Nigrostriatal tract: Cell bodies in substantia nigra → D-2 receptors in the corpus striatum (predominant receptor)

Mesolimbic tract: Cell bodies in ventral tegmental (VTA) area → D-4 receptors of the limbic system

Mesocortical tract: Cell bodies in VTA → cerebral cortex (predominantly frontal cortex)

Tubero-infundibular tract: Cell bodies in arcuate nucleus and periventricular area of the hypothalamus → pituitary gland and infundibulum

---

FIGURE 1. The Dopamine Pathway

Phenylalanine → tyrosine → DOPA → dopamine → norepinephrine → epinephrine whereas increased dopaminergic neurotransmission has enhancing effects on sexual drive (Baum & Starr, 1980; Everitt & Bancroft, 1991; Ferguson, Henriksen, & Cohen, 1970; Mas, 1995). The catecholamines have also been implicated in the etiology of sexual deviancy. A group of Dutch researchers administered the postsynaptic 5-HT2 receptor agonist, meta-chlorophenylpiperazine (mCPP), to pedophiles and normal controls. Plasma epinephrine and norepinephrine concentrations were determined prior and subsequent to the administration of the agonist. Results were quite intriguing in that norepinephrine and especially epinephrine levels were significantly elevated in the index group but not in the controls. These data, though preliminary, suggest a dysregulation at the level of the sympathoadrenal system in pedophilic patients.

THE ROLE OF SEX HORMONES IN THE PARAPHILIAS

Given that paraphilias are very rare in women, the following discussion on endogenous sex hormones will be limited to the male gender. Approximately five to six weeks after conception and under the influence of systemic androgens, in particular dihydrotestosterone, a male fetus begins to develop and differentiate as such. In the postpartum period, testosterone levels remain initially elevated but then decline progressively to prepubertal levels. The maturation of the hypothalamic-pituitary-gonadal axis is usually preceded by an increased secretion of adrenal androgens into the bloodstream (Griffin & Wilson, 1980). All through adolescence and in response to hypothalamic-releasing hormones as well as circulating sex hormones (via a feedback mechanism), the anterior lobe of the pituitary gland synthesizes and releases hormones such as luteinizing hormone (LH), follicle stimulating hormone (FSH), and adrenocorticotropic hormone (ACTH).

After reaching their target organs (e.g., the testes), they induce processes called testicular steroidgenesis and spermatogenesis. In fact, in the testicular interstitial (Leydig) cells, the bulk of testosterone, an androgen and anabolic steroid, is synthesized and secreted into the blood. Once secreted, it firmly binds to steroid-binding proteins. As soon as testosterone diffuses from the blood into the cytoplasma of somatic and neuronal cells, it is converted by the enzyme 5-alpha reductase to the more active dihydrotestosterone. A smaller amount is converted peripherally to oestradiol. At the time of puberty, this dramatic upsurge in the synthesis of sex hormones is responsible for the physical maturation and development of primary and secondary sex organs. Besides their influence on reproductive organs, androgens also manipulate, through their effects on the brain, mood, and sexual behavior (Bancroft, 1989; Liang, Tymoczko, Chan, Hung, & Liao, 1977).

In line with the aforesaid, data from pharmacological and castration studies provide evidence in support of the regulatory effects of androgens on sexual drive, interest, and behavior. Indeed, a group of more than 900 convicted and orchidectomized (surgical removal of testes) sex offenders were studied and followed longitudinally for several years. Following surgery, many patients reported a significant reduction in sex drive. These subjective reports were supported by the relatively low recidivism rate of less than 3% (Sturup, 1972). Data on serum testosterone levels and their significance in relation to deviant sexual behaviors continue to be conflicting. Some investigators found elevated plasma testosterone levels among sexually violent rapists (Rada, Laws, & Kellner, 1976, 1983). Davidson, Canargo, and Smith (1979) showed that testosterone administered to a group of men with baseline plasma testosterone levels of below 150ng/100ml led to an increase in sex drive.

Along the same lines, Bradford and Bourget (1987) noted a relationship between serum testosterone levels and sexual appetite and/or sexual aggression. A group of investigators examined testosterone levels in adolescents who had engaged in violence, including sexual violence. Subjects (total $N = 194$, ages 15-17) were subdivided into three groups and were classified according to their index offense in violent ($n = 75$), non-violent ($n = 102$), and sex offenders ($n = 17$). Serum testosterone levels (a.m. blood draw) were compiled and compared among the three groups. Testosterone levels were comparable in those subjects who had committed a sexual offense or a non-violent offense, but differed from those who had perpetrated a violent but non-sexual offense. Indeed serum testosterone levels were significantly higher in this latter group (Brooks & Reddon, 1996). In contrast to the above findings, these researchers could not establish a clear link between serum testosterone levels and sexual violence. Other research has fallen short in demonstrating any correlation between serum testosterone levels and sexual drive or desire (Brown, Monti, & Carrivean, 1978; Kravitz, Haywood, Kelly, & Cavanaugh, 1996; Lang, Langevin, & Bain, 1989). With these basic principles in mind, we will now shift focus to a discussion on psychopharmacological treatments in the paraphilias.

PHARMACOLOGICAL TREATMENTS

Whenever cravings for socially unacceptable and unconventional sexual acts become intense and overpowering, afflicted individuals may pose not only a risk to the targets of their paraphilic focus but also to their own welfare. Indeed, if left untreated, patients have considerably higher recidivism rates than those who undergo treatment (Alexander, 1997). Over the last few decades a number of treatment modalities have been proposed, including the psychologically based therapies such as psychodynamic psychotherapies (Peters & Roether, 1972; Salzman, 1971), behavioral therapies (i.e., aversion therapy, masturbatory satiation), and cognitive behavior therapy (Laws & Marshall, 1991; Marks, Gelder, & Bancroft, 1970; Marks, 1981). The biological based treatments encompass the surgical procedures (i.e., orchidectomy [Ortmann, 1980] and stereotaxic neurosurgery [Roeder, Muller, & Orthner, 1972]), and the pharmacotherapeutic interventions (the focus of this section).

In view of the very nature of the paraphilias, the approach to treatment should always be broad and multifaceted. In the authors' judgment, most patients diagnosed with a paraphilic or sexually related disorder do benefit from cognitive behavioral group psychotherapy. The principal goal of therapy is to help patients learn to control inappropriate sexual thoughts and behaviors, to gain empathy for victims, and to develop effective relapse prevention strategies.

Psychopharmacological therapies have not only proven to be valuable but are sometimes indispensable in the treatment and management of paraphilic patients. Notwithstanding the value of pharmacological treatments, the reader should be cognizant of the fact that all currently employed medications are not approved by the U.S. Food and Drug Administration (FDA). Yet using psychopharmacological agents off-label does not imply that such use is experimental or investigative; it only denotes that the drug has not been adequately studied in patients afflicted with the specific disorder in question for which it is prescribed. The treating psychiatrist or licensed physician should, therefore, carefully document his or her clinical observation, diagnosis, and rationale before the prescription of an off-label medication. Because of inherent medical, ethical, and legal impediments and quandaries, randomized double-blind placebo-controlled research studies continue to be scarce in the paraphilias (Berlin, 1989; Walker, Meyer, Emory, & Rubin, 1984).

The drugs used in the treatment of the paraphilias can be divided into two groups: (a) the testosterone-lowering medications, and (b) the serotonergic antidepressants. Both will be discussed here.

Testosterone-Lowering Agents

Although technically not an antiandrogen, given its inability to bind to intracellular androgen receptors (Southren, Gordon, Vittek, & Altman, 1977), medroxyprogesterone acetate (MPA) continues to play an important role in the management and treatment of sexual deviation syndromes (Meyer, Cole, & Emory, 1992). MPA is a potent synthetic progestational agent that through its manifold combined pharmacological effects reduces serum and tissue concentrations of testosterone. Its primary pharmacological effect is the hepatic induction of testosterone-A-reductase. It also increases testosterone's metabolic clearance rate by interfering with its binding to plasma globulins (Albin, Vittek, & Gordon, 1973). MPA also inhibits the secretion of gonadotropin from the pituitary gland, and thereby decreases spermatogenesis and testicular testosterone synthesis (Albin, Vittek, & Gordon, 1973; Berlin & Schaerf, 1985; Camacho, Williams, & Montalvo, 1972).

MPA is available in a parenteral (intramuscular) and oral form. Its suspension, when given orally, has been shown to be bioequivalent to MPA pills. Indeed, Antal, Gillespiem, and Albert (1983) demonstrated in a randomized, crossover study that serum plasma levels in 19 adult subjects were comparable after the administration of either the intramuscular or the oral formulation. MPA is primarily metabolized in the liver by the human hepatic cytochrome enzyme system (CYP P450). Contraindications of its use are manifold and include severe hepatic disease, cancerous processes involving the breast or genitalia, thromboembolic disorders, such as thrombophlebitis, pulmonary embolism, and cerebral vascular apoplexy, hypersensitivity to the drug, and undiagnosed vaginal bleeds. MPA can cause a number of potentially serious and less serious adverse effects, including depressive symptoms, breast tenderness and galactorrhea, Cushing's syndrome (Dux, Bishara, Marom, Blum, & Pitlik, 1998; Shotliff & Nussey, 1997), weight gain–apparently secondary to increased fat deposition (Amatayakul, Sivasomboon, & Thanangkul, 1980), nausea, abdominal pain, nightmares, hot flashes, acne, alopecia, hirsutism, hyperglycemia, diabetes mellitus, gallstones (Meyer, Walker, Emory, & Smith, 1985), hypogonadism, hypospermatogenesis, and hypertension.

Despite these potential adverse effects, MPA is considered a relatively safe and efficacious drug in the treatment of the paraphilias. Through the multitude of its pharmacological actions, it suppresses sexual drive and thereby reduces the intensity and frequency of deviant sexual urges and cravings (Berlin, 1983; Berlin & Meinecke, 1981; Gagne, 1981; Kierch,

1990; Kravitz et al., 1995; Meyer et al., 1992). Since the oral and the intramuscular formulation are pharmacologically equivalent, either one can be prescribed to a patient. Gottesman and Schubert (1993), using groups of adult male subjects with both "noncontact" and "contact" paraphilias, conducted an open non-blind study on the efficacy of low-dose oral MPA. The average trial period for low-dose MPA was 15.33 months. All subjects, except one, received MPA at a daily dosage of 60 mg. All subjects were considered treatment responders (serum testosterone levels declined by as much as 75%). Throughout the trial period none of the participants engaged in sexually deviant and offending behaviors.

The depot preparation (matrix that incorporates the parent compound) is injected into an area of large muscle, from where it is slowly absorbed into the bloodstream. Despite substantial clinical data on MPA, the starting dose for the depot form is not established. Indeed, based on the clinician's preference and the individual's case, the recommended dosages for the acute treatment phase can range from 200 to 500 mg/week (Berlin, 1983; Berlin & Meinecke, 1981; Gagne, 1981; Meyer et al., 1992). Hucker, Langevin, and Bain (1988) conducted a small double-blind placebo-controlled study, and found that MPA, at a dose of 200 mg, was effective in ameliorating paraphilic symptoms in a cohort of pedophilic patients.

Once inappropriate sexual thoughts are adequately suppressed and sexually deviant urges are controlled, tapering of the initial active phase dose can be considered (Walker & Meyer, 1981; Walker et al., 1984). The clinically effective maintenance dose can be as low as 100 mg/week. Some clinicians discontinue antiandrogen treatment altogether. Data presented by Cooper (1987) showed that discontinuing MPA does not necessarily result in a recurrence of sexually inappropriate behaviors. On the other hand, in spite of adequate androgen suppression, some patients continue to remain symptomatic (Gagne, 1981). Before prescribing one of the less conventional and less studied agents (e.g., serotonergic medications), a trial with another testosterone-lowering agent, with different pharmacodynamic properties, should be considered.

Cyproterone acetate (CPA), a progestogen with "true" antiandrogenic characteristics, is predominantly used in Canada and Europe (CPA is not available in the United States). The antiandrogenic effects of CPA are primarily mediated through competitive antagonism of intracellular androgen receptors (Goldenberg & Bruchovsky, 1991; Jurzyk, Spielvogel, & Rose, 1992). For that reason, testosterone and dihydrotestosterone are precluded from exercising their pharmacological effects at the level of their target tissues. CPA's inhibitory effect at the level of the pituitary gland leads to a suppression of gonadotropine secretion, and ultimately results in a reduction of serum androgen levels (Bradford & Pawlak, 1987; Goldenberg & Bruchovsky, 1991; Liang et al., 1977).

In contrast to previous data (Schering, 1983), more recent studies suggest that oral CPA is slowly and poorly absorbed from the gastrointestinal tract (Jurzyk et al., 1992). After its absorption, the bulk of CPA binds to plasma proteins. CPA is metabolized in the liver in part to its main metabolite, 15 beta-hydroxycyproterone. Its side effects are dose dependent (Laschet & Laschet, 1975) and include hypochromic anemia, thromboembolic phenomena, myocardial ischemia, cardiac insufficiency, depression, gastrointestinal symptoms, hepatotoxicity, fatal hepatitis (Blake, Sawyerr, Dooley, Scheuer, & McIntyre, 1990; Levesque et al., 1989), lipid abnormalities, breast tenderness, gynecomastia, decreased spermatogenesis, headaches, weight gain, fatigue, hot flashes, night sweats, and ophthalmologic symptoms (Goldenberg & Bruchovsky, 1991; Jurzyk et al., 1992).

CPA is available in either the oral or alternatively in the long-acting intramuscular form. Oral dosages in the range of 50 to 200 mg/day have been shown to be effective in treating aberrant sexual symptoms. The intramuscular formulation can be administered weekly or biweekly with effective doses ranging from 300 to 700 mg/injection (Reilly, Delva, & Hudson, 2000).

As noted above, CPA has proven to be efficient in the treatment of paraphilic patients (Cooper, 1986; Cooper, Cernosvsky, & Magnus, 1992). Cooper, Sandhu, Losztyn, and Cernovsky (1992) demonstrated in a 28-week double-blind placebo-controlled study that MPA and CPA are equally effective in alleviating sexually deviant (pedophilic) symptoms. Noteworthy is the case of a patient with sadistic male-to-male pedophilia whose sexual arousal patterns changed quantitatively, qualitatively, and differentially while being treated with CPA (Bradford & Pawlak, 1987). The only double-blind placebo-controlled study using CPA not only confirmed its beneficial effects on paraphilic symptoms (range: 50 to 200 mg/day), but more interestingly, replicated its aforementioned differential effects on sexual arousal (Bradford & Pawlak, 1993).

Leuprolide acetate (leuprolide), a luteinizing hormone-releasing-hormone agonist (LHRH-A), has been used in patients with central precocious puberty, prostate cancer and endometriosis (Smith, 1986; Williams et al., 1983). Since the early '90s, leuprolide has been employed in the management and treatment of paraphilic patients. Due to leuprolide's proven antilibidinal effects and its relative tolerability, some physicians regard it as a viable alternative to MPA and/or CPA (Briken, Nika, & Berner, 2001; Krueger & Kaplan, 2001). Indeed, leuprolide has been shown to be effective in those paraphiliacs who did not respond to previous treatments with MPA or CPA (Cooper & Cernovsky, 1994; Rousseau, Couture, Dupont, Labrie, & Couture, 1990). Dickey (1992) for example, reported the case of a young man with multiple paraphilias who continued to be symptomatic despite treatments with depot-MPA (maximum dose 550 mg/week, testosterone levels as low as 0.9 nmol/L) and depot-CPA (200 to maximum dose of 500 mg/week). In an attempt to alleviate this patient's debilitating paraphilic symptoms, leuprolide was prescribed at a dose of 7.5 mg/month. One month into the treatment, masturbation to deviant sexual thoughts declined, and more importantly, all overt and abusive sexual behaviors ceased.

Though long term and continuous treatment with leuprolide will eventually result in a net decrease in testosterone and dihydrotestosterone, the first two to four weeks are marked by a paradoxical increase in testicular steroidogenesis, and therefore sex hormone production (Bradford, 1985; Vance & Smith, 1984). The first segment of leuprolide's biphasic effect on the hypothalamic-pituitary-gonadal axis can be antagonized and attenuated by the nonsteriodal, nonhormonal, antiandrogen flutamide (Crawford, Eisenberger, & McLeod, 1989; Dickey, 1992; Rousseau et al., 1990).

Leuprolide's active phase dose is 7.5 mg/month or 22.5 mg/q3months. Given its lack of oral bioavailability, leuprolide is injected into an area of large muscle. After its parenteral administration, the parent compound exerts its pharmacodynamic actions at the level of its target tissues (see below). After being metabolized to inactive peptides, leuprolide is excreted to some extent via the kidneys (Prod Info Lupron Depot ®-7.5 mg, 1997). Pre-existing congestive heart failure and gastrointestinal ulcers are contraindications for its use. Precautions should be taken whenever a patient presents with a history of cardiovascular disease, thromboembolism, osteoporosis, and urinary tract obstruction. Leuprolide can cause leukopenia, pure red cell aplasia, pulmonary embolism, thrombosis, myocardial infarction, arrhythmias, anaphylaxis (Dickey, 1992), gastrointestinal bleed, erythema multiforme, demineralization, and osteopenia. More common though less serious adverse effects are hot flashes, headaches, peripheral edema, headaches, dizziness, anorexia, nausea, vomiting, diarrhea, constipation, hypertriglyceridemia, hyperphosphatemia, muscle and bone pain, blurred vision, paresthesias, acne, rash, seborrhea, alopecia, gynecomastia, breast tenderness, testicular atrophy, and urinary dysfunction.

Triptorelin (now available in the United States), a long-acting agonist analogue of gonadotropin-releasing hormone, has been shown to be effective in the treatment of paraphilic patients (Rosler & Witztum, 1998; Thibaut, Cordier, & Kuhn, 1993). Despite these data, more studies are needed before triptorelin can be considered an alternative to the already established agents.

The aforementioned paragraphs clearly demonstrate that antiandrogens and the hormonal agents can reduce within a relatively short period of time, both frequency and intensity of deviant sexual desire and sexual arousal. Indeed, paraphilic patients who are treated with testosterone-lowering agents usually show recidivism rates similiar to those patients who underwent orchidectomy (Berlin & Meinecke, 1981; Berlin et al., 1991; Ortman, 1980). Given the invasive and intrusive nature of the treatment and the potential for serious side effects, more "benign" pharmacotherapeutic treatments have been proposed and are employed in the management of paraphilic patients.

The Serotonergic Agents

As mentioned earlier, basic science and pharmacological data provide ample evidence in support of the involvement of central monoamine neurotransmission in the pathophysiology of the paraphilias. In fact, a steadily rising number of researchers have studied the effects of the tricyclic antidepressants (TCA) and the serotonin-specific reuptake inhibitors (SSRIs) on sexual deviancy. The results are promising. Clomipramine, for instance, a TCA with potent serotonin reuptake inhibitor properties, abated sexually inappropriate thoughts and behaviors in paraphiliacs at doses ranging from 125-200 mg/day (Leo & Kim, 1995; Rubey, Brady, & Norris, 1993). Kruesi, Fine, Valladares, Phillips, and Rapoport (1992) alternatively conducted a double-blind crossover study, using clomipramine and desipramine (noradrenergic), in a heterogeneous group of patients with paraphilic disorders (entrees $n = 15$, completers $n = 8$). Methodological limitations notwithstanding (small sample size, heterogeneous patient population), the study results were interesting in that desipramine proved to be equally effective as clomipramine in reducing paraphilic symptoms.

Fluoxetine (SSRI) has been used with some success in the treatment of paraphilic patients (Coleman, Cesnik, Moore, & Dwyer, 1992; Emmanuel, Lydiard, & Ballenger, 1991; Galli, Raute, McConville, & McElroy, 1998; Jorgensen, 1990; Kafka, 1992; Kafka & Prentky, 1992). Perilstein and colleagues (1991), for example, reported the successful treatment of paraphilia-like phenomena in three men using fluoxetine at doses ranging from 20 mg/day to 40 mg twice a day. As early as 10 days into the treatment, deviant sexual symptoms diminished. Improvements were sustained for up to six months of follow-up. Anorgasmia and retarded ejaculation were the only reported side effects.

Other SSRIs have also been found to be effective. Abouesh and Clayton (1999) used paroxetine with satisfactory results in a voyeur and in an exhibitionist. Zohar, Kaplan, and Benjamin (1994) reported on the beneficial effects of fluvoxamine in controlling aberrant sexual behaviors in an exhibitionist. In a retrospective study Greenberg, Bradford, Curry, and O'Rourke (1996) showed that fluvoxamine (n = 16), sertraline (n = 25), and fluoxetine (n = 17) were all equally effective in ameliorating paraphilic symptoms.

Kafka (1994) conducted an open trial in 24 men with paraphilias or paraphilia-related disorders (PRD), using sertraline as the primary SSRI. Doses ranged from 25-250 mg/day (trial period 4-64 weeks). Four patients required augmentation with lithium, methylphenidate, or trazodone, respectively. Ten patients did not adequately respond to sertraline and were therefore tried on fluoxetine (9/10) with doses ranging from 10-80 mg/day. One-third (3/9) necessitated methylphenidate augmentation. Interestingly, and in line with data presented by Brown and Harrison (1992), the majority of patients treated with fluoxetine showed a subsequent reduction in their target symptoms, despite their previous inadequate response to sertraline. The results of this study provide further evidence in support of the use of either sertraline or fluoxetine in the treatment of paraphilic patients.

More recently, Greenberg and Bradford (1997) conducted, in a group of 18 pedophiles, an open-label dose study, using sertraline at a mean daily dose of 131 mg/day. Results of this study, in concordance with previous and later published data, were very promising. Improvements were noted on almost all outcome measures.

Few anecdotal case reports and open clinical trials have detailed the use of somewhat unconventional treatments for the paraphilias. Though different pharmacodynamically and less established than the aforementioned medications, these agents (e.g., buspirone hydrochloride, nefazodone, lithium, phenothiazine, quetiapine, risperidone) seemed to be effective in attenuating sexually deviant and deviant-like symptoms (Bartholomew, 1968; Bourgeois & Klein, 1996; Coleman, Gratzer, Nesvacil, & Raymond, 2000; Fedoroff, 1992, 1993; MacKnight & Rojas-Fernandez, 2000; Rubenstein & Engel, 1996). More clinical trials are needed to substantiate the efficacy and tolerability of these psychoactive medications before membership in the pharmacopoeia of first-line or even second-line agents can be considered.

Since many of the above mentioned medications have the potential to induce serious adverse effects, it would be prudent for patients to submit themselves to a thorough medical examination prior to the commencement of such treatments. This should include a complete physical and, if indicated, neurological examination. Laboratory studies should include a complete blood count, comprehensive metabolic panel (serum electrolytes, liver and renal function test), plasma reagin test (RPR), and endocrine assays (thyroid-stimulating-hormone [TSH], free and total serum testosterone, progesterone, estradiol, prolactin, serum FSH and serumLH) (Bradford, 2001). Urine should also be collected for urinalysis and β-Human-Chorionic-Gonadotropin (BHCG, pregnancy test) surveys. Given leuprolide's propensity to cause demineralization of bony structures, patients with risk factors for osteoporosis should be referred for Dual Energy X-Ray Absorptiometry (DEXA).

In conclusion, the treatment of paraphilic patients should always be broad and multifaceted, and ought to include psychosexual therapies and, if indicated, pharmacologically based treatments.

REFERENCES

Abouesh, A., & Clayton, A. (1999). Compulsive voyeurism and exhibitionism: A clinical response to paroxetine. *Archives of Sexual Behavior, 28*(1), 23-30.

Albin, J., Vittek, J., & Gordon, G. (1973). On the mechanism of the antiandrogenic effect of medroxyprogesterone acetate. *Endocrinology, 93*, 417-422.

Alexander, M. A. (1997). *Sexual offender treatment probed ANGW*. Madison, WI: Wisconsin Department of Corrections Sex Offender Treatment Program.

Amatayakul, K., Sivasomboon, B., & Thanangkul, O. (1980). A study of the mechanism of weight gain in medroxyprogesterone acetate users. *Contraception, 22*(6), 605-622.

American Psychiatric Association. (2000). *Diagnostic and statistical manual of mental disorders* (text revision). Washington, DC: Author.

Antal, E. J., Gillespie, W. R., & Albert, K. S. (1983). The bioavailability of an orally administered medroxyprogesterone acetate suspension. *International Journal of Clinical Pharmacologic Therapy Toxicology, 21*(5), 257-259.

Asberg, M., Schalling, D., & Traskman, L. (1987). Psychobiology of suicide, impulsivity and related phenomenon. In H.Y. Meltzer (Ed.), *Psychopharmacology: Third generation of progress* (pp. 655-688). New York: Raven Press.

Bancroft, J. (1989). The biological basis of human sexuality. In J. Bancroft (Ed.), *Human sexuality and its problems* (pp. 12-145). Edinburgh: Churchill Livingstone.

Bartholomew, A. A. (1968). A long-term phenothiazine as a possible agent to control deviant sexual behavior. *American Journal of Psychiatry, 123*, 917-923.

Baum, M. J., & Starr, M. S. (1980). Inhibition of sexual behavior by dopamine antagonists or serotonin agonist drugs in castrated male rats given estradiol or dihydrotestosterone. *Pharmacologic Biochemistry and Behavior, 13*, 47-67.

Berlin, F. S. (1983). Sex offenders: A biomedical perspective and a status report on biomedical treatment. In J. B. Greer, & I. R. Stuart (Eds.), *The sexual aggressor: Current perspectives on treatment* (pp. 83-123). New York: Van Nostrand Reinhold Co.

Berlin, F. S. (1989). The paraphilias and Depo-Provera: Some medical, ethical and legal considerations. *Bulletin American Academy of Psychiatry and the Law, 17*(3), 233-239.

Berlin, F. S., Frost, J. J., Mayberg, H. S., Behal, R., Daniels, R. F., Links, J. M. et al. (1988). *Endogenous opiate secretion in the brain during sexual arousal detectible by PET scanning.* Unpublished Data.

Berlin, F. S., & Meinecke, C. F. (1981). Treatment of sex offenders with antiandrogenic medication: Conceptualization, review of treatment modalities, and preliminary findings. *American Journal of Psychiatry, 138*, 601-607.

Berlin, F. S., & Schaerf, F. W. (1985). Laboratory assessment of the paraphilias and their treatment with antiandrogenic medication. In R. C. W. Hall, & T. P. Beresford (Eds.), *Handbook of psychiatric diagnostic procedures* (pp. 273-305). New York: Spectrum Publications.

Berlin, F. S., Wayne, H. P., Martin, M. M., Dyer, A., Gregory, L. K., & Sharon, D. (1991). A five-year plus follow-up survey of criminal recidivism within a treated cohort of 406 pedophiles, 111 exhibitionists and 109 sexual aggressives: Issues and outcome. *American Journal of Forensic Psychiatry, 12*(3), 5-28.

Blake, J. C., Sawyerr, A. M., Dooley, J. S., Scheuer, P. J., & McIntyre, N. (1990). Severe hepatitis caused by cyproterone acetate. *Gut, 31*(5), 556-557.

Bourgeois, J. A., & Klein, M. (1996). Risperidone and fluoxetine in the treatment of pedophilia with comorbid dysthymia. *Journal of Clinical of Psychopharmacology, 16*(3), 257-258.

Bradford, J. M. W. (1985). Organic treatment for the male sex offender. *Behavioral Sciences & the Law, 3*(4), 355-375.

Bradford, J. M. W. (1996). The role of serotonin in the future of forensic psychiatry. *Bulletin American Academy of Psychiatry and the Law, 24*(1), 57-72.

Bradford, J. M. W. (1999). The paraphilias, obsessive-compulsive spectrum disorder and the treatment of sexually deviant behavior. *Psychiatry Quarterly, 70*, 209-19.

Bradford, J. M. W. (2001). The neurobiology, neuropharmacology, and pharmacological treatment of the paraphilias and compulsive sexual behaviour. *Canadian Journal of Psychiatry, 46*(1), 26-34.

Bradford, J. M. W., & Bourget, D. (1987). Sexually aggressive men. *Psychiatric Journal of the University of Ottawa, 12*, 169-175.

Bradford, J. M. W., Greenberg, D., Gojer, J., Martindale, J. J., & Goldberg, M. (1995, May). *Sertraline in the treatment of pedophilia: An open label study.* Paper presented at the meeting of the American Psychiatric Association, Miami, FL.

Bradford, J. M. W., & Pawlak, A. (1987). Sadistic homosexual pedophilia: Treatment with cyproterone acetate; A single case study. *Canadian Journal of Psychiatry, 32*, 22-31.

Bradford, J. M. W., & Pawlak, A. (1993). Effects of cyproterone acetate on sexual arousal patterns of pedophiles. *Archives of Sexual Behavior, 22*(6), 629-641.

Briken, P., Nika, E., & Berner, W. (2001). Treatment of paraphilia with luteinizing hormone-releasing hormone agonists. *Journal of Sex and Marital Therapy, 27*(1), 45-55.

Brooks, J. H., & Reddon, J. R. (1996). Serum testosterone in violent and nonviolent young offenders. *Journal of Clinical Psychology, 52*(4), 475-483.

Brown, W. A., & Harrison, W. (1992). Are patients who are intolerant to one SSRI intolerant to another? *Psychopharmacology Bulletin, 28*, 253-256.

Brown, W. A., Monti, P. M., & Carrivean, D. P. (1978). Serum testosterone and sexual activity and interest in men. *Archives of Sexual Behavior, 7*(7), 97-103.

Camacho, A. M., Williams, L. D., & Montalvo, J. M. (1972). Alterations of testicular histology and chromosomes in patients with constitutional sexual precocity treated with medroxyprogesterone acetate. *Journal of Clinical Endocrinology Metabolism, 34*, 279-286.

Coleman, E., Cesnik, J., Moore, A. M., & Dwyer, S. M. (1992). An exploratory study of the role of psychotropic medications in the treatment of sexual offenders. *Journal of Offender Rehabilitation, 18*, 75-88.

Coleman, E., Gratzer, T., Nesvacil, L., & Raymond, N. C. (2000). Nefazodone and the treatment of nonparaphilic compulsive sexual behavior: A retrospective study. *Journal of Clinical Psychiatry, 61*(4), 282-284.

Cooper, A. J. (1986). Progestogens in the treatment of male sex offenders: A review. *Canadian Journal of Psychiatry, 31*(1), 73-79.

Cooper, A. J. (1987). Medroxyprogesterone acetate (MPA) treatment of sexual acting out men suffering from dementia. *Journal of Clinical Psychiatry, 48*, 368-370.

Cooper, A. J., & Cernovsky, Z. Z. (1994). Comparison of cyproterone acetate (CPA) and leuprolide acetate (LHRH agonist) in a chronic pedophile: A clinical case study. *Biological Psychiatry, 36*, 269-271.

Cooper, A. J., Cernosvsky, Z., & Magnus, R. V. (1992). The long-term use of cyproterone acetate in pedophilia: A case study. *Journal of Sex and Marital Therapy, 18*(4), 292-302.

Cooper, A. J., Sandhu, S., Losztyn, S., & Cernovsky, Z. (1992). A double-blind placebo controlled trial of medroxyprogesterone acetate and cyproterone acetate with seven pedophiles. *Canadian Journal of Psychiatry, 37*(10), 687-693.

Crawford, E. D., Eisenberger, M. A., & McLeod, D. G. (1989). A controlled trial of leuprolide with and without flutamide in prostatic carcinoma. *New England Journal of Medicine, 321*, 419-424.

Davidson, J. M., Canargo, C. M., & Smith, E. R. (1979). Effects of androgen on sexual behavior in hypogonadal men. *Journal of Clinical Endocrinological Metabolism, 48*, 995-958.

Dickey, R. (1992). The management of case of treatment-resistant paraphilia with a long-acting LHRH agonist. *Canadian Journal of Psychiatry, 37*(8), 567-9.

Dux, S., Bishara, J., Marom, D., Blum, I., & Pitlik, S. (1998). Medroxyprogesterone acetate-induced secondary adrenal insufficiency. *Annals of Pharmacotherapy, 32*(1), 134.

Emmanuel, N. P., Lydiard, R. B., & Ballenger, J. C. (1991). Fluoxetine treatment of voyeurism. *American Journal of Psychiatry, 148*(7), 950.

Everitt, B. J., & Bancroft, J. (1991). Of rats and men: The comparative approach to male sexuality. *Annual Review of Sex Research, 2*, 77-118.

Fedoroff, J. P. (1992). Buspirone hydrochloride in the treatment of an atypical paraphilia. *Archives of Sexual Behavior, 21*(4), 401-406.

Fedoroff, J. P. (1993). Buspirone hydrochloride in the treatment of transvestic fetishism. *Journal of Clinical Psychiatry, 54*(5), 182-188.

Fedoroff, J. P., Peyser, C., Franz, M. L., & Folstein, S. E. (1994). Sexual disorders in Huntington's disease. *Journal of Neuropsychiatry Clinical Neurosciences, 6*(2), 147-153.

Ferguson, J., Henriksen, S., & Cohen, H. (1970). "Hypersexuality" and behavioral changes in cats caused by administration of p-chlorophenylalanine. *Science, 168*, 499-501.

Gaffney, G. R., & Berlin, F. S. (1984). Is there hypothalamic-pituitary-gonadal dysfunction in pedophilia? A pilot study. *British Journal of Psychiatry, 145*, 657-660.

Gagne, P. (1981). Treatment of sex offenders with medroxyprogesterone acetate. *American Journal of Psychiatry, 138*, 644-646.

Galli, V. B., Raute, N. J., McConville, B. J., & McElroy, S. L. (1998). An adolescent male with multiple paraphilias successful treated with fluoxetine. *Journal of Child and Adolescent Psychopharmacology, 8*(3), 195.

Goldenberg, S. L., & Bruchovsky, N. (1991). Use of cyproterone acetate in prostate cancer. *Urologic Clinics of North America, 18*(1), 111-122.

Gottesman, H. G., & Schubert, D. S. P. (1993). Low-dose oral medroxyprogesterone acetate in the management of the paraphilias. *Journal of Clinical Psychiatry, 54*(5), 182-188.

Greenberg, D. M., & Bradford, J. M. W. (1997). Treatment of the paraphilic disorders. A review of the role of the selective serotonin reuptake inhibitors. *Sexual Abuse: A Journal of Research and Treatment, 9*, 349-361.

Greenberg, D. M., Bradford, J. M. W., Curry, S., & O'Rourke, A. (1996). A comparison of treatment of paraphilias with three serotonin reuptake inhibitors: A retrospective study. *Bulletin American Academy of Psychiatry and the Law, 24*(4), 525-532.

Griffin, J. E., & Wilson, J. D. (1980). Disorders of the testes and male reproductive tract. In J. D. Wilson, & D. W. Foster (Eds.), *Textbook of endocrinology* (7th ed.) (pp. 259-311). Philadelphia: Saunders.

Hendricks, S. E., Fitzpatrick, D. F., Hartman, K., Quaife, M. A., Stratbucker, R. A., & Graber, B. (1988). Brain structure and function in sexual molesters of children and adolescents. *Journal of Clinical Psychiatry, 49*(3), 108-112.

Hucker, S., Langevin, R., & Bain, J. (1988). A double-blind trial of sex drive reducing medication in pedophiles. *Annals Review of Sex Research, 1*, 227-242.

Jeffcoate, J. W., Matthews, R. W., Edwards, C. R., Field, L. H., & Besser, G. M. (1980). The effect of cyproterone acetate on serum testosterone, LH, FSH, and prolactin in male sex offenders. *Clinical Endocrinology, 13*(2), 189-195.

Jorgensen, V. T. (1990). Cross-dressing successfully treated with fluoxetine (letter). *NY State Journal of Medicine, 90*, 5667.

Jurzyk, R. S., Spielvogel, R. L., & Rose, L. I. (1992). Antiandrogens in the treatment of acne and hirsutism. *American Family Physician, 45*(4), 1803-1806.

Kafka, M. P. (1992). Successful treatment of paraphilic coercive disorder (a rapist) with fluoxetine hydrochloride. *British Journal of Psychiatry, 53,* 351-358.

Kafka, M. P. (1994). Sertraline pharmacotherapy for paraphilias and paraphilia-related disorders: An open trial. *Annals Clinical Psychiatry, 6*(3), 189-195.

Kafka, M. P. (1997). A monoamine hypothesis for the pathophysiology of paraphilic disorders. *Archives of Sexual Behavior, 26*(4), 343-358.

Kafka, M. P., & Prentky, R. (1992). Fluoxetine treatment of non-paraphilic sexual addictions and paraphilias in men. *Journal of Clinical Psychiatry, 53,* 351-358.

Kierch, T. A. (1990). Treatment of sex offenders with Depo-Provera. *Bulletin American Academy of Psychiatry and the Law, 18,* 179-187.

Kravitz, H. M., Haywood, T. W., Kelly, J., & Cavanaugh, J. L., Jr. (1996). Medroxy- progesterone and paraphiles: Do testosterone levels matter? *Bulletin American Academy of Psychiatry and the Law, 24*(1), 73-83.

Kravitz, H. M., Haywood, T. W., Kelly, J., Wahlstrom, C., Liles, S., & Cavanaugh, J. L. (1995). Medroxyprogesterone treatment for paraphiliacs. *Bulletin American Academy of Psychiatry and the Law, 23*(1), 19-33.

Krueger, R. B., & Kaplan, M. S. (2001). Depot-leuprolide acetate for treatment of paraphilias: A report of twelve cases. *Archives of Sexual Behavior, 30*(4), 409-422.

Kruesi, M. J., Fine, S., Valladares, L., Phillips, R. A. Jr., & Rapoport, J. L. (1992). Paraphilias: A double-blind crossover comparison of clomipramine versus desipramine. *Archives of Sexual Behavior, 21*(6), 587-593.

Lang, R. A., Langevin, R., & Bain, J. (1989). Sex hormone profiles in genital exhibitionists. *Annals of Sex Research, 2,* 67-75.

Laschet, U., & Laschet, L. (1975). Antiandrogens in the treatment of sexual deviations of men. *Journal Steroid Biochemistry, 6*(6), 821-826.

Laws, D. R., & Marshall, W. L. (1991). Masturbatory reconditioning with sexual deviates: An evaluative review. *Advances in Behavior Research and Therapy, 13,* 13-25.

Lee, R., & Coccaro, E. (2001). The neuropsychopharmacology of criminality and aggression. *Canadian Journal of Psychiatry, 46*(1), 35-44.

Leo, R. J., & Kim, K. Y. (1995). Clomipramine treatment of paraphilias in elderly demented patients. *Journal of Geriatric Psychiatry and Neurology, 8*(2), 123-124.

Levesque, H., Trivalle, C., Manchon, N. D., Vinel, J. P., Moore, N., Hemet, J. et al. (1989). Fulminant hepatitis due to cyproterone acetate. *Lancet, 1*(8631), 215-216.

Liang, T., Tymoczko, J. L., Chan, K. M. B., Hung, H. C., & Liao, S. (1977). Androgen action: Receptors and rapid responses. In L. Martini, & M. Motta (Eds.), *Androgens and antiandrogens* (pp. 77-89). New York: Raven Press.

MacKnight, C., & Rojas-Fernandez, C. (2000). Quetiapine for sexually inappropriate behavior in dementia. *Journal American Geriatric Society, 48*(6), 707.

Maes, M., De Vos, N., Van Hunsel, F., Van West, D., Westenberg, H., Cosyns, P. et al. (2001). Pedophilia is accompanied by increased plasma concentrations of catecholamines, in particular epinephrine. *Psychiatry Research, 103*(1), 43-49.

Mann, J. J., Arango, V., Marzuk, S., Theccanat, S., & Rtes, D. J. (1989). Evidence of the 5-ht hypothesis of suicide: A review of post mortem studies. *British Journal of Psychiatry, 155,* 7-14.

Marks, I. M. (1981). Review of behavior psychotherapy, II: Sexual disorders. *American Journal of Psychiatry, 138*, 750-756.

Marks, I., Gelder, M., & Bancroft, J. (1970). Sexual deviants two years after electric aversion. *British Journal of* Psychiatry, *117*, 173-185.

Mas, M. (1995). Neurobiological correlates of masculine sexual behavior. *Neuroscience Biobehavior Rev*iew, *19*, 261-277.

Mendez, M. F., Chow, T., Ringman, J., Twitchell, G., & Hinkin, C. H. (2000). Pedophilia and temporal disturbances. *Journal of Neuropsychiatry Clinical Neuroscience, 12*(1), 71-76.

Meyer, W. J., Cole, C., & Emory, E. (1992). Depo provera treatment for sex offending behavior: An evaluation of outcome. *Bulletin American Academy of Psychiatry and the Law, 20*, 249-259.

Meyer, W. J., Walker, P. A., Emory, L. E., & Smith, E. R. (1985). Physical, metabolic, and hormonal effects on men of long-term therapy with medroxyprogesterone acetate. *Fertility and Sterility, 43*(1), 102-109.

Ortman, J. (1980). The treatment of sexual offenders. Castration and antihormone therapy. *International Journal of Law and Psychiatry, 3*, 443-451.

Perilstein, R. D., Lipper, S., & Friedman, L. J. (1991). Three cases of paraphilias responsive to fluoxetine treatment. *Journal of Clinical Psychiatry, 52*(4), 169-170.

Peters, J. J., & Roether, H. A. (1972). Group psychotherapy for probationed sex offenders. In L. P. Resnik, & M. E. Wolfgang (Eds.), *Sexual behaviors: Some clinical and legal aspects* (pp. 167-185). Boston: Little Brown.

Rada, R. T., Laws, D. R., & Kellner, R. (1976). Plasma testosterone and the rapist. *Psychosomatic Medicine, 38*, 257-268.

Rada, R. T., Laws, D. R., & Kellner, R., (1983). Plasma androgens in violent and nonviolent sex offenders. *Bulletin American Academy of Psychiatry and the Law, 11*, 149-158.

Reilly, D. R., Delva, N. J., & Hudson, R. W. (2000). Protocols for the use of cyproterone, medroxyprogesterone, and leuprolide in the treatment of paraphilia. *Canadian Journal of Psychiatry, 45*(6), 559-563.

Roeder, F. D., Muller, D., & Orthner, H. (1972). The stereotaxic treatment of pedophilic homosexuality and other sexual deviations. In E. Hitchcock, L. Laitienn, & K. Vaernet (Eds.), *Psychosurgery* (pp. 87-111). Springfield, IL: Charles C. Thomas.

Rosler, A., & Witztum, E. (1998). Treatment of men with paraphilia with a long acting analogue of gonadotropin-releasing hormone. *New England Journal of Medicine, 338*, 416-65.

Rosler, A., & Witztum, E. (2000). Pharmacotherapy of paraphilias in the next millennium. *Behavioral Sciences & the Law, 18*(1), 43-56.

Rousseau, L. R., Couture, M., Dupont, A., Labrie, F., & Couture, N. (1990). Effect of combined androgen blockade with an LHRH agonist and flutamide in one severe case of male exhibitionism. *Canadian Journal of Psychiatry, 35*, 338-341.

Rubenstein, E. B., & Engel, N. L. (1996). Successful treatment of transvestic fetishism with sertraline and lithium. *Journal of Clinical Psychiatry, 57*(2), 92.

Rubey, R., Brady, K. T., & Norris, G. T. (1993). Clomipramine treatment of sexual preoccupation. *Journal of Clinical Psychopharmacology, 13*, 158-159.

Salzman, L. (1971). The psychodynamic approaches to sex deviations. *International Psychiatry Clinics, 8,* 20-40.

Schering, A. G. (1983). *Androcur.* Berlin, Germany: Berlin/Bergkamen.

Shotliff, K., & Nussey, S. S. (1997). Medroxyprogesterone acetate induced Cushing's syndrome. *British Journal of Clinical Pharmacology, 44*(3), 304.

Sjoerdsma, A., & Palfreyman, M. G. (1990). History of serotonin and serotonin disorders. In P. M. Whitaker-Azuitia, & S. J. Peroutka (Eds.), *The neuropharmacology of serotonin* (pp. 600:1-8). New York: Annals of the New York Academy of Sciences.

Smith, J. A. (1986). Luteinizing hormone-releasing hormone (LH-RH) analogs in treatment of prostatic cancer. *Urology, 27,* 9-15.

Southren, A. L., Gordon, G. G., Vittek, J., & Altman, K. (1977). Effect of progestagens on androgen metabolism. In L. Martini, & M. Motta (Eds.), *Androgens and antiandrogens* (pp. 263-279). New York: Raven Press.

Sturup, G. K. (1972). Castration: The total treatment. In H. P. L. Resnik, & M. E. Wolfgang (Eds.), *Sexual behaviors: Social, clinical and legal aspects* (pp. 361-382). Boston: Little Brown & Co.

Thibaut, F., Cordier, B., & Kuhn, J. M. (1993). Effect of a long-lasting gonadotropin hormone-releasing hormone agonist in sex cases of severe male paraphilia. *Acta Psychiatrica Scandinavica, 87,* 445-450.

Tucker, J. C., & File, S. E. (1983). Serotonin and sexual behavior. In D. Weathley (Ed.), *Psychopharmacology and sexual disorders* (pp. 22-49). New York: Oxford University Press.

Vance, M. A., & Smith, J. A., Jr. (1984). Endocrine and clinical effects of leuprolide in prostate cancer. *Clinical Pharmacology & Therapeutics, 36*(3), 350-354.

Van Praag, H. M. (1984). CSF 5-HIAA and suicide in non-depressed schizophrenics. *Lancet, 2,* 977-978.

Walker, P. A., & Meyer, W. J. (1981). Medroxyprogesterone acetate treatment for paraphilic sex offenders. In J. R. Hayes, T. K. Roberts, & K. S. Soloway (Eds.), *Violence and the violent individual* (pp. 353-373). New York: Spectrum Publications.

Walker, P. A., Meyer, W. J., Emory, L. E., & Rubin, A. L. (1984). Antiandrogen treatment of the paraphilias. In H. C. Stancer, P. E. Garfinkel, & V. M. Rakoff (Eds.), *Guidelines for the use of psychotropic drugs* (pp. 427-443). Jamaica, NY: Spectrum Publications.

Williams, G., Allen, J. M., O'Shea, J. P., Mashiter, K., Doble, A., & Bloom, S. R. (1983). Prostatic cancer: Treatment with long-acting LHRH analogue. *British Journal of Urology, 55*(6), 743-746.

Zohar, J., Kaplan, Z., & Benjamin, J. (1994). Compulsive exhibitionism successfully treated with fluvoxamine: A controlled case study. *Journal Clinical Psychiatry, 55*(3), 86-88.

Enhancing Victim Empathy for Sex Offenders

Mark S. Carich
Carole K. Metzger
Mirza S. A. Baig
Joseph J. Harper

SUMMARY. Victim empathy is a widely used component of sex offender treatment throughout North America and Great Britain. Yet, it has been controversial over the past few years. One of the complications involves giving empathy a solid definition. Empathy was defined as the capacity to express compassion for victims. A multi-level system was developed to help specify the definition. The second issue concerns which methods to use in enhancing victim empathy. A variety of techniques are provided as specific ways in which clinicians can help enhance an offender's empathy level. *[Article copies available for a fee from The Haworth Document Delivery Service: 1-800-HAWORTH. E-mail address: <docdelivery@haworthpress.com> Website: <http://www.HaworthPress.com> © 2003 by The Haworth Press, Inc. All rights reserved.]*

KEYWORDS. Victim empathy, empathy techniques, levels of empathy, responsibility, distortions, victim impact

Address correspondence to: Mark S. Carich, PhD, Big Muddy Correctional Center, P.O. Box 1000, Ina, IL 62846-1000.

[Haworth co-indexing entry note]: "Enhancing Victim Empathy for Sex Offenders." Carich, Mark S. et al. Co-published simultaneously in *Journal of Child Sexual Abuse* (The Haworth Maltreatment & Trauma Press, an imprint of The Haworth Press, Inc.) Vol. 12, No. 3/4, 2003, pp. 255-276; and: *Identifying and Treating Sex Offenders: Current Approaches, Research, and Techniques* (ed: Robert Geffner et al.) The Haworth Maltreatment & Trauma Press, an imprint of The Haworth Press, Inc., 2003, pp. 255-276. Single or multiple copies of this article are available for a fee from The Haworth Document Delivery Service [1-800-HAWORTH, 9:00 a.m. - 5:00 p.m. (EST). E-mail address: docdelivery@haworthpress.com].

http://www.haworthpress.com/web/JCSA
© 2003 by The Haworth Press, Inc. All rights reserved.
Digital Object Identifier: 10.1300/J070v12n03_10

For many years, victim empathy has been a component of sex offender treatment (Freeman-Longo, Bird, Stevenson, & Fiske, 1995; Knopp, Freeman-Longo, & Stevenson, 1992; Marshall, 1999). According to Webster and Beech (2000), the promotion of empathy among sex offenders is a core component in the majority of programs in Britain and the United States. From the late 1970s until the 1990s, many professionals utilized a shamed-based approach to address victim empathy in sex offender treatment (Baker & Price, 1997). In recent years, however, a more compassionate treatment approach has emerged with emphasis on respect, compassion, and individuality (Blanchard, 1995; Carich, Kassel, & Stone, 2001; Carich, Newbauer, & Stone, 2001; Freeman-Longo & Blanchard, 1998; Marshall, 1996).

Over the years, controversies have arisen concerning the use of victim empathy and treatment itself. Some researchers (Quinsey, personal communication, June 6, 2000) have argued against using victim empathy in treatment, denying its effectiveness. Quinsey and associates base most of their criticism on a program at a Canadian maximum-security psychiatric program in the 1970s. This program was considered a "state of the art" program based on a "therapeutic community" concept. There appeared to be a lack of supervision, with a highly confrontational environment. Elements of the program included the use of LSD and sexual "orgies." The outcome results, based on recidivism, demonstrated higher recidivism rates with the treated sample as opposed to the untreated.

Another basis for criticism is that victim empathy was not a factor correlated with recidivism in a meta-analysis of 61 sex offender recidivism studies (e.g., Hanson & Bussiere, 1998). One reason for this is that most of the correlated factors were static or unchangeable in nature. Thus, the vast majority of validated risk assessment instruments and statistically oriented research into dynamic risk factors (including victim empathy as a factor) is now underway and in its infancy (Hanson, personal communication, March 7, 2000).

Many critics allege that victim empathy reinforces or even increases deviant sexual behaviors. They also believe that psychopathic offenders cannot learn victim empathy, and there is a tendency to generalize this belief to all sex offenders. Others hold the belief that victim empathy does not influence treatment outcomes or recidivism. The next issue is that it is difficult for therapists to enhance empathy, and it is likewise too difficult for offenders to learn empathy. However, all of these complaints have been refuted and discussed (Carich, 2002). In actuality, most sex offenders are not extremely antisocial or psychopathic. Only a small percentage of sex offenders meet the criteria for these diagnoses.

Victim empathy can be viewed as a multi-level skill and process that can be learned by most sexual abusers. However, these researchers do make a point in that if victim empathy is conducted inappropriately, negative outcomes will result.

The thrust of this article is based on the assumption that treatment can result in effective outcomes if done effectively and the offender wants to make the necessary changes, as indicated by Hanson (1997), Marshall, Anderson, and Fernandez (1999), and Marshall and Pithers (1994). Likewise, victim empathy can be learned and is a useful component of treatment.

DEFINING EMPATHY

There are many different definitions of empathy, including a multiple level analysis of skills. According to Hennessy, Walter, and Vess (2002), the construct of empathy and its definition have been discussed in the professional literature for decades without consensus. Empathy is the capacity to understand and identify with another's perspective and the capacity to experience the same emotions as another. Historically, empathy has been defined as a "cognitive ability to understand and identify with another's perspective, an emotional capacity to experience the same feelings as another . . . or an interplay of cognitive and affective factors" (Pithers, 1994, p. 565).

Within a therapeutic context, empathy has been defined by a number of writers. George and Cristiani (1990) define empathy as "the ability to tune in to the client's feelings and to be able to see the client's world as it truly seems to be to the client . . . The ability to be empathetic in a relationship requires that the counselor respond sensitively and accurately to the clients' feelings and experiences as they were his own" (p. 130). Egan (1986) defined empathy as "the ability to enter into and understand the world of another person and communicate this understanding to him or her" (p. 95). He goes on to differentiate several types of empathy such as emotional empathy, which is the ability to understand or communicate another's state, condition, or point of view. Specific elements include listening, observing, understanding, and communicating that understanding.

Victim empathy is defined in contemporary sex offender treatment as the offender's understanding of the victim's pain or the impact of his offenses. Hanson (1997) notes that many treatment professionals strive to help the offender develop the ability to accurately perceive the victim's suffering or victim impact and to respond in a compassionate manner.

A MULTI-LEVEL MODEL OF VICTIM EMPATHY

Victim empathy can be viewed multi-dimensionally and in levels. The highest level consists of the offender's spontaneous, compassionate understanding and emotional expression of that understanding at both intellectual and emotional levels, of the victim(s) situation (i.e., victim impact) created by the offender. The offender understands what he did to the victim, understands the victim's suffering, and can emotionally express those feelings spontaneously. We have defined a five-point model of victim empathy and delineated the specific characteristics of each level (see Table 1).

Level 0 indicates that the offender is devoid of victim empathy and perhaps global empathy. Research shows that most offenders may not be devoid of global empathy, but have difficulties empathizing with their own victims (Marshall, Jones, Hudson, & McDonald, 1993). Level 0 would include a very limited number of offenders. These offenders enjoying distressing and/or victimizing others. They are more psychopathic in nature and tend to have severe antisocial and narcissistic personality characteristics. They appear to others as being cold, callous, non-caring, and apathetic.

A low level of empathy appears in Level 1. This level is characterized by superficial understanding and false remorse. Although the offender still appears to enjoy distressing others, he at least displays a superficial level of empathy. At this level, one can still generate victim empathy. This is based on the premise described by Fernandez, Marshall, Lightbody, and O'Sullivan (1999), who indicate that child molesters are not generally devoid of empathy. They state: "These results suggest the possibility that child molesters have learned to inhibit their empathetic responses toward victims of sexual abuse and most particularly their own victims. This inhibition of empathy would permit molesters to continue abusing children without feeling remorse since they could maintain that they had not harmed their victims" (p. 27).

In Level 2, the offender intellectually understands the victim's perspective. The offender cognitively recognizes the impact on the victim but has problems with emotional recognition. Research suggests that many offenders, particularly child molesters, have difficulty with emotional recognition and emotional expression (Hansen & Scott, 1995;

TABLE 1. The Five-Point Multi-Level Model of Victim Empathy

Level 0–Nonexistence

Characteristics:

- Psychopathic tendencies
- Lacks conscience (no remorse displayed)
- Self-centered or out for self
- Victimizes
- Very manipulative
- Appears apathetic, cold, callous, non-caring
- Lacks global empathy
- Shallow and superficial
- Severe antisocial and narcissistic personality disorders
- Enjoys victimizing and distressing others
- Does not care for victims at all

Level 1–Superficial Understanding and False Remorse

Characteristics:

- Superficial empathy at best, with false remorse
- Cognitive distortions in offense disclosure
- Self-centered, does not consider others
- May try to act like he has victim empathy
- Enjoys distressing others and/or offending
- May pretend to care for victims and others only for ulterior motives
- Very insincere responses
- Limited global empathy

Level 2–Intellectual Understanding Only

Characteristics:

- Intellectually understands victim perspective at best
- Limited use of some cognitive distortions
- Fluctuates on responsibility/accountability
- Lacks emotional recognition and expression
- Fluctuates on victim perspective (intellectual at best)
- Increased but still limited global empathy
- Victim stances and self-pity
- Recognizes victim harm at intellectual level only
- Continues to victimize others (non-sexually or even perhaps sexually)

Level 3–Generates Occasional Emotional Victim Empathy Responses

Characteristics:

- Emotional recognition
- Occasional emotional victim empathy responses
- Does tend to feel for victims, but has difficulty expressing feelings occasionally
- Struggles with being vulnerable
- Has obtained a victim perspective
- Fluctuates from self-centered to other-centered

TABLE 1 (continued)

- Remains somewhat self-centered
- Has developed perspective taking skills
- Takes responsibility for offenses
- May have emotional global empathy for crisis situations, however not concerning specific victims
- Gets distracted when focus in on victim empathy
- Recognizes victim harm
- Conscience fluctuates

Level 4–Generates Consistent Emotional Victim Empathy Responses

Characteristics:

- Generates emotional victim empathy response consistently
- Victim perspective
- Can be vulnerable
- Obtains responsibility on an emotional level
- Holds self accountable/responsible
- Does not use cognitive distortions/defenses to block victim empathy
- Does not victim stance
- Not self-centered and tends to stay other-centered
- Has developed some level of self-worth/adequacy/esteem and remorse
- Deep sense of conscience
- Tends to stay focused on victim empathy
- Realizes victim impact on both primary and secondary victims
- Emotional recognition

Level 5–Spontaneous Emotional Victim Empathy

Characteristics:

- Higher and deepest levels
- Spontaneous emotional victim empathy expression
- Consistent victim perspective/generates victim empathy
- Consistent global empathy
- Deep sense of remorse
- Balances self-worth/esteem with adequate sense of remorse
- Doesn't fear vulnerability
- Assumes responsibility/accountability
- Other-centered
- Has fully developed consciences
- When focused on victims/victim impact, stays focused
- Understands full impact of behavior

Hennessy et al., 2002; Hudson et al., 1993; Marshall et al., 1999). An intellectual grasp on harm recognition is necessary to fully experience victim empathy at emotional levels in Levels 4 and 5 of this model.

Level 3 is reached when the offender is able to generate occasional victim empathy responses. In this level, the offender achieves emotional recognition of the impact of the offense with occasional emotional expressions. The offender has gained perspective-taking skills and takes responsibility for the offense. However, the offender still has problems with emotional expression on a consistent basis and continues to exhibit self-centered behaviors.

Level 4 is achieved when the offender generates consistent emotional victim empathy responses, which is the primary goal of sex offender treatment. At this level, the offender holds himself responsible and accountable for his offenses. This means that he does not harbor any offense-specific cognitive distortions and has restructured previously held distortions. This level is further characterized by the development of an appropriate level of self-worth, esteem, or sense of adequacy balanced with healthy remorse. Instead of being suppressed, the affect domains are fully connected with self, and they are consistently expressed.

Level 5, spontaneous emotional victim empathy, is the highest and deepest level of empathy obtainable. Few offenders reach this level. The offender is vulnerable and offers outreach when necessary. He spontaneously expresses victim empathy and remorse. Yet, he balances self-worth/esteem with victim empathy. His conscience is fully developed, as the offender fully understands the victim impact.

The therapeutic goal in victim empathy work is to reach Level 4 and, if possible, Level 5. Level 4 provides enough emotional glue to bind treatment. Victim empathy also encompasses a variety of experiential domains including cognitive (perceptual), affective, behavioral, social (communicational), and bio-physiological. These are addressed throughout this article either directly or indirectly. In essence, ". . . empathy is multi-dimensional and includes not only the cognitive and emotional components, but also communicative and relational elements" (Marshall, Hudson, Jones, & Fernandez, 1995, p. 101). Although the particulars are not yet refined, this level perspective can be used as an assessment process.

Victim empathy can be categorized in terms of offender specific empathy and global victim empathy. Treatment professionals use several terms to distinguish victim empathy. These terms include remorse, conscience, and false-remorse. Remorse can be defined as the painful guilt and regret of violating another. The conscience is the part of the human mind/brain that registers when one violates another and/or does something wrong, and generates a bad feeling regarding that behavior. False remorse is described as remorse that does not have meaning, or remorse that is superficial in nature.

Not all offenders are devoid of empathy. Marshall and colleagues (1993) suggest that empathy deficits may not pertain globally; in fact, they assert that empathetic response deficits appear to be victim specific and not representative of global deficiencies.

KEY ELEMENTS AND PROCESSES OF VICTIM EMPATHY

Victim empathy is a complex and difficult concept to grasp. Several authors (Carich, 1999; Carich & Cadler, 2003; Carich & Harper, 2003; Carich, Kassel, & Stone, 2001; Hanson, 1997; Marshall & Fernandez, 2001) have attempted to analyze it in terms of components of processes and elements. Marshall and Maric (1996) emphasize highly cognitive and emotional deficits.

Hanson and Scott (1995) discuss empathy and outline three major components: (a) perspective taking ability, (b) emotional responding to others, and (c) caring. They define perspective taking as the ability or capacity to accurately identify the emotional state of another person and respond to particular situations. They see empathy primarily as a cognitive ability. Later, Hanson (1997) outlined three components of victim empathy or what he called sympathy. The first is what he termed the "offender victim relationship" which refers to the degree to which the offender can develop a caring relationship with the victim. The second is termed "perspective taking ability" which is the degree to which one can cognitively understand another's thoughts and feelings; it is the ability to describe facial expression, body language, voice tone, and other non-verbal behavior, and recognize the victim's suffering from his/her sexual transgression. The third component is termed "sympathy training" which refers to working through distortions.

Marshall and Fernandez (2001) outlined four components of empathy. The first is emotional recognition of another's emotional state. The second is "perspective taking" or seeing the world as the other person. The third is identifying with another person or experiencing the same emotional state as another person. The fourth involves the offender feeling the need to stop victimizing and to comfort others.

Carich, Kassel, and Stone (2001) identified six key elements of empathy. The first element is *emotional recognition* as identified by Marshall and Fernandez (2001). This is the ability to recognize one's own emotions and emotions of others or identifying feelings. Hudson and colleagues (1993) suggest that child molesters may have more difficulty with emotional recognition.

The second element is *victim harm recognition* as identified by Marshall and Fernandez (2001). Victim harm recognition is the ability to identify and recognize the harm inflicted upon the victim through the offender's transgression or acknowledging the violation of the victim.

The third element is *assuming responsibility*. This means that the offender accepts full responsibility for his offenses. This involves ownership of one's behavior without distortions. Empathy has been linked to cognitive distortions (Hanson, 1997; Marshall et al., 1995; Marshall & Fernandez, 2001; McGrath, Cann, & Konopasky, 1998). Ward, Hudson, Johnston, and Marshall (1997) and Webster and Beech (2000) suggest a direct link between sexual offenders' cognitive distortions and their victim specific empathy.

The fourth element is *perspective taking*. This is identifying with one's victim and developing a compassionate understanding of the victim. In other words, it is understanding the victim impact and what the victim went through and/or goes through. This includes experiencing the same feelings as the victim.

The fifth element is a *guilt response*. This is feeling bad for violating the victim. Marshall and Fernandez (2001) emphasize experiencing a sad emotional state. Here the offender cannot only identify, but experiences the victim's emotional state.

The final element is *emotional expression*. This means the emotional expression of the victim's pain and hurt is experienced by the offender as the offender struggles with victim impact issues (Marshall & Fernandez, 2001).

The basic process of developing empathy consists of five distinct steps. The first is offense disclosure and responsibility. The second step is recognizing emotional cues from another. The third step is perspective taking. The fourth step is the ability to experience similar emotions. The final step is expressing and using emotional experiences.

CLINICAL JUSTIFICATIONS FOR USING VICTIM EMPATHY

There are a number of clinical justifications for using victim empathy. Victim empathy is just as critical as basic perspective taking and communication skills. It helps offenders learn to identify feelings and express them, become vulnerable, and be emotionally integrated. It becomes an effective arousal control by taking the form of an internal inhibition for offenders. It also provides the internal motivation for the offender not to re-offend. It has been successfully used as a relapse intervention because it solidifies cognitive restructuring processes. Most of all, victim empathy enhances the offender's level of social interest and conscience (Carich, Kassel et al., 2001).

Victim empathy and remorse are some of the most difficult elements (i.e., skills and experiences) for the offender to generate. Yet, both are common goals in treatment plans and components of programs (Association for the Treatment of Sexual Abusers, 1997; Carich & Mussack, 2001; Marshall et al., 1999; Metzger & Carich, 1999).

Schwartz and Canfield (1998) best described the importance of victim empathy by pointing out the need to supplement cognitive-behavioral therapy with emotional work that would enhance an offender's motivation not to re-offend. They state:

> Developing empathy for the victim as well as for the others in their life is a prime method of motivating sex offenders. Sex offenders have difficulty empathizing with others . . . Empathy is a crucial component of all interpersonal relations. It is perhaps the most vital component of sex offender treatment. If one can learn to appreciate and care about the harm one has done to another human, this appreciation can provide the motivation to engage in the difficult process of therapy. (pp. 240-241)

Longo (2002) also expressed the importance of learning to express emotional responses appropriately. He states:

> Most sexual abusers entering treatment programs suffer from a lack of or deficit of health emotions. Like unhealthy thinking, unhealthy emotions serve as a block to developing empathy. Helping clients develop a healthy emotional self should include learning about feelings and how to recognize them in oneself and in others, emotional expression and empathy training and development. (p. 16)

The key in victim empathy is helping the offender maintain it consistently across a variety of contexts. Thus, it can be viewed as a state that must be generalized or anchored across states.

VICTIM EMPATHY TECHNIQUES

A number of techniques designed to build or foster victim empathy have been used by clinicians. A group context is considered to be the best treatment modality to utilize these techniques and enhance victim empathy (Carich & Cadler, 2003; Marshall et al., 1999). However, several group contextual factors must be present in order to obtain effective treatment outcomes. First there must be no victimizing. Group cohesion helps to foster the treatment process and promote honesty. Therapeutic rapport is also essential to the treatment process. The offender needs to view treatment as beneficial and view the treatment as a source of support. The ideal group environment involves vulnerability, support, cohesion, and compassion, and includes 6 to 12 group members. Several group techniques have been selected for review in the following sections.

Utilizing Readings and Videos

The use of readings and videos encompasses instructing offenders to read selected written victim impact materials and viewing selected videos/movies, etc., that illustrate victim impact issues (Marshall & Fernandez, 2001). Videos can come from television documentaries, talk shows, movies, etc., that demonstrate the devastating experiences of the victim. For example, the Safer Society's modules have a "911" victim empathy segment, in which the actual sounds from the rape of a woman were taped during her 911 call for help. Offenders are instructed to identify or recognize their own feelings and the feelings of the victim (emotional recognition). Victim harm and impact are emphasized, and empathetic responses are encouraged.

Since offenders are at different places, arousal to victim distress and sexual deviancy safeguards need to be in place, or else it can be a reinforcing experience. Deviant arousal needs to be addressed, probed, and crashed. This can be done through probing questions, cognitive restructuring tactics, confrontation, selecting aversive elements (for that client), and then pairing them with the victim's distress and paraphilia. Quickly review a time when the offender was wronged and link this to this victim(s) experience to avoid victim stancing. Victim stancing is a situation in which the perpetrator engages in self-pity or sorrow for himself rather than feeling empathy for victims. In essence, the offender engages in playing the victim role usually to avoid experiencing feeling sorry for victims.

Victim Clarification Letters

Victim clarification responsibility letters are letters written by the offender to their victim(s) but not mailed (unless under therapeutic direction), in which the offender takes full responsibility for the offense(s). There are no excuses, minimizations, blaming, etc. (Freeman-Longo &

Pithers, 1992; Marshall et al., 1999; Marshall, O'Sullivan, & Fernandez, 1996). These letters are discussed in a group setting to invoke empathetic and remorseful responses. Letters are only sent to the victim based upon the survivor's needs, level of stability, therapeutic focus and direction. Take caution that offenders who want to send out letters could be doing so to feel better about himself and/or to control the victim. These letters can also be used with resistant offenders to challenge their current perspective of minimizing the impact of the offenses, and to avoid secrecy in disclosing offenses.

Victim Letters

Victim letters are written by the victim and directed at a "specific" offender or offenders in general (Carich, 1996, 1997). These letters can have a great impact because they are the victim's views and experience(s) of the offense(s) and its impact. The most significant impact is made when the offender receives a letter from his victim specifically outlining the devastating experiences or victim impact. Offenders identify what the victim is/was feeling (victim impact). Offenders are expected to identify and share their feelings concerning victim(s) experience. These experiences are processed in the group.

Role Playing

There are a number of useful role-play tactics and variations. Role-playing techniques involve instructing the offender to re-enact the offense (without actually perpetrating), utilizing another offender as a victim (Pithers, 1999). Safeguards are taken to avoid placing anyone in physical danger. The goal is to create a strong reaction in which the offender feels disgusted perpetrating against the victim. The offender can distinguish between how he is feeling now versus during the offense. These feelings of disgust can be linked to feelings of empathy and remorse. Specific cognitive distortions can be countered and defused and empathetic feelings explored.

Reverse role-playing techniques involve instructing the offender to play the role of his victim. The offender is then able to enhance his awareness of the victim's harm, and practice perspective taking, emotional recognition, and expression. These tactics break down distortions and defenses. Safeguards need to be taken into consideration to ensure that offenders playing the perpetrator role do not become aroused or that no one is re-victimized.

As with any of these tactics, offenders may need assistance in emotional recognition.

Answering Victim Questions

Normally victims of sex offenses have numerous questions. They tend to blame themselves, feel shameful, dirty, or guilty. These questions can be addressed in role-play situations by instructing one or more offenders to play the victim and then ask them questions that a victim would ask. Stick with one offender/victim at a time to help him visualize speaking to the victim. Typical questions might include the following:

1. Why me?
2. What did I do to deserve this?
3. Is this my fault?
4. What do I feel so dirty, shameful, and guilty?
5. How could I have prevented it?
6. Did he/she love me?
7. Why did he/she do it?

Basic Confrontational Techniques

Basic confrontation involves bringing specific issues to the client's attention. Confrontation is exploring at one level and challenging at another level. Specific areas that can be targeted include: incongruencies, inconsistencies, lack of empathy/remorse, denial, cognitive distortions (minimizations, blame, justifications, victim stancing, etc.), supporting offenses, and blocking empathy. Intense and rigorous confrontation tactics can be used only in the appropriate context, or one in which rapport is strong and the offender feels the group's support and concern. Confrontation is best used when challenging offenders on the above issues and behaviors while being supportive. Supportive behaviors from the therapist can be expressed both verbally and nonverbally. For example, softer voice tones at a key moment can make the difference in the offender's perception of support. Confrontation is not a license to victimize offenders in the name of therapy.

Victim Impact Statements

Victim impact statements are specific statements from the victim concerning the offense. This is the victim's version of what happened.

This usually accompanies court files or may be contained in the statement of facts. Quite often the offender's version is much different than the victim's. When presented with the victim's version, it can be quite emotional for the offender. The offender's emotions are linked back to what the victim experienced. Any offender distortions and inconsistent counts are challenged.

Using Statements of Facts

These are the facts of the offense as presented in court that can be accessed in legal files. These facts are compared to the offender's story in a way that presents the victim's view. A variety of issues can be addressed including distortions, responsibility, victim impact, etc. Emotional experiences are linked to the victim.

Focusing on When the Offender Was Wronged

One intense method used to enhance empathy is focusing on specific times or events in which the offender was violated or wronged and experienced trauma. The offender's own abuse or personal trauma can be used. Once the offender is at an emotional level, the offender's reactions are explored and linked to their specific victim(s) experiences. Emphasis is placed on the victim's experience and victim impact issues. The offender's own abusive experiences are linked to their own specific victims and victims in general. One should avoid victim stancing (the offender playing the victim role). This leads to self-pity and justifications to offend. It also creates a victim perpetrator cycle, or the offender viewing himself as the victim, and this justifies perpetration. It is strongly recommended that offender trauma and related core issues be resolved or worked through to a less intense level (but not at this time). Victim empathy groups are not considered the appropriate time or place to work on offender trauma issues. Focus here should be on the victim's trauma. As a general rule, the offender's traumatic experiences are linked to victim empathy (Schwartz, 1995). This prevents victim stancing.

Personalizing the Victim

Typically, the offender depersonalizes the victim into a non-person or may re-personalize (mentally place) the victim into another identity. Thus, in the offender's mind, the victim loses his/her true identity and takes on characteristics of another. Perhaps the offender places the victim as an object of his fantasy or connects the victim to significant figures from the past. Re-personalizing the victim is removing the victim from being the symbolic representation of someone/something else. Emphasis is placed on viewing the victim as a real person with an identity. Distortions are challenged as the victim takes on "real" personal characteristics.

Victim Voice Technique

Victim voice techniques consist of the offender describing his offense from the victim's perspective. The perpetrator writes out the offense from the victim's perspective using the victim's words. In the group, the offender then verbalizes the offense using the victim's words describing each event and reaction. This technique helps offenders elicit intense feelings of empathy and remorse.

Victim Impact Collages

A collage is a collection of pictures, sayings, images, etc., pasted together on a poster board. Victim impact collages are collected pictures, sayings, etc., involving victim impact themes. For example, this might include pictures of sad eyes, sad faces, or any devastating scenes that relate to victim harm and sadness. This reminds the perpetrator of the devastating impact of offending. The trauma and pain that the victim felt at the time, along with other short- and long-term behavior can be displayed in a collage of pictures or words.

"As If" Technique

The "as if" technique was originally developed by Adler and has many variations (Ansbacher & Ansbacher, 1956; Carich, 1989, 1991, 1997). It is a futuristic tactic in which the client projects himself into the future and responds accordingly. The client is instructed to pretend or enact a scenario using the framework of "act as if you . . ." or "what if you . . ." or "what if the victim experienced . . ." Applied to victim empathy or remorse, offenders are instructed to project themselves into the future by psychologically enacting a "what if/as if" scenario. These scenarios usually involve victim impact themes by placing the offender in the victim role. For example, the offender may experience being the victim of his perpetration or perhaps another victim. The offender's immediate feelings and experiences are linked to the offender's specific victim's experiences. Another version of this technique is to instruct the offender to pretend as if he has experienced victim empathy, emphasizing specific feelings of sadness for victims, victim impact, remorse, etc. This experience is highlighted and connected to the offender's current position.

Victim/Survivor Interactional Group

Victim/offender interactional groups consist of therapeutic groups with both survivors (victims) and offenders. With adult offenders, groups are composed of both adult survivors and offenders. These groups can have very powerful impacts. These types of groups have to be constructed in a way that survivors do not get victimized. Likewise, it is just as important to minimize the offenders getting victimized by survivors. However, survivors may tend to ventilate their feelings toward offenders, and offenders need to utilize those experiences to enhance empathy and remorse as a form of restitution. For optimal results, both offenders and survivors need to be at a certain level of stability and recovery. Survivors need to be stable and not self-destructive. Likewise, offenders need to be at a certain level (i.e., motivated and committed toward recovery, willing to take some responsibility, less distorted, etc.), or they may react with anger, defensiveness, and deviant arousal and try to re-victimize their survivors. Although some survivors may want to face their perpetrators, usually in these groups, survivors are unknown to offenders.

Specific group parameters must be established. Group themes involve survivors discussing their experiences and victim impact issues. Survivors may ask offenders why they were assaulted and offenders encouraged to answer. A basic group rule of no victimizing needs to be in place and enforced. Violators of the rule should be confronted. If survivors ventilate their feelings toward the offenders, the offenders need to link up their reactions along with the survivors' reactions to empathy and remorse.

Offender/survivor groups provide the offender with an opportunity to take responsibility, feel for their victims, and provide emotional restitution. In essence, offenders witness the pain of their victims, and survivors observe the painful struggle of the offender. There is no known data on this technique. It may be considered controversial; however, it was often used in the 1970s and 1980s.

Guided Imagery Apologetic Technique

The guided imagery apologetic technique, otherwise known as the apologetic imagery technique, is based on Cloe Madanes' (1990) work on reparations with sex offenders. This is applied to restorative justice. Apology refers to the expression of regret for violating another person. In this context, it is expressing regret for sexually violating another person through mental representations or imagery. In essence, the offenders imagine apologizing to their victims in a certain way described below. The purpose is to experience empathy and remorse at both intellectual and emotional levels, to acknowledge wrongs, feel the pain, accentuate responsibility and accountability, and to initiate restitution. The contextual parameters of the techniques include developing an image of the victim sitting down and the offender apologizing to them (individually) while the offender is on their knees. The image and structure has to be vividly mentally constructed. The formula for the apology includes the following: (a) acknowledgment–of violating the victim (victim harm), (b) ownership–of the offense, (c) responsibility–taking the offender off of the "hook," (d) apologizing–apologizing on the knees, to the victim, at the victim's age at the time of the assault(s), (e) re-affirming a commitment–to having no more victims, and (f) restitution–making up behaviors.

Other factors that should be considered include size differential; it is important that the victim appear the same size. The offender should be humble. The offender must give up control of the victim. The offender must also relinquish his sense of entitlement that he had a right to assault. The offender must not ask for forgiveness. This process is for the victim, not the offender. The sequence must be continuously cycled until all goals are adequately met.

Refocusing on the Victim's Eyes

Refocusing on the victim's eyes is a reframing imagery technique used to facilitate both victim empathy and remorse. It is an imagery (internal visualizing) tactic with a metaphoric reframe associated with the image. The procedure has nine distinct steps.

Step 1: Offense/case review. The most significant (most meaningful) offenses are selected. They are reviewed in detail. Offenders are often instructed to write out these offenses and then discuss them in group.

Step 2: Scale the problem. Scaling the problem originated with Rossi (1993), in which he emphasizes scaling the symptoms within the healing process. Offenders are instructed to scale the following items: (a) their ability to identify and express affect, (b) their ability to visualize the offense and the clarity of these images, and (c) their level of distress arousal (arousal surrounding hurting the victim; i.e., sadistic arousal) and their level of arousal associated with the pain in the victim's eyes. Scales consist of numbers 0 to 10, with 10 being the highest. This allows the therapist and offender to assess the client's level of empathy.

Step 3: Identify key cognitive distortions. The offender identifies his own key cognitive distortions including: (a) specific distortions associated with the victim's eyes and (b) the general distortions associated with his offending. This is taken from Step 1 and processed in the group.

Step 4: Develop an image of victim's eyes. The offender is then instructed to develop an image of the victim's eyes. The image is typically of sadness.

Step 5: Select a reframing metaphor. A metaphor or therapeutic theme is selected. It may include cognitive restructuring counters relating to specific distortions involving the victim's eyes. Metaphors may also include pain, shock, sadness, stealing the victim's soul or life, etc. It has to be meaningful to the offender.

Step 6: Access to feelings or related affective states.

Step 7: Affective expression. It is important for the offender to express empathetic feelings in this step and to enhance the offender's expression of feelings.

Step 8: Futuristic projection. To generalize the experience across contexts, the offender is projected into the future. More specifically, the offender is projected into the future experiencing sadness and empathy when looking into the victim's eyes. The therapist provides suggestions so that when the offender visualizes the victim's eyes, he will generate feelings of compassion.

Step 9: Generalize this experience to other victims. This experience is then generalized to other victims and victims in general. Experience of what a particular victim felt is linked to other victim's experiences.

Some precautions should be taken when using this technique. Do not use the techniques if the outcome will reinforce the victim's pain with deviant patterns, arousal, or offending. Do not use the techniques if the offender has high distress arousal that cannot be "crashed" or defused by using this technique. Do not leave the offender suicidal.

CONCLUSION

According to Marshall and Maric (1996), "It may be better to view empathy as an unfolding staged process with each stage involving both emotional and cognitive futures" (p. 108). Although many of the most effective components of sex offender treatment are still under investigation, victim empathy has been considered a critical as well as necessary component of such treatment (Hennessy et al., 2002). It is not difficult to facilitate once the professional understands the processes, principles, and tactics involved.

Two important factors are knowing the skills and developing the appropriate treatment context. It is acknowledged that not all sex offenders can learn victim empathy; for example, highly psychopathic/antisocial serial offenders or sexual abusers cannot learn victim empathy as suggested by Quinsey (personal communication, June 7, 2000), Salter (personal communication, June 7, 2000), and Hare (personal communication, September 6, 2001). Brain damaged offenders also really do not have the physiological capabilities to learn empathy skills. Although clinical experience indicates that over time some have learned it, these individuals must have the desire to let go of the deviancy.

Victim empathy work is counterproductive for any sex offender who only desires satisfaction or gratification from distressing others and who is unwilling to let go of his deviancy. In these cases, empathy work can reinforce offending patterns by allowing the offender to use therapeutic material as deviant fantasy material. Thus, the deviant pattern must be broken down first with arousal control. Arousal control tactics of covert sensitization may be used in combination with victim empathy techniques. Covert sensitization involves pairing or associating undesirable images or covert events with deviant arousal stimuli/responses. Yet, victim empathy is an excellent inhibitor of arousal when an abuser is able to grasp the concepts and emotional levels of empathy for others.

The remaining issue for clinicians and offenders is developing effective bridges from the therapeutic context to everyday life. The victim empathy experience needs to be generalized throughout life. Paradoxically, it is important for the offender to feel empathy for victims and maintain an adequate self-concept.

REFERENCES

Ansbacher, H., & Ansbacher, R. (Eds.). (1956). *The individual psychology of Alfred Adler*. New York: Basic Books.

Association for the Treatment of Sexual Abusers. (1997). *Ethical standards and principles for the management of sexual abusers*. Beaverton, OR: Author.

Baker, D., & Price, S. (1997). Developing therapeutic communities for sex offenders. In B. Schwartz, & H. Cellini (Eds.), *The sex offender: New insights, treatment innovations, and legal development, Volume II* (pp. 19-1-19-14). Kingston, NJ: Civic Research Institute.

Blanchard, G. T. (1995). *The difficult connection*. Brandon, VT: Safer Society Press.

Carich, M. S. (1989). Variations of the "as if" technique. *Individual Psychology, 45*(4), 538-545.

Carich, M. S. (1991). The hypnotic "as if" technique: An example of beyond Adler. *Individual Psychology, 46*(4), 509-514.

Carich, M. S. (1996). Facilitating and developing victim empathy and remorse: Basic goals and tactics. *INMAS Newsletter, 4*(4), 3-6.

Carich, M. S. (1997). Utilizing victim empathy techniques in sex offender treatment: Training module. In M. S. Carich (Ed.), *Sex offender treatment and overview: Training for the mental health professional* (Appendix). Springfield, IL: Illinois Department of Corrections.

Carich, M. S. (1999, September). *Enhancing victim awareness and empathy*. Paper presented at the meeting of the Association for the Treatment of Sexual Abusers, Orlando, FL.

Carich, M. S. (2002). Pros and cons of teaching victim empathy in treatment. *The IL-ATSA Review, 5*(1), 5.

Carich, M. S., & Cadler, M. (2003). *Contemporary treatment of adult male sex offenders*. Dorset, England: Russell House Press.

Carich, M. S., & Harper, J. (2003). An outline of the key elements of victim empathy. *The Illinois ATSA Review, 6*(1), 4-5.

Carich, M. S., Kassel, M., & Stone, M. (2001). Enhancing social interest in sex offenders. *Journal of Individual Psychology, 57*(1), 18-25.

Carich, M. S., & Mussack, S. (Eds.). (2001). *A handbook for sexual offender assessment and treatment*. Brandon, VT: The Safer Society Press.

Carich, M. S., Newbauer, J., & Stone, M. (2001). Sex offenders and contemporary treatment. *The Journal of Individual Psychology, 57*(1), 3-17.

Egan, G. (1986). *The skilled helper: A systematic approach to effective helping*. Monterey, CA: Brooks/Cole Publishing.

Fernandez, Y. M., Marshall, W. L., Ligthbody, S., & O'Sullivan, C. (1999). The child molester empathy measure. *Sexual Abuse: A Journal of Research and Treatment, 11*, 17-31.

Freeman-Longo, R. E., Bird, S., Stevenson, W. F., & Fiske, J. A. (1995). *1994 national survey of treatment programs and models: Serving abuse-reactive children and adolescent and adult sex offenders*. Brandon, VT: The Safer Society Press.

Freeman-Longo, R. E., & Blanchard, G. (1998). *Sexual abuse in America: Epidemic of the 21st century*. Brandon, VT: Safer Society Press.

Freeman-Longo, R. E., & Pithers, W. D. (1992). *Client's manual: A structured approach to preventing relapse: A guide to sex offenders.* Brandon, VT: Safer Society Press.

George, R. L., & Cristiani, T. S. (1990). *Counseling theory and practice.* Englewood Cliffs, NJ: Allyn and Bacon.

Hanson, R. K. (1997). Invoking sympathy: Assessment and treatment of empathy deficits among sexual offenders. In B. K. Schwartz, & H. R. Cellini (Eds.), *The sex offender: New insights, treatment, innovations, and legal developments, volume II* (pp. 1-12). Kingston, NJ: Civic Research Institute.

Hanson, R. K., & Bussiere, M. T. (1998). Predicting relapse: A meta-analysis of sexual offender recidivism studies. *Journal of Clinical and Consulting Psychology, 66,* 348-362.

Hanson, K., & Scott, H. (1995). Assessing perspective taking among sexual offenders, nonsexual criminals, and nonoffenders. *Sexual Abuse: A Journal of Research and Treatment, 7,* 259-277.

Hennessy, M., Walter, J., & Vess, J. (2002). An evaluation of the empathy as a measure of victim empathy with civilly committed sexual offenders. *Sexual Abuse: A Journal of Research and Treatment, 14,* 241-252.

Hudson, W. L., Marshall, W. L., Wales, D. S., McDonald, E., Bakker, L. W., & McLean, A. (1993). Emotional recognition skills for sex offenders. *Annals of Sex Research, 6,* 199-211.

Knopp, F. H., Freeman-Longo, R., & Stevenson, W. (1992). *Nationwide Survey of Juvenile and Adult Sex Offender Treatment Programs.* Brandon, VT: Safer Society Press.

Longo, R. E. (2002). A holistic/integrated approach to treating sexual offenders. In B. L. Schwartz (Ed.), *The sex offender: Current treatment modalities and systems issues volume IV* (pp. 2-1-2-19). Kingston, NJ: Civic Research Institute.

Madanes, C. (1990). *Sex, love, and violence.* New York: W. W. Norton.

Marshall, W. L. (1996). Assessment, treatment, and theorizing about sexual offenders: Developments over the past 20 years and future decisions. *Criminal Justice and Behavior, 23*(1), 162-199.

Marshall, W. L. (1999). Current status of North American assessment and treatment programs for sexual offenders. *Journal of Interpersonal Violence, 14*(3), 221-239.

Marshall, W. L., Anderson, D., & Fernandez, Y. (1999). *Cognitive behavioral treatment of sexual offenders.* New York: John Wiley and Sons.

Marshall, W. L., & Fernandez, Y. M. (2001). Empathy training. In M. S. Carich, & S. Mussack (Eds.), *A handbook on the sexual abuser* (pp. 141-148). Brandon, VT: Safer Society Press.

Marshall, W. L., Hudson, S. M., Jones, R., & Fernandez, Y. M. (1995). Empathy in sexual offenders. *Clinical Psychology Review, 15,* 99-113.

Marshall, W. L., Jones, R., Hudson, S. M., & McDonald, E. (1993). Generalized empathy in child molesters. *Journal of Child Sexual Abuse, 2,* 61-69.

Marshall, W. L., & Maric, A. (1996). Cognitive and emotional components of generalized empathy deficits in child molesters. *Journal of Child Sexual Abuse, 5,* 101-110.

Marshall, W. L., O'Sullivan, C., & Fernandez, Y. M. (1996). The enhancement of victim empathy among incarcerated child molesters. *Legal and Criminological Psychology, 1,* 95-102.

Marshall, W. L., & Pithers, W. D. (1994). A reconsideration of treatment outcome with sex offenders. *Criminal Justice and Behavior, 21*(1), 10-27.

McGrath, M., Cann, S., & Konopasy, R. (1998). New measures of defensiveness, empathy, and cognitive distortions for sexual offenders against children. *Sexual Abuse: A Journal of Research and Treatment, 10*(1), 25-36.

Metzger, C., & Carich, M. S. (1999). Eleven point comprehensive sex offender treatment plan. In M. Calder (Ed.), *Assessing risk in adult males who sexually abuse children* (pp. 293-311). Dorset, England: Russell House Publishing Limited.

Pithers, W. D. (1994). Process evaluation of a group therapy component designed to enhance sex offender's empathy for sexual abuse survivors. *Behaviour Research and Therapy, 32*(5), 565-570.

Pithers, W. D. (1999). Empathy: Definition, enhancement, and the relevance to the treatment of sexual abusers. *Journal of Interpersonal Violence, 14*(3), 257-284.

Rossi, E. L. (1993). *The psychobiology of mind-body healing: New concepts of therapeutic hypnosis.* New York: W.W. Norton.

Schwartz, B. K. (1995). Characteristics and typologies of sex offenders. In B. K. Schwartz, & H. R. Cellini (Eds.), *Correction, the sex offender: Treatment and legal practice* (pp. 3-1-3-36). Kingston, NJ: Civic Research Institute.

Schwartz, B. K., & Canfield, G. M. S. (1998). Treating the sexually dangerous person: The Massachusetts treatment center. In W. L. Marshall, Y. M. Fernandez, S. M. Hudson, & T. Ward (Eds.), *Sourcebook of treatment programs for sexual offenders* (pp. 235-245). New York: Plenum Press

Ward, T., Hudson, S., Johnston, L., & Marshall, W. L. (1997). Cognitive distortions in sex offenders: An integrative review. *Clinical Psychology Review, 17*, 479-507.

Webster, S., & Beech, A. (2000). The nature of sexual offender's affective empathy: A grounded theory analysis. *Sexual Abuse: A Journal of Research and Treatment, 12*, 249-256.

Index

"A Brief Review of Contemporary
    Sex Offender Treatment,"
    xiv
Abel Assessment for Sexual Interest
    Screen, 61,155
Abel, G.G., 35,134,142,152
Abel Screening Test, 85,145,147
Abel-Becker Cognitions Scale, 9,10,
    155
Abnormality(ies), mental, 36
Abouesh, A., 246
Abrams, J.B., 180
Abrams, S., 180
Abuse, child. *See* Child abuse
Actuarial risk assessment, of sex
    offenders, 86-89
Adler School of Professional
    Psychology, xiii
Affiliated Psychologists, Ltd., xv-xvi
Albert, K.S., 241
Alexander, R., 36-37
Alliant International University,
    California School of
    Professional Psychology at,
    in San Diego, xiv
American Academy of Forensic
    Sciences, xvi
American Polygraph Association, 187
American Psychiatric Association
    (APA), 42,129,131,234
American Psychological Association,
    140
Anderson, D., 257
Anderson, P.B., 59
Antal, E.J., 241
APA. *See* American Psychiatric
    Association (APA)
Arizona Judicial Department, 39

"As if" technique, in victim empathy,
    269-270
Assessment and Treatment of Sex
    Offenders Research Team, at
    Muriel McQueen Fergusson
    Centre for Family Violence
    Research, at University of
    New Brunswick, xvi
Association for the Treatment of
    Sexual Abusers (ATSA), 11,
    33,177
Association for the Treatment of
    Sexual Abusers (ATSA) 21st
    Annual Research and
    Treatment Conference, xiv,
    xv
ATSA. *See* Association for the
    Treatment of Sexual
    Abusers (ATSA)
Atteberry-Bennett, J., 107
"Attention, sexualized," 105
Attitudes Towards Women Scale, 155
Ault, H.S., 23-24

Baig, M.S.A., xiii,12,255
Bailey, R., 106
Bain, J., 242
Barabee, H.E., 83,95
Barland, 182
Basic confrontation, in victim
    empathy, 267
BDI-II. *See* Beck Depression
    Inventory-II (BDI-II)
Beck Depression Inventory-II
    (BDI-II), 154
Becker, J.V., 35
Beech, A., 256,263

5-Hydroxytryptamine, in sexual
behaviors, 236

Illinois Department of Corrections, xv
at Big Muddy River CC, xiii
Illinois Department of Human
Services, xiii
"Incest, emotional," 105
Informed consent, in sex offender
evaluation, 141
Integrated Theory of Sexual Deviancy,
83
Internet, 135
Internet Websites, 21
Intimacy, in cognitive-behavioural
treatment of adult sex
offenders, 207-208

Jacob Wetterling Crimes Against
Children and Sexually
Violent Offender Registration
Act, 19
Jamieson, D.W., 181
Janus, E.S., 33,39,41,45
Johns Hopkins Hospital, xvi
Johns Hopkins Sexual Disorders
Clinic, xiii
Johns Hopkins University School of
Medicine, xvi
Johnson, T.C., xiv,9,103,105
Johnston, L., 263
Jones, K.D., 23-24,24
Jones, L., 187

Kafka, M.P., 134,135,246
Kanka, M., 19
Kansas Supreme Court, 32,33
Kansas v. Crane, 33
Kansas v. Hendricks, 32,37
Kaplan, Z., 246
Kassel, M., 262

Kaufman Brief Intelligence Test
(K-BIT), 153
K-BIT. *See* Kaufman Brief
Intelligence Test (K-BIT)
Kennedy, H., 147
Kerbeshian, J., 64
Klinefelter's syndrome, 64
Klüver-Bucy syndrome, 68
Knight, R.A., 135,160,161
Koch, S., 80
Kohlberg, 190
Kokish, R., xv,10,175,179,186,190
Koss, M.P., 2
Krusei, M.J., 245

LaFond, J.Q., 39
Lalumiere, M., 86,95
Langevin, R., 137,147,242
Lanyon, R., 155
Law enforcement, 27
Law of Parsimony, 79
Lee, A., 160,161
Legal issues
in sex offender evaluation, 143-145
sex offender-related, 4-7
Letter(s)
victim, in victim empathy, 266
victim clarification, in victim
empathy, 265-266
Leuprolide acetate, for paraphilic
disorders, 243-245
Levenson, J.S., xv,8,17
LH. *See* Luteinizing hormone (LH)
LHRH. *See* Luteinizing
hormone-releasing hormone
(LHRH)
Lieb, R., 20,26
Lightbody, S., 258
Limbic-hypothalamic-pituitary-
gonadal axis,
in sexual deviancy,
62-63,62t
Longo, R.E., 264
Losztyn, S., 243

testosterone-lowering agents in,
241-245
triptorelin in, 245
TSH in, 247
Parent/child interactions, overreactions
to, caution regarding,
108-109
Paroxetine, for paraphilic disorders,
246
PCL-R. *See* Psychopathy
Checklist-Revised (PCL-R)
PCSOT. *See* Post-conviction Sex
Offender (polygraph)
Testing (PCSOT)
Pedophile(s), 34
Peitgan, H., 92
Penile plethysmography, 155
People v. Stoll, 144
Perilstein, R.D., 245
*Personal Sentence Completion
Inventory,* 155
Perspective taking, 262,263
PET. *See* Positron emission
tomography (PET)
Petrila, J., 140
Petrosino, A.J., 28-29
Petrosino, C., 28-29
Peyser, C., 64
Phenylethanolamine-*N*-methyl-
transferase (PNMT),
in sexual behaviors, 236
Phillips, R.A., Jr., 245
Plasma reagin test (RPR), 247
Plaud, J., 179
Plethysmography, penile, 155
PNMT. *See* Phenylethanolamine-*N*-
methyl-transferase
(PNMT)
Podlesny, 182
"Policy Interventions Designed to
Combat Sexual Violence:
Community Notification and
Civil Commitment," 8
Polygraph, in context, 186-189

Polygraph testing
in context, 186-189
sex offender
accuracy estimates of, 181-186
base rates of truthfulness and
attempted deception in,
183-186
current status of, 189-192
eliciting increased information
with, 178-179
examinees in, 182
examiners in, 112
future directions in, 189-192
increased treatment and
supervision compliance with,
180
laboratory *vs.* field data in,
181-182
post-conviction, 175-194
post-conviction sex offender
polygraph testing in,
175-194. *See also* Polygraph
testing, sex offender,
post-conviction
tests in, 182-183
treatment goals, 176-177
Polygraphy, described, 176
Portland State University, xiv
Positron emission tomography (PET),
65
in human sexuality, 66-67
Post-conviction Sex Offender
(polygraph) Testing
(PCSOT), 177,178,179,181,
183,185,189,190,192
Poythress, N.G., 140
"Practical Considerations in the
Interview and Evaluation of
Sexual Offenders," 9,10
PRDs. *See* Paraphilia-related
disorders (PRDs)
Predator(s), sexually violent, civil
commitment of, 30-47
Prentky, R.A., 21,83,95,135,160,161

practical considerations in,
127-173
psychological testing in,
153-155
review existing available data in,
148
risk assessment in, 139,157-168,
158t,161t,167t
methods in, 161-166,161t
overall approach to, 166-168,
167t
research related to,
158-161,158t
interviewing of, practical
considerations in, 127-173.
See also Sex offenders,
evaluation of, practical
considerations in
legal issues related to, 4-7
psychopathy in, 85-86
public policies related to, 4-7
treatment of, 139
goals in, 176-177
victim empathy for, enhancement
of, 255-276
Sex Offender Needs Assessment
Rating (SONAR), 46,89,94,
95,165,201
Sex offender notification outcome
research, 25-28
Sex Offender Programs at the
Correctional Service of
Canada, xvi
Sex Offender Risk Appraisal Guide
(SORAG), 153,164,165
Sex offender treatment (SOT), 186,
187
Sex offender treatment programs
(SOTPs), 177,183,184,185,
186,188,190
Sex offending, understanding of,
integrative approaches to,
82-83
Sex offense recidivism, 21-22

Sexual behaviors, neurotransmitters in,
role of, 235-238,237t
Sexual deviance
defined, 129-131,130t
in sex offender evaluation, 129-131,
130t
Sexual deviancy, 53-76
assessment of, importance of, 60-62
brain pathology in, 67-69
case examples, 54-56
definitions associated with, 56-58,
57t
differential diagnosis of, 62t
epidemiological data related to,
59-60
genes in, role of, 64-65
limbic-hypothalamic-pituitary-
gonadal axis in,
role of, 62-63,62t
neuroradiological concepts in,
75-76
neuroradiological findings in, 65-66
"Sexual Deviancy: Diagnostic and
Neurobiological
Considerations," 8
Sexual Offenders Committee, of
American Academy of
Psychiatry and the Law, xvi
Sexual offense(s), in sex offender
evaluation, 131-133,132t
Sexual offense recidivism
civil commitment on, impact of,
40-41
prediction of, 44-45
Sexual preference, deviant, in
cognitive-behavioural
treatment of adult sex
offenders, 209-211
Sexual violence
combatting of, policy interventions
in, 17-52
future research in, implications
for, 29-30
implications for, 46-47
community notification of, 17-52.
See also Sexual violence,